Postoperative Complications

Editors

AMY L. LIGHTNER
PHILLIP R. FLESHNER

SURGICAL CLINICS OF NORTH AMERICA

www.surgical.theclinics.com

Consulting Editor
RONALD F. MARTIN

October 2021 • Volume 101 • Number 5

ELSEVIER

1600 John F. Kennedy Boulevard • Suite 1800 • Philadelphia, Pennsylvania, 19103-2899

http://www.surgical.theclinics.com

SURGICAL CLINICS OF NORTH AMERICA Volume 101, Number 5
October 2021 ISSN 0039–6109, ISBN-13: 978-0-323-81361-7

Editor: John Vassallo, j.vassallo@elsevier.com
Developmental Editor: Arlene Campos

Photocopying

Single photocopies of single articles may be made for personal use as allowed by national copyright laws. Permission of the Publisher and payment of a fee is required for all other photocopying, including multiple or systematic copying, copying for advertising or promotional purposes, resale, and all forms of document delivery. Special rates are available for educational institutions that wish to make photocopies for non-profit educational classroom use. For information on how to seek permission visit www.elsevier.com/permissions or call: (+44) 1865 843830 (UK)/(+1) 215 239 3804 (USA).

Derivative Works

Subscribers may reproduce tables of contents or prepare lists of articles including abstracts for internal circulation within their institutions. Permission of the Publisher is required for resale or distribution outside the institution. Permission of the Publisher is required for all other derivative works, including compilations and translations (please consult www.elsevier.com/permissions).

Electronic Storage or Usage

Permission of the Publisher is required to store or use electronically any material contained in this periodical, including any article or part of an article (please consult www.elsevier.com/permissions). Except as outlined above, no part of this publication may be reproduced, stored in a retrieval system or transmitted in any form or by any means, electronic, mechanical, photocopying, recording or otherwise, without prior written permission of the Publisher.

Notice

No responsibility is assumed by the Publisher for any injury and/or damage to persons or property as a matter of products liability, negligence or otherwise, or from any use or operation of any methods, products, instructions or ideas contained in the material herein. Because of rapid advances in the medical sciences, in particular, independent verification of diagnoses and drug dosages should be made.

Although all advertising material is expected to conform to ethical (medical) standards, inclusion in this publication does not constitute a guarantee or endorsement of the quality or value of such product or of the claims made of it by its manufacturer.

Surgical Clinics of North America (ISSN 0039–6109) is published bimonthly by Elsevier Inc., 360 Park Avenue South, New York, NY 10010-1710. Months of publication are February, April, June, August, October, and December. Business and Editorial Offices: 1600 John F. Kennedy Blvd., Suite 1800, Philadelphia, PA 19103-2899. Periodicals postage paid at New York, NY and additional mailing offices. Subscription prices are $443.00 per year for US individuals, $1198.00 per year for US institutions, $100.00 per year for US & Canadian students and residents, $547.00 per year for Canadian individuals, $1270.00 per year for Canadian institutions, $536.00 for international individuals, $1270.00 per year for international institutions and $250.00 per year for foreign students/residents. To receive student/resident rate, orders must be accompanied by name of affiliated institution, date of term, and the *signature* of program/residency coordinator on institution letterhead. Orders will be billed at individual rate until proof of status is received. Foreign air speed delivery is included in all *Clinics* subscription prices. All prices are subject to change without notice. POSTMASTER: Send address changes to *Surgical Clinics*, Elsevier Health Sciences Division, Subscription Customer Service, 3251 Riverport Lane, Maryland Heights, MO 63043. **Customer Service (orders, claims, online, change of address): Telephone: 1-800-654-2452 (U.S. and Canada); 314-447-8871 (outside U.S. and Canada). Fax: 314-447-8029. E-mail: journalscustomerservice-usa@elsevier.com (for print support); journalsonlinesupport-usa@elsevier.com (for online support).**

Reprints. For copies of 100 or more, of articles in this publication, please contact the Commercial Reprints Department, Elsevier Inc., 360 Park Avenue South, New York, New York 10010-1710. Tel. 212-633-3874, Fax: 212-633-3820, E-mail: reprints@elsevier.com.

The *Surgical Clinics of North America* is also published in Spanish by McGraw-Hill Interamericana Editores S.A., P.O. Box 5-237 06500 Mexico D.F. Mexico; and in Portuguese by Interlivros Edicoes Ltda., Rua Comandante Coelho 1085, CEP 21250, Rio de Janeiro, Brazil; and in Greek by Paschalidis Medical Publications, Athens Greece.

The *Surgical Clinics of North America* is covered in *MEDLINE/PubMed (Index Medicus), EMBASE/Excerpta Medica, Current Contents/Clinical Medicine, Current Contents/Life Sciences, Science Citation Index*, and *ISI/BIOMED*.

Contributors

CONSULTING EDITOR

RONALD F. MARTIN, MD, FACS
Colonel (Retired), United States Army Reserve, Department of General Surgery and
Surgical Oncology, Madigan Army Medical Center, Tacoma, Washington

EDITORS

AMY L. LIGHTNER, MD
Director, Center for Regenerative Medicine and Surgery, Associate Professor of
Colorectal Surgery, Digestive Disease Institute, Associate Professor of Inflammation and
Immunity, Lerner Research Institute, Core Member in the Center for Immunotherapy,
Cleveland Clinic, Cleveland, Ohio

PHILLIP R. FLESHNER, MD
Department of Colorectal Surgery, Digestive Disease and Surgical Institute, Cleveland
Clinic, Cleveland, Ohio; Division of Colon and Rectal Surgery, Cedars-Sinai, Los Angeles,
California

AUTHORS

ZAHRAA AL-HILLI, MD, FRCSI, FACS
Assistant Professor of Surgery, Department of General Surgery, Digestive Diseases and
Surgery Institute, Cleveland Clinic, Cleveland, Ohio

RACHEL R. BLITZER, MD
Department of Surgery, UC San Diego Health System, San Diego, California

MIGUEL BURCH, MD
General Surgery, Cedars Sinai Medical Center, Los Angeles, California

DAVID C. CHEN, MD
Professor of Clinical Surgery, Department of Surgery, David Geffen School of Medicine at
UCLA, Lichtenstein Amid Hernia Clinic at UCLA, Santa Monica, California

JASON A. CORRELL, MS
University of Michigan Medical School, Ann Arbor, Michigan

SAMUEL EISENSTEIN, MD
Associate Professor, Department of Surgery, UC San Diego Health System, San Diego,
California

OLIVER J. FACKELMAYER, MD
Clinical Instructor, Section of Endocrine Surgery, UCLA David Geffen School of Medicine
at UCLA, UCLA Endocrine Center, Los Angeles, California

XIAOXI (CHELSEA) FENG, MD, MPH
Department of Surgery, Cedars Sinai Medical Center, Los Angeles, California

DAVID N. HANNA, MD
Division of General Surgery, Section of Colon and Rectal Surgery, Vanderbilt University, Vanderbilt University Medical Center, Nashville, Tennessee

ALEXANDER T. HAWKINS, MD, MPH
Division of General Surgery, Section of Colon and Rectal Surgery, Vanderbilt University, Vanderbilt University Medical Center, Nashville, Tennessee

LORRAINE I. KELLEY-QUON, MD, MSHS
Division of Pediatric Surgery, Children's Hospital Los Angeles, Department of Surgery, Keck School of Medicine of USC, Department of Preventive Medicine, University of Southern California, Los Angeles, California

DANNY LASCANO, MD
Division of Pediatric Surgery, Children's Hospital Los Angeles, Department of Surgery, Keck School of Medicine of USC, Los Angeles, California

CHRISTOPHER V. LAVIN, BS
Research Fellow, Hagey Laboratory for Pediatric Regenerative Medicine, Stanford University School of Medicine, Stanford, California

YANG LU, MD
Resident Physician, Department of Surgery, David Geffen School of Medicine at UCLA, Los Angeles, California

IAN T. MACQUEEN, MD
Assistant Professor of Clinical Surgery, Department of Surgery, David Geffen School of Medicine at UCLA, Lichtenstein Amid Hernia Clinic at UCLA, Santa Monica, California

TRAVIS J. MILLER, MD
Resident, Division of Plastic and Reconstructive Surgery, Department of Surgery, Stanford University School of Medicine, Stanford, California

ARASH MOMENI, MD
Assistant Professor of Surgery, Division of Plastic and Reconstructive Surgery, Department of Surgery, Stanford University School of Medicine, Hagey Laboratory for Pediatric Regenerative Medicine, Stanford University School of Medicine, Stanford, California

EDWARD PHILLIPS, MD
Department of Surgery, Cedars Sinai Medical Center, Los Angeles, California

MOHAMMAD QRAREYA, MD
Cardiovascular Surgery Department, Mayo Clinic, Rochester, Minnesota

SHA'SHONDA L. REVELS, MD
Assistant Professor, Division of Thoracic Surgery, David Geffen School of Medicine at UCLA, Los Angeles, California

MICHAEL J. ROSEN, MD
Cleveland Clinic Foundation, Cleveland, Ohio

DANIEL SHOUHED, MD
Department of Surgery, Cedars Sinai Medical Center, Los Angeles, California

ROBERT SIMON, MD
Clinical Staff, General Surgery, Department of Hepatopancreaticobiliary Surgery,
Digestive Disease and Surgery Institute, Cleveland Clinic Foundation, Cleveland, Ohio

JOSHUA D. SMITH, MD
Department of Otolaryngology–Head and Neck Surgery, University of Michigan, Ann
Arbor, Michigan

CHAZ L. STUCKEN, MD
Department of Otolaryngology–Head and Neck Surgery, University of Michigan, Ann
Arbor, Michigan

EMILY Z. STUCKEN, MD
Department of Otolaryngology–Head and Neck Surgery, University of Michigan, Ann
Arbor, Michigan

PAUL A. TOSTE, MD
Assistant Professor, Division of Thoracic Surgery, David Geffen School of Medicine at
UCLA, Ronald Reagan UCLA Medical Center, Los Angeles, California

DERRICK C. WAN, MD
Professor of Surgery, Hagey Family Faculty Scholar in Stem Cell Research and
Regenerative Medicine, Division of Plastic and Reconstructive Surgery, Department of
Surgery, Stanford University School of Medicine, Stanford, California

AVIA WILKERSON, MD
Department of General Surgery, Digestive Diseases and Surgery Institute, Cleveland
Clinic, Cleveland, Ohio

JAMES X. WU, MD
Assistant Professor, Section of Endocrine Surgery, UCLA David Geffen School of
Medicine at UCLA, UCLA Endocrine Center, Los Angeles, California

MICHAEL W. YEH, MD
Professor, Section of Endocrine Surgery, David Geffen School of Medicine at UCLA,
UCLA Endocrine Center, Los Angeles, California

SAMUEL J. ZOLIN, MD
Cleveland Clinic Foundation, Cleveland, Ohio

BARA ZUHAILI, MD, FACS
Michigan Vascular Center, Michigan State University, Flint, Michigan

Contents

> The complications encountered in colorectal surgery can be categorized into early and late. The most consequential early complication is anastomotic leak, which can be managed with percutaneous drainage or reoperation, depending on the patient's clinical status. Other early complications include anastomotic bleeding, surgical site infection, ileus, postoperative urinary retention, and stoma-related complications. Most stoma-related complications can be managed without reoperation. Late complications, such as bowel dysfunction, sexual dysfunction, and anastomotic stricture, are usually managed expectantly and should be discussed in the preoperative setting. There is growing interest in prevention of postoperative outcomes with preoperative nutritional supplementation and prehabilitation.

> Bariatric and metabolic surgery is a safe and effective treatment of morbid obesity, a disease that continues to increase in prevalence in the United States and worldwide. The two most commonly performed operations are the sleeve gastrectomy and the gastric bypass. Early and late complications can occur, and although referral to a bariatric surgeon or center is ideal, emergency management of acute problems is relevant to all general surgeons. Bariatric surgery can have surgical and metabolic consequences. An understanding of the altered anatomy and physiology helps to guide management of morbidities. This article discusses surgical postoperative complications and metabolic complications.

> Ventral and inguinal hernia repairs are some of the most commonly performed general surgery operations worldwide. This review focuses on the management of postoperative complications, which include surgical site infection, hernia recurrence, postoperative pain, and mesh-related issues. In each section, we aim to discuss classifications, risk factors,

Cervical endocrine operations include parathyroidectomy, thyroid lobectomy, thyroidectomy, central neck dissection, and lateral neck dissection. The vital structures at risk include the recurrent laryngeal nerves to the intrinsic muscles of the larynx, additional cranial nerves, parathyroid glands essential for calcium homeostasis, aerodigestive structures, and great vessels. Here, the authors discuss complications of endocrine neck surgery, including cervical hematoma and other fluid collections, hypocalcemia from hypoparathyroidism, and nerve injuries, along with their prevention, mitigation, and management. Significant and permanent morbidity can result, but fortunately the overall rate of complications remains low, especially when surgery is performed by high-volume surgeons.

Endovascular aneurysm repair (EVAR) is a minimally invasive therapeutic approach to manage abdominal aortic pathologies (eg, aneurysm and dissection). EVAR was first introduced in 1991. In 1994, endovascular technique was also applied for thoracic aorta, thoracic endovascular aortic repair (TEVAR). In recent decades, EVAR has become an acceptable first-line treatment with 50% utilization rate across most practices, especially in high-risk patients. The safety profile of EVAR is comparable to the open approach, with superiority in terms of perioperative mortality and morbidity. This article summarizes the most common complications following EVAR/TEVAR and the most current treatment modalities across practices.

This review discusses complications unique to pediatric surgical populations. Here the authors focus primarily on five of the most common procedures performed in children: appendectomy, central venous catheterization, pyloromyotomy, gastrostomy, and inguinal/umbilical hernia repair.

In this article, we discuss 4 common free flaps performed in reconstructive surgery: the anterolateral thigh flap, the radial forearm flap, the fibula flap, and the transverse rectus abdominis myocutaneous/deep inferior epigastric perforator flap. Donor and recipient complications for each flap type and strategies on how to prevent and manage such complications are discussed.

Joshua D. Smith, Jason A. Correll, Chaz L. Stucken, and Emily Z. Stucken

Unanticipated complications of ENT surgeries may have profound functional and esthetic consequences for patients. Herein, we provide a broad overview of postoperative complications after ENT surgery, illustrating their unique nature, impact, and principles of management. The discussion is organized by subspecialty to highlight the great anatomic complexity of the head and neck and the importance of critical neurovascular and sensory structures that make ENT an impactful, yet challenging surgical specialty.

Zahraa Al-Hilli and Avia Wilkerson

Breast cancer surgery is associated with low rates of surgical morbidity. Postoperative complications related to breast surgery include seroma, infection, hematoma, mastectomy flap necrosis, wound dehiscence, persistent postsurgical pain, Mondor disease, fat necrosis, reduced tactile sensation after mastectomy, and venous thromboembolism. Postoperative complications related to axillary surgery include seroma, infection, lymphedema, nerve injury, and reduced shoulder/arm mobility. The overall rate of complication related to axilla surgery may be confounded by the type of breast surgery performed. The management of postoperative complications related to oncologic breast and axillary surgery independent of reconstruction is reviewed here.

Robert Simon

The most common complications after a pancreaticoduodenectomy are delayed gastric emptying, pancreatic fistulae, hemorrhage, chyle leaks, endocrine and exocrine pancreatic insufficiency, and surgical site infections. Understanding the potential complications and recognizing them are imperative to taking great care of these complex patients. Taking care of these patients postoperatively requires a team approach including experienced nursing staff combined with robust gastroenterology and interventional radiology.

Samuel J. Zolin and Michael J. Rosen

This article reviews evidence-based techniques for abdominal closure and management strategies when abdominal wall closures fail. In particular, optimal primary fascial closure techniques, the role of prophylactic mesh, considerations for combined hernia repair, closure techniques when the fascia cannot be closed primarily, and management approaches for fascial dehiscence are reviewed.

Xiaoxi (Chelsea) Feng, Edward Phillips, and Daniel Shouhed

Cholecystectomy is one of the most common general surgery procedures performed worldwide. Complications include bile duct injury, strictures, bleeding, infection/abscess, retained gallstones, hernias, and postcholecystectomy syndrome. Obtaining a critical view of safety and following the other tenets of the Safe Cholecystectomy Task Force will aid in the prevention of bile duct injury and other morbidity associated with cholecystectomy.

Paul A. Toste and Sha'shonda L. Revels

Lung resections are associated with a variety of potential postoperative complications. Not surprisingly, pulmonary complications are most frequent after lung surgery. Cardiac and thromboembolic complications are also important. It is essential that surgeons anticipate the possibility of these complications and take preventative measures whenever possible. When complications do occur, prompt recognition and treatment is required to assure optimal patient outcomes.

Rachel R. Blitzer and Samuel Eisenstein

Perioperative venous thromboembolism (VTE) is a common complication within the surgical patient population. Perioperative mechanical and chemoprophylaxis have been shown to reduce the incidence of both deep venous thrombosis and pulmonary embolism. Prophylactic regimen must be tailored to the patient's individual risk factors as well as the nature of the procedure. In the event of VTE, treatment most commonly includes long-term anticoagulation, whereas more severe cases may require lytic or mechanical interventions.

SURGICAL CLINICS
OF NORTH AMERICA

FORTHCOMING ISSUES

December 2021
Controversies in General Surgery
Sean J. Langenfeld, *Editor*

February 2022
Surgical Critical Care
Brett H. Waibel, *Editor*

April 2022
Head and Neck Surgery
Brian J. Mitchell and Kyle Tubbs, *Editors*

RECENT ISSUES

August 2021
Education and the General Surgeon
Paul J. Schenarts, *Editor*

June 2021
Management of Esophageal Cancer
John A. Federico, Thomas Fabian, *Editors*

April 2021
Emerging Bariatric Surgical Procedures
Shanu N. Kothari, *Editor*

SERIES OF RELATED INTEREST

Advances in Surgery
https://www.advancessurgery.com/
Surgical Oncology Clinics
https://www.surgonc.theclinics.com/
Thoracic Surgery Clinics
http://www.thoracic.theclinics.com/

Foreword

Complications

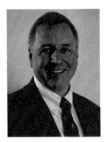

Ronald F. Martin, MD, FACS
Consulting Editor

Nobody likes complications. Nobody. Not surgeons. Not patients. Not families. Not hospital administrators. Not insurers. Nobody.

Yet, there always have been complications, and there likely always will be. There will be complications if we intervene. There will be complications if we fail to intervene. The only way one might avoid complications in the world of surgery is to not be in it—not be a surgeon and probably not be a patient.

All the above sentiments recognized and understood, we must seriously consider complications. We must also recognize that there is, or should be, a well-understood difference between complications, mal-outcomes, medical negligence, errors in judgment, misdiagnosis, and a whole host of other potentially undesirable occurrences. While there may be substantial overlap among and between the above referenced concerns, they are not synonymous.

I submit that complications may be considered as any untoward event that may occur during a patient's clinical course. Some of these may be the result of intervention, and some may be due to the lack of intervention or of intervention at an improper time. That a complication occurred does necessarily imply that something inappropriate was done nor does it imply that nothing inappropriate was done—in and of itself, the recognition of a complication is not a judgmental process; it is observational. We may choose to make a such judgments of appropriateness after the factors that are involved are considered. I would suggest that the more we link the recognition that a complication occurred to the concept that something wrong was done, the less likely we make it for people to accurately report when something has gone awry. And subsequently, we diminish our ability to learn from our mistakes.

It has been said that good judgment comes from experience and experience comes from bad judgment. There is more than a grain of truth to that. What isn't explicitly stated in this aphorism is that we are not limited to gain experience solely from our own bad judgment—we can learn from others. I might agree that lessons learned

Surg Clin N Am 101 (2021) xiii–xv
https://doi.org/10.1016/j.suc.2021.07.003
0039-6109/21/© 2021 Published by Elsevier Inc.

seem to be more immediate and long lasting when they are learned in the first person, but there are plenty of lessons to be learned from seeing events from nearby or even the cheap seats.

We surgeons invented our morbidity and mortality (M&M) conferences in large part to allow this communal education. To be certain, M&M conferences are variably effective and serve varied functions, but it's a start. These meetings are usually more effective when they are conducted systematically and with reliable processes. They are generally effective for those who are present but are frequently of little to no use to those who are not physically present. Due to the nature of the material discussed—in particular, the discoverable nature—we rarely distribute or rediscuss these specific situations outside of limited and protected meetings. As a result, the learning that takes place rarely amplifies and disseminates.

Attempts have been made to catalog and distribute the information and occurrences that lead to M&M discussions. Databases have been created for dissemination of some parts of the material with either tight controls of distribution or careful deidentification of information. While that is laudable and provides a good effort, it rarely is as useful as being involved in the actual discussions in real time.

The intent in developing this specific issue of the *Surgical Clinics* was twofold. First, people are far more likely to publish their successes than their failures. We wanted a forum to look at the "underrepresented" side of the literature. Second, we wanted a group of thoughtful people to provide us a resource of not only what things can go wrong but also how we can take adequate measures to treat, mitigate, or prevent these undesirable events. We are deeply indebted to Dr Lightner, Dr Fleshner, and their colleagues for generating this unflinching compendium of topics we wish to never encounter but know we will.

I have had the opportunity to lead M&M conferences and other various risk management or QA meetings for longer than I care to recall. One observation has always stood out: almost all complications are a result of a failure in something simple or basic and are rarely the result of something extraordinarily complex. Also, many if not most complications are preventable—in theory. Presentations of complications and the discussions that ensue occasionally follow the stages of grief starting with plaintive attempts at denial and eventually arriving at acceptance.

The process acknowledging and analyzing our errors is not just an intellectual exercise but also a means of catharsis. The value and power of catharsis in these situations should not be taken lightly. Even the coolest-headed surgeon needs to recover emotionally from unintentionally causing harm to effectively get back in the game. I have tried to counsel my residents and other trainees that a crucial step in developing surgical maturity is to develop the ability to be critical of an action that one took without being critical of the person. It is necessary to separate the two constructs to protect the integrity of the person confronting an error and to maximize the likelihood that people would be forthcoming in reporting complications.

The concept of "zero complications" or "never events" may be admirable but it is unrealistic in many ways. At the risk of being called defeatists, we are humans taking care of humans within the limits of systems created by and paid for by humans. No matter what lofty and aspirational goals are set for us by governments, insurers, or other bodies, sometimes things are going to go less well than hoped for. The preceding disclaimer aside, we can and should strive to reduce our adverse outcome rate to the smallest that it can be. To do so, we must rely on reliable content put into context by those who understand these topics very well. This is what we hope to have compiled for you. I hope you enjoy reading it and live a life sufficiently charmed that you can avoid mishaps that you otherwise may have encountered.

Ronald F. Martin, MD, FACS
Colonel (retired), United States Army Reserve
Department of General Surgery and
Surgical Oncology
Madigan Army Medical Center
9040 Jackson Avenue
Tacoma, WA 98431, USA

E-mail address:
rfmcescna@gmail.com

Preface

Introducing the Management of Postoperative Complications

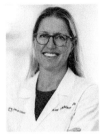 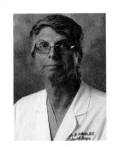

Amy L. Lightner, MD   Phillip R. Fleshner, MD
Editors

As surgeons, we do our best to prevent postoperative complications by optimizing perioperative patient care. Investigations have long focused on how we can better optimize the perioperative period, underscoring the desire to minimize any adverse events for our patients. However, postoperative complications remain throughout all surgical subspecialties. Thus, we must do our best to acknowledge and treat the complications in an expedient, safe, and effective manner. We herein discuss the management of postoperative complications across the most common general surgery subspecialties in hopes that our readers become better equipped to manage complications when they occur.

Colorectal complications, including infectious complications, anastomotic leaks, and dehiscence, are discussed by David Hanna and Alexander Hawkins. Complications following elective operations for bariatric surgery, a patient population fraught with significant morbidity, are discussed by Xiaoxi Feng and Miguel Burch. The optimal management of postoperative complications following ventral and inguinal hernia repair, some of the most common operations we perform, is taught by Yan Lu, David Chen, and Ian Macqueen. Endocrine surgery, which has the potential for life-threatening complications with an operative field in the neck, is described by Oliver Fackelmayer, James Wu, and Michael Yeh. The management of postoperative complications following aortic aneurysm repair, most of which needs to be quickly recognized and addressed, is discussed by Mohammed Qrareya and Bara Zuhaili. The management of postoperative complications in pediatric surgery, a variable array of surgical interventions, is described by Danny Lascanao and Lorrain Kelly-Quon. Tissue flaps, often used to fill dead space in many of our surgical subspecialities, including colorectal and breast, are fraught with potential breakdown and necrosis; the prevention and management of these complications are discussed by Travis

Surg Clin N Am 101 (2021) xvii–xviii
https://doi.org/10.1016/j.suc.2021.07.002
0039-6109/21/© 2021 Published by Elsevier Inc.

Miller, Christopher Lavin, Arash Momeni, and Derrick Wan. Infectious, vascular, and airway complications may be lethal in ENT surgery; management of these complications in an expedient fashion is illustrated by Joshua Smith, Jason Correll, Chaz Stucken, and Emily Stucken. Breast surgery, complicated by lymphovascular dissection and flap creation, has potential side effects that contribute to significant morbidity; these are highlighted by Zahraa Al-Hilli and Avia Wilkerson. Pancreaticoduodenectomy has many potential side effects in the postoperative period, which are illustrated by Robert Simon. The prevention and management of abdominal wall closures, often seen in general surgery and its subspecialties, are discussed by Samuel Zolin and Michael Rosen. Cholecystectomy, one of the most common operations performed in general surgery, has several potential postoperative complications, including common bile duct injury biloma, which are highlighted by Xiaoxi Feng, Daniel Shouhed, and Edward Philliops. Following lung resection in thoracic surgery, patients may experience significant pulmonary morbidity, all of which is highlighted by Paul Toste and Sha'shonda Revels. Last, the prevention and management of venous thromboembolic events and pulmonary embolism, seen across all surgical subspecialties, are discussed by Rachel Blitzer and Samuel Eisenstein.

While not entirely comprehensive of all complications across general surgery and its subspecialties, we hope that this underscores key preventative and management strategies across several subspecialities.

Amy L. Lightner, MD
Center for Regenerative Medicine and Surgery
Digestive Disease Institute
Lerner Research Institute
Cleveland Clinic
9500 Euclid Avenue
Cleveland, OH 44195, USA

Phillip R. Fleshner, MD, FASCRS
Division of Colon and Rectal Surgery
Cedars-Sinai Medical Center
8737 Beverly Boulevard
Los Angeles, CA 90048, USA

E-mail addresses:
Lightner.amy@mayo.edu; ghtna@ccf.org (A.L. Lightner)
phillip.fleshner@cshs.org (P.R. Fleshner)

Colorectal

Management of Postoperative Complications in Colorectal Surgery

David N. Hanna, MD[a], Alexander T. Hawkins, MD, MPH[b],*

KEYWORDS

• Colorectal surgery • Anastomotic leak • Urinary retention • Anastomotic stricture

KEY POINTS

- There is a growing body of evidence that prehabilitation can improve postoperative outcomes.
- Anastomotic leak is the most dreaded complication in colorectal surgery, but most patients do not require reoperation.
- Anastomotic bleeding is usually self-limited or can be managed nonoperatively.
- Stoma-related complications can be usually managed with noninvasive measures, with reoperation reserved for patients with significant pouching issues or strangulated parastomal hernias.
- Late complications in colorectal surgery include bowel and sexual dysfunction, as well as anastomotic stricture.

INTRODUCTION

Colorectal surgery is performed for a variety of diseases, including cancer, inflammatory bowel disease, and diverticulitis. There has been growing interest in the prevention of postoperative compilations in colorectal surgery, with a focus on preoperative nutrition and rehabilitation. Although the risks of colorectal surgery are similar to other major abdominal operations, there are some that are of particular interest, including anastomotic leak, stoma-related complications, anastomotic bleeding, and later bowel and sexual dysfunction. Anastomotic leaks are a source of significant morbidity and are managed based on the patient's clinical status and degree of leakage. Stoma-related complications are typically managed nonoperatively in most cases. Later complications are managed for the most part expectantly and should be discussed in the preoperative

[a] Division of General Surgery, Section of Colon and Rectal Surgery, Vanderbilt University, Vanderbilt University Medical Center, 1161 21st Avenue South, CCC-4322B MCN, Nashville, TN 37232, USA; [b] Division of General Surgery, Section of Colon and Rectal Surgery, Vanderbilt University, Vanderbilt University Medical Center, 1161 21st Avenue South, Room D5248 MCN, Nashville, TN 37232, USA
* Corresponding author.
E-mail address: alex.hawkins@vumc.org

Surg Clin N Am 101 (2021) 717–729
https://doi.org/10.1016/j.suc.2021.05.016
0039-6109/21/Published by Elsevier Inc.
surgical.theclinics.com

setting. This article highlights some of the most common and clinically significant complications of colorectal surgery.

PERIOPERATIVE CONSIDERATIONS AND PREDICTION IN POSTOPERATIVE COMPLICATIONS

One of the best ways to manage postoperative complications is to prevent them from happening in the first place. Over the past decades, a large amount of research has been put into predicting postoperative complications. Although this is a broad field, there are several important themes.

Preoperative malnutrition in the patient has been strongly linked to postoperative complications, including death. Patients being considered for colorectal surgery should be assessed for malnutrition. Based on expert consensus, a diagnosis of malnutrition requires that the patient exhibit 2 or more of the following: insufficient energy intake, weight loss, loss of muscle mass, loss of subcutaneous fat, localized or generalized fluid accumulation that may sometimes mask weight loss, and/or diminished functional status as measured by handgrip strength.[1] In any patient with suspected malnutrition, protein status should be assessed with serum albumin, transferrin, and prealbumin. Low serum albumin (<2.2 g/dL) is a marker of a negative catabolic state and a predictor of poor outcome.[2] For any patient with identified malnutrition, supplementation should be initiated. The first choice for supplementation is enteral. Perioperative immunonutrition seems to be the best approach to support malnourished patients with cancer, with an observed reduction in complications and length of stay.[3] Consultation with a nutritionist is recommended. For patients with identified malnutrition who need to undergo urgent or emergent surgery, avoidance of an anastomosis (via Hartmann procedure) or protection of the anastomosis (via diverting loop ileostomy) should be strongly considered. This group of patients should be screened early for postoperative total parenteral nutrition (TPN).

The concept of frailty has emerged as a more accurate description of age-related physiologic decline than age itself. The concept of frailty and the risk for complications has been well described.[4] Frailty is easily screened for with several easy-to-administer assessment tools, including the Fried Frailty Tool, the FRAIL scale and The Study of Osteoporotic Fractures (SOF) frailty tool. Once identified, there are several emerging strategies to try and improve postoperative outcomes. The most popular of these is the concept of prehabilitation, where a combination of nutritional supplementation, physical exercise and cognitive exercise is used to improve postoperative outcomes. Studies have shown improved aerobic capacity and fewer complications (eg, cardiovascular events, perioperative infection, or paralytic ileus) in high-risk patients engaging in prehabilitation.[5]

Finally, several novel risk calculators allow surgeons to give an accurate expectation of a patient's postoperative course. The most robust of these is the American College of Surgeons National Surgical Quality Improvement Program (NSQIP) Surgical Risk Calculator (https://riskcalculator.facs.org/RiskCalculator/). This Web site allows for a realistic assessment of risk for postoperative complications. This can be used not only to provide data to inform a discussion of risk and benefits of surgery, but also to motivate patients to undertake lifestyle changes to reduce risk.

EARLY COMPLICATIONS IN COLORECTAL SURGERY
Anastomotic Leak

Anastomotic leak (AL) is the most feared complication in colorectal surgery, resulting in significant morbidity, mortality, hospital length of stay, medical cost, and even cancer recurrence.[6] Generally, the risk of AL increases with more distal anastomoses. In a prospective study of almost 2000 patients who underwent colorectal resections, the AL rate for rectal anastomoses was 6.7%, compared with a 2.6% leak rate for colonic anastomoses, and even lower for ileocolic anastomoses.[7] Patient-specific risk factors include obesity, smoking, ASA status, corticosteroid use, male sex, and malnutrition. Patients with inflammatory bowel disease (IBD) are commonly on immunosuppressive medications, such as anti-tumor necrosis factor (TNF) agents and corticosteroids. A large systematic review that included almost 10,000 patients found that the AL rate was approximately 2 times higher in patients receiving corticosteroids than those who did not (6.8% vs 3.3%).[8] Although there are conflicting data regarding the use of anti-TNF agents and their effect on AL, cessation of such agents should be considered prior to surgery.

New technology has allowed surgeons to assess proximal limb perfusion, including Doppler ultrasonography and fluorescence angiography with indocyanine green. These technologies have been shown to be safe and can help determine perfusion, but there are limited data to suggest that these technologies can prevent AL. Intraoperative endoscopic assessment of left-sided anastomoses is recommended to assess for bleeding and anastomosis integrity. An air leak test should be performed by filling the pelvis with saline and occluding the bowel proximal to the anastomosis prior to insufflating the rectum with an endoscope.[9] One prospective randomized study showed a significant reduction in AL between patients who underwent an air leak test compared with those who did not (4% vs 14%).[10] If the surgeon observes a potentially questionable aspect of the anastomosis, it should be recreated or repaired, with or without diverting stoma.9 Two metanalyses within the last 10 years, both involving almost 1000 patients, showed that defunctioning stomas are associated with lower incidence of AL and reoperation in patients who underwent low anterior resection.[11,12] The decision to perform a diverting stoma should incorporate preoperative patient risk factors, such as prior radiation, use of corticosteroids, and malnutrition, as well as intraoperative assessment of the anastomosis.

Given the significant morbidity and increased patient mortality in the setting of AL, prompt diagnosis and intervention are imperative. Computed tomography (CT) with intravenous contrast is helpful in identifying the presence of an abscess. Additionally, rectal contrast provides evaluation of low colorectal anastomoses and should be administered by a member of the surgical team using a pliable catheter. An emerging clinical technique involves the postoperative measurement of biomarkers to provide cost-effective immediate monitoring of a potential AL. A recent meta-analysis demonstrated that CRP is a useful negative predictive test for postoperative AL, with a negative predictive value of 97%.[13]

The management of AL relies largely on the patient's clinical status. A recent retrospective study using the National Surgical Quality Improvement Program (NSQIP) database of over 30,000 patients demonstrated that 43.9% of patients with anastomotic leak do not require reoperation.[14] The extent of leakage and patient's physiologic status dictate the need for operation or percutaneous drainage (**Figs. 1** and **2**). For patients with hemodynamic stability and radiographic evidence of a fluid collection near the anastomosis, percutaneous drainage may be appropriate. Alternatively, endoscopic or transanal drainage can be performed for leaks associated with pelvic anastomoses, particularly if the leak is small.[15] Finally, covered stents with proximal diversion are an option for colorectal or distal colo-colo anastomoses. Regardless of the nonoperative method pursued, if a patient does not clinically improve or develops sepsis or peritonitis, reoperation is needed. The principles of reoperation

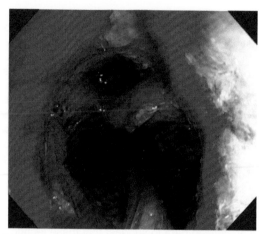

Fig. 1. Endoscopic image of a disrupted ileal pouch anal anastomosis (IPAA). The pouch is seen at the top of the image. The operative drain is seen coursing through the leak at the bottom of the image.

include washout and fecal diversion via end stoma or diverting stoma with or without anastomosis repair or reconstruction.

Anastomotic Bleeding

Postoperative bleeding after colorectal surgery is typically minor, self-limited, and caused by intraluminal bleeding from a newly created anastomosis. Fortunately, this complication is rare, comprising 0.5% to 1.8% of all patients undergoing elective colorectal surgery.[16] Several large prospective studies have demonstrated consistent risk factors associated with postoperative hemorrhage requiring transfusion, including the need for an emergent operation, longer operative times, and age.[17–19]

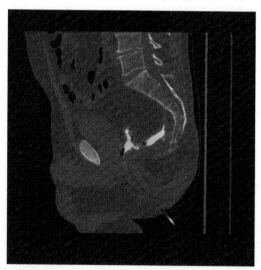

Fig. 2. Radiographic image of AL of IPAA. There is extravasation of contrast through the posterior aspect of the anastomosis. An operative drain is seen near the anastomosis.

Side-to-side stapled anastomoses are inspected for bleeding at the time of anasto-mosis creation. Surgeons typically assess their colorectal or ileorectal anastomotic lines with intraoperative endoscopy. In a prospective study of about 1000 patients, postoperative anastomotic bleeding was observed in 4.3% patients who did not un-dergo intraoperative endoscopy, most of whom required postoperative endoscopic clipping.[20] In the event that a procedural intervention is needed, endoscopic evalua-tion with electrocoagulation, submucosal epinephrine injection, or endoscopic clip-ping can be used safely.[16] In the rare event that anastomotic bleeding cannot be controlled via those measures or causes significant hemodynamic instability, laparot-omy with oversewing of the anastomosis or resection and recreation of the anasto-mosis is needed. Overall, anastomotic hemorrhage requiring intervention is rare, and endoscopic techniques have largely replaced laparotomy.

Ileus

Postoperative ileus after colorectal surgery remains a significant cause of prolonged hospital stay, hospital costs, and delayed recovery.[21,22] Although the exact mecha-nism by which postoperative ileus develops remains unknown, the prevailing theory revolves around edema and inflammation.[21] The reported incidence ranges from 3% to 30% after elective colorectal surgery.[23] In a prospective study of over 300 pa-tients, male gender, decreased preoperative albumin, open surgical technique, increased intravenous fluid administration, and blood transfusion were independent predictors of prolonged postoperative ileus.[24] Other prospective and retrospective studies have found prior abdominal operations, obesity, intraoperative hypothermia, and opioid use to be associated with increased risk of prolonged postoperative ileus.[25,26]

There have been several new therapeutic strategies to minimize postoperative ileus, such as the administration of prokinetic agents, dopamine agonists, and opioid ago-nists. However, these have not been shown to prevent postoperative ileus in random-ized trials.[27] Patients with a postoperative ileus should be allowed nothing by mouth and started on maintenance intravenous fluids. In the setting of persistent nausea, emesis, and concern for aspiration, a nasogastric tube should be placed and losses replaced with intravenous fluids. In the setting of prolonged ileus, TPN should be initiated.

Ostomy Complications

Complications related to stomas are usually minor and can be managed with local sto-mal therapy, with reoperation reserved for significant or devastating complications. Ostomy support groups and involvement of wound ostomy continence nurses (WOCNs) have been shown to reduce complication rates and improve long-term qual-ity of life.[28] Additionally, choosing a proper stoma site should be done preoperatively, if possible. The patient should be examined while supine, sitting, and standing. The stoma site should be clear of old incisions, skin creases, and should be surrounded by healthy skin for appropriate appliance application.

Dehydration and electrolyte derangements from high-volume output are the most common causes of readmission in patients with a newly created stoma, which occur as frequently as in 17% of cases.[29] These readmissions are more common in patients with an ileostomy. Prior to initial discharge, patients should undergo intensive educa-tion that emphasizes proper water and salt balance, recording the quantity and quality of output, and adequate food consumption. Typically, the target daily output of less than 1200 mL is desired for ileostomies.[30] Prevention and initial strategies to reduce high ostomy output include avoiding fatty meals while also increasing fiber intake to at least 20 g/d. Additionally, pharmacologic agents such as supplemental soluble fiber, loperamide, or diphenoxylate can be used.

Local anatomic stomal complications include retraction, necrosis, and prolapse. Stomal retraction is defined as a stoma that terminates at least 0.5 cm below the skin surface (**Fig. 3**).[31] These stomas can be managed with convex appliance systems that flatten the peristomal skin and stoma belts or binders. If continued associated complications occur, surgical revision or resiting must be considered. Stomal necrosis, which occurs because of local or mechanical ischemia, is relatively rare. If the necrosis proceeds lower than the abdominal wall fascia, immediate surgical revision is warranted. Stomal stenosis is usually self-limited and resolves as postoperative bowel edema subsides and can be aided with decompressive rubber catheter or serial dilation. Stomal prolapse, which is more common with colostomies, is a full-thickness telescoping of the bowel through the fascial and skin opening (**Fig. 4**). Acute prolapse is often managed by gentle bedside reduction with the aid of sugar or other osmotic gents. Additionally, stoma binders can aid in preventing recurrent prolapse. However, chronic prolapse can lead to stoma incarceration, or strangulation, which requires resection and revision.

Parastomal hernias are defined as incisional hernias that occur through the created abdominal wall defect of the stoma site (**Fig. 5**). Parastomal hernias are most prevalent among end colostomies and generally occur within the first 2 years after stoma creation.[32] The incidence of clinically significant parastomal hernias ranges from 25% to 40%, while incidentally detected parastomal hernias occur with greater than 75% of stomas.[33] Risk factors for parastomal hernias are consistent with risk factors for other stoma-related complications as well as steroid use, ascites, and constipation. Parastomal hernias are frequently asymptomatic and are often well tolerated, even when

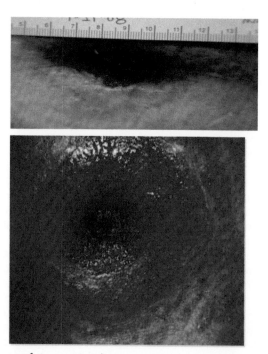

Fig. 3. Patient images of stoma retraction.

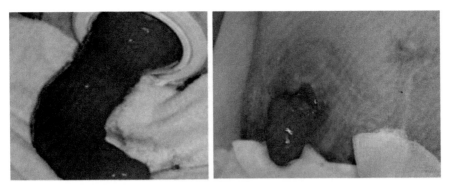

Fig. 4. Patient image of stoma prolapse.

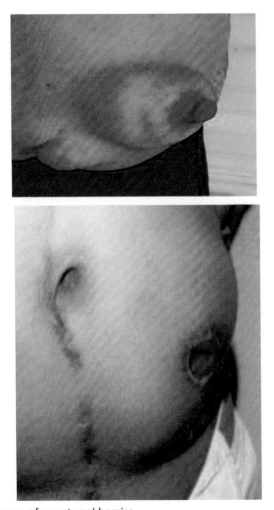

Fig. 5. Patient images of parastomal hernias.

symptoms of abdominal pain and skin irritation occur. However, strangulation of the hernia contents warrants reoperation.

The use of prophylactic intraperitoneal mesh to reduce the incidence of parastomal hernias has been extensively studied. Several studies have shown that that placement of synthetic or biologic mesh in the sublay position is safe.[34] A recent meta-analysis of about 500 patients found a significant reduction in parastomal hernia formation and need for reoperation in patients who underwent prophylactic mesh placement without an increase in the surgical or soma-specific complications.[35] However, the benefits of placing a prophylactic mesh need to be weighed against the risks of increased operative time, complications, and technical success. Fewer than 25% of patients with parastomal hernias require repair, including patients with a strangulated parastomal hernia or those with chronic debilitating symptoms. The 3 methods of repair include local repair, mesh repair, or stomal relocation.

Surgical Site Infections

Surgical site infections (SSIs) are the most common source of morbidity for patients undergoing colorectal surgery. They are associated with increased hospital stay, readmission, and cost utilization.[36] Given the oftentimes contaminated nature of colorectal surgeries, these surgeries have high rates of SSI, ranging from 5% to 30%.[37] Patient and disease factors that contribute to SSI include higher ASA class, obesity, tobacco use, chronic obstructive pulmonary disease (COPD), diabetes, age, and IBD. Surgical risk factors include intraoperative blood transfusion, operative time, open operation, and contamination. The principles of the treatment for SSIs in colorectal surgery are similar to those of other surgical specialties, including antibiotics and source control as clinically indicated. The most studied preoperative measure to reduce SSI is mechanical bowel prep (MBP). The landmark randomized controlled trial (RCT), which compared MBP to MBP with oral antibiotics, showed a significant decrease in SSI with the addition of antibiotics.[38] Further studies have shown that the benefits of MBP and antibiotics extend beyond just SSI, but also to rates of AL, readmission rates, and hospital length of stay.[39,40]

Genitourinary Complications

The use of indwelling urinary catheters after abdominal operations is commonplace. Cather-associated urinary tract infections (CAUTIs) are a common, costly, and preventable condition that has been the subject of much attention. The push for early urinary catheter removal has led to the increased postoperative urinary retention (POUR). POUR is most common among patients undergoing APR, which can be as high as 40% in men and 35% in women.[41] The rate of POUR in colon resection is about 2% and up to 24% for rectal resections.[42] Risk factors for POUR include older age, male sex, longer operative time, pelvic dissection, and low rectal cancers.[42,43]

When urinary retention does occur after urinary catheter removal, it is replaced, and an alpha-1 blocker or a 5-alpha reductase inhibitor is prescribed, such as tamsulosin and finasteride. Much attention has been given to prevention of POUR, which relies heavily on duration of urinary catheterization. Several randomized trials have been unable to demonstrate an optimal time to remove the urinary catheter.[44,45]

LATE COMPLICATIONS–ISSUES THAT PERSIST LONGER THAN 6 MONTHS
Bowel Dysfunction

Colorectal surgery, especially those procedures that involve a partial proctectomy with a colorectal anastomosis, introduce new physiology into the act of defecation.

Functional disturbances constitute a major problem for many patients following partial or complete proctectomy, with symptoms ranging from incontinence to obstructed defecation and constipation to clustering. Although these symptoms have an impact on the patient's quality of life, there is presently no universal treatment. Instead, management is empiric and uses existing therapies for fecal incontinence, fecal urgency, and rectal evacuatory disorders. It is estimated that 25% to 80% of patients develop some degree of bowel dysfunction following rectal surgery. About 50% of patients still report symptoms more than 10 years after surgery.[46,47] A detailed history is necessary to identify the exact manifestation of dysfunction. Work-up may include a barium enema or colonoscopy to rule out an anastomotic stricture as well as defecography and anorectal manometry to assess obstructed defecation and/or incontinence. Minor dysfunction can usually be treated medically with fiber therapy, an antidiarrheal agent, and/or pelvic floor physical therapy. More severe cases may require neurostimulation or fecal diversion.

Sexual Dysfunction and Fertility

For both men and women, sexual dysfunction and fertility issues can be significant long-term concerns after proctectomy. Male sexual dysfunction can manifest in a wide range of issues, including issues with both erection and ejaculation. Studies report that following treatment for rectal cancer, as many as 63% of men will have some measure of erectile dysfunction, and that 60% will have difficulty with ejaculation.[48] It is important to differentiate acute from long-term dysfunction. Generally, it takes approximately 6 months for symptoms to plateau. Evaluation and treatment should generally be guided by a urologist. The potential for sexual dysfunction should be addressed in preoperative counseling. Sperm banking should be considered in men of childbearing age.

Because of the proximity of autonomic nerves necessary for sexual function to the rectum, women undergoing proctectomy are at increased risk for sexual dysfunction. Female sexual dysfunction is primarily manifested in vaginal dryness, dyspareunia, and reduced sexual desire. Over 50% of women report some level of sexual dysfunction following resection for rectal cancer. Abdominal perineal resection is an independent risk factor for sexual dysfunction. Treatment should be guided by symptoms, and preoperative counseling should be an integral part of the consent process.

Women undergoing pelvic procedures should undergo preoperative discussion of the potential risk for fertility problems. This is most important in women of childbearing age and mostly includes women undergoing proctectomy for IBD or polyposis syndromes. A meta-analysis revealed a postoperative infertility rate of 48% after restorative proctocolectomy for ulcerative colitis, compared with 15% preoperatively.[49] Preoperative counseling should focus on both education and consideration of delaying any pelvic procedure until after the patient has completed plans for motherhood. Egg freezing and/or embryo cryopreservation should also be discussed.

Anastomotic Stricture

Depending on definition, the incidence of an anastomotic stricture or stenosis after a colorectal anastomosis ranges from 0% to 30%.[50] Anastomotic stricture may arise because of tissue ischemia, inflammation, radiation, anastomotic leak, or recurrent disease. Treatment should be tailored to patient symptoms. All strictures should be biopsied, but asymptomatic strictures generally do not require intervention. First-line treatment for benign anastomotic stricture is endoscopic balloon dilation, with long-term success rates of 88% balanced against relatively low complications rates of around 10%.[51] Should conservative measures fail, resection and repeat anastomosis should be considered. Patients with a coloanal anastomosis may need to be converted to a permanent colostomy.

CLINICS CARE POINTS

- The optimal choice for preoperative nutritional supplementation is enteral.
- Preoperative "pre-habilitation" may prevent postoperative complications in high-risk or frail patients.
- While the management of anastomotic leaks rely on the patient's clinical status, the principles of reoperation include washout and fecal diversion.
- When caring for a patient with a prolonged ileus, consider insertion of a nasogastric tube if there is concern for aspiration as well as administration of total parenteral nutrition.
- Parastomal hernias are frequently asymptomatic and are usually well tolerated when symptoms do occur. However, hernia strangulation warrants reoperation.
- Bowel dysfunction after colorectal surgery can be evaluated with barium enema, colonoscopy, defecography, or anorectal manometry and can usually be treated medically.
- It is important to discuss potential risk of fertility issues with female patients of childbearing age undergoing pelvic procedures.
- All anastomotic strictures should be biopsied.

DISCLOSURE

Dr. Hawkin's work on this manuscript was supported by the National Institute of Diabetes and Digestive and Kidney Disease of the National Institutes of Health under award number K23DK118192. Dr. Hanna's work on this manuscript was supported by an NIH T32 training grant (T32CA10618).

REFERENCES

1. White JV, Guenter P, Jensen G, et al. Consensus statement: Academy of Nutrition and Dietetics and American Society for Parenteral and Enteral Nutrition: characteristics recommended for the identification and documentation of adult malnutrition (undernutrition). JPEN J Parenter Enteral Nutr 2012;36(3):275–83.
2. van Stijn MF, Korkic-Halilovic I, Bakker MS, et al. Preoperative nutrition status and postoperative outcome in elderly general surgery patients: a systematic review. JPEN J Parenter Enteral Nutr 2013;37(1):37–43.
3. Braga M, Gianotti L, Nespoli L, et al. Nutritional approach in malnourished surgical patients: a prospective randomized study. Arch Surg 2002;137(2):174–80.
4. Fagard K, Leonard S, Deschodt M, et al. The impact of frailty on postoperative outcomes in individuals aged 65 and over undergoing elective surgery for colorectal cancer: a systematic review. J Geriatr Oncol 2016;7(6):479–91.
5. Barberan-Garcia A, Ubre M, Roca J, et al. Personalised Prehabilitation in High-risk Patients Undergoing Elective Major Abdominal Surgery: A Randomized Blinded Controlled Trial. Ann Surg 2018;267(1):50–6.
6. Chambers WM, Mortensen NJ. Postoperative leakage and abscess formation after colorectal surgery. Best Pract Res Clin Gastroenterol 2004;18(5):865–80.
7. Branagan G, Finnis D, Wessex Colorectal Cancer Audit Working G. Prognosis after anastomotic leakage in colorectal surgery. Dis Colon Rectum 2005;48(5):1021–6.

8. Eriksen TF, Lassen CB, Gogenur I. Treatment with corticosteroids and the risk of anastomotic leakage following lower gastrointestinal surgery: a literature survey. Colorectal Dis 2014;16(5):O154–60.

9. Thomas MS, Margolin DA. Management of Colorectal Anastomotic Leak. Clin Colon Rectal Surg 2016;29(2):138–44.

10. Beard JD, Nicholson ML, Sayers RD, et al. Intraoperative air testing of colorectal anastomoses: a prospective, randomized trial. Br J Surg 1990;77(10):1095–7.

11. Huser N, Michalski CW, Erkan M, et al. Systematic review and meta-analysis of the role of defunctioning stoma in low rectal cancer surgery. Ann Surg 2008; 248(1):52–60.

12. Chen J, Wang DR, Yu HF, et al. Defunctioning stoma in low anterior resection for rectal cancer: a meta- analysis of five recent studies. Hepatogastroenterology 2012;59(118):1828–31.

13. Singh PP, Zeng IS, Srinivasa S, et al. Systematic review and meta-analysis of use of serum C-reactive protein levels to predict anastomotic leak after colorectal surgery. Br J Surg 2014;101(4):339–46.

14. Moghadamyeghaneh Z, Hanna MH, Alizadeh RF, et al. Contemporary management of anastomotic leak after colon surgery: assessing the need for reoperation. Am J Surg 2016;211(6):1005–13.

15. Sirois-Giguere E, Boulanger-Gobeil C, Bouchard A, et al. Transanal drainage to treat anastomotic leaks after low anterior resection for rectal cancer: a valuable option. Dis Colon Rectum 2013;56(5):586–92.

16. Cirocco WC, Golub RW. Endoscopic treatment of postoperative hemorrhage from a stapled colorectal anastomosis. Am Surg 1995;61(5):460–3.

17. Pribelsky M, Porubsky J, Schnorrer M. [The effect of age and risk factors on postoperative complications and mortality in patients with surgery for colorectal carcinoma]. Bratisl Lek Listy 1996;97(1):50–3.

18. Hida K, Yamaguchi T, Hata H, et al. Risk factors for complications after laparoscopic surgery in colorectal cancer patients: experience of 401 cases at a single institution. World J Surg 2009;33(8):1733–40.

19. Santoro E, Carboni F, Ettorre GM, et al. Early results and complications of colorectal laparoscopic surgery and analysis of risk factors in 492 operated cases. Updates Surg 2010;62(3–4):135–41.

20. Shamiyeh A, Szabo K, Ulf Wayand W, et al. Intraoperative endoscopy for the assessment of circular-stapled anastomosis in laparoscopic colon surgery. Surg Laparosc Endosc Percutan Tech 2012;22(1):65–7.

21. Mattei P, Rombeau JL. Review of the pathophysiology and management of postoperative ileus. World J Surg 2006;30(8):1382–91.

22. Baig MK, Wexner SD. Postoperative ileus: a review. Dis Colon Rectum 2004; 47(4):516–26.

23. van Bree SH, Nemethova A, Cailotto C, et al. New therapeutic strategies for postoperative ileus. Nat Rev Gastroenterol Hepatol 2012;9(11):675–83.

24. Vather R, Josephson R, Jaung R, et al. Development of a risk stratification system for the occurrence of prolonged postoperative ileus after colorectal surgery: a prospective risk factor analysis. Surgery 2015;157(4):764–73.

25. Choi JW, Kim DK, Kim JK, et al. A retrospective analysis on the relationship between intraoperative hypothermia and postoperative ileus after laparoscopic colorectal surgery. PLoS One 2018;13(1):e0190711.

26. Rybakov EG, Shelygin YA, Khomyakov EA, et al. Risk factors for postoperative ileus after colorectal cancer surgery. Colorectal Dis 2017;20(3):189–94.

27. Traut U, Brugger L, Kunz R, et al. Systemic prokinetic pharmacologic treatment for postoperative adynamic ileus following abdominal surgery in adults. Cochrane Database Syst Rev 2008;(1):CD004930.

28. Salvadalena G, Hendren S, McKenna L, et al. WOCN Society and ASCRS position statement on preoperative stoma site marking for patients undergoing colostomy or ileostomy surgery. J Wound Ostomy Continence Nurs 2015;42(3):249–52.

29. Steinhagen E, Colwell J, Cannon LM. Intestinal stomas-postoperative stoma care and peristomal skin complications. Clin Colon Rectal Surg 2017;30(3):184–92.

30. Nagle D, Pare T, Keenan E, et al. Ileostomy pathway virtually eliminates readmissions for dehydration in new ostomates. Dis Colon Rectum 2012;55(12):1266–72.

31. Kwiatt M, Kawata M. Avoidance and management of stomal complications. Clin Colon Rectal Surg 2013;26(2):112–21.

32. Krishnamurty DM, Blatnik J, Mutch M. Stoma Complications. Clin Colon Rectal Surg 2017;30(3):193–200.

33. Whitehead A, Cataldo PA. Technical Considerations in Stoma Creation. Clin Colon Rectal Surg 2017;30(3):162–71.

34. Janes A, Cengiz Y, Israelsson LA. Preventing parastomal hernia with a prosthetic mesh: a 5-year follow-up of a randomized study. World J Surg 2009;33(1):118–21 [discussion: 122-3].

35. Wijeyekoon SP, Gurusamy K, El-Gendy K, et al. Prevention of parastomal herniation with biologic/composite prosthetic mesh: a systematic review and meta-analysis of randomized controlled trials. J Am Coll Surg 2010;211(5):637–45.

36. Keenan JE, Speicher PJ, Thacker JK, et al. The preventive surgical site infection bundle in colorectal surgery: an effective approach to surgical site infection reduction and health care cost savings. JAMA Surg 2014;149(10):1045–52.

37. Tanner J, Khan D, Aplin C, et al. Post-discharge surveillance to identify colorectal surgical site infection rates and related costs. J Hosp Infect 2009;72(3):243–50.

38. Nichols RL, Schumer W, Nyhus LM. Technique of preoperative bowel sterilisation. Lancet 1973;2(7831):735.

39. Bellows CF, Mills KT, Kelly TN, et al. Combination of oral non-absorbable and intravenous antibiotics versus intravenous antibiotics alone in the prevention of surgical site infections after colorectal surgery: a meta-analysis of randomized controlled trials. Tech Coloproctol 2011;15(4):385–95.

40. Cannon JA, Altom LK, Deierhoi RJ, et al. Preoperative oral antibiotics reduce surgical site infection following elective colorectal resections. Dis Colon Rectum 2012;55(11):1160–6.

41. Luna-Perez P, Rodriguez-Ramirez S, Vega J, et al. Morbidity and mortality following abdominoperineal resection for low rectal adenocarcinoma. Rev Invest Clin 2001;53(5):388–95.

42. Tekkis PP, Cornish JA, Remzi FH, et al. Measuring sexual and urinary outcomes in women after rectal cancer excision. Dis Colon Rectum 2009;52(1):46–54.

43. Kin C, Rhoads KF, Jalali M, et al. Predictors of postoperative urinary retention after colorectal surgery. Dis Colon Rectum 2013;56(6):738–46.

44. Benoist S, Panis Y, Denet C, et al. Optimal duration of urinary drainage after rectal resection: a randomized controlled trial. Surgery 1999;125(2):135–41.

45. Hakvoort RA, Elberink R, Vollebregt A, et al. How long should urinary bladder catheterisation be continued after vaginal prolapse surgery? A randomised controlled trial comparing short term versus long term catheterisation after vaginal prolapse surgery. BJOG 2004;111(8):828–30.

46. Chen TY, Wiltink LM, Nout RA, et al. Bowel function 14 years after preoperative short-course radiotherapy and total mesorectal excision for rectal cancer: report of a multicenter randomized trial. Clin Colorectal Cancer 2015;14(2):106–14.
47. Sturiale A, Martellucci J, Zurli L, et al. Long-term functional follow-up after anterior rectal resection for cancer. Int J Colorectal Dis 2017;32(1):83–8.
48. Hendren SK, O'Connor BI, Liu M, et al. Prevalence of male and female sexual dysfunction is high following surgery for rectal cancer. Ann Surg 2005;242(2): 212–23.
49. Waljee A, Waljee J, Morris AM, et al. Threefold increased risk of infertility: a meta-analysis of infertility after ileal pouch anal anastomosis in ulcerative colitis. Gut 2006;55(11):1575–80.
50. Schlegel RD, Dehni N, Parc R, et al. Results of reoperations in colorectal anastomotic strictures. Dis Colon Rectum 2001;44(10):1464–8.
51. Suchan KL, Muldner A, Manegold BC. Endoscopic treatment of postoperative colorectal anastomotic strictures. Surg Endosc 2003;17(7):1110–3.

Management of Postoperative Complications Following Bariatric and Metabolic Procedures

Xiaoxi (Chelsea) Feng, MD, MPH, Miguel Burch, MD*

KEYWORDS

- Bariatric • Complications • Morbidity • Gastric bypass • Gastric sleeve
- Metabolic surgery • Weight loss surgery

KEY POINTS

- Bariatric and metabolic surgeries, including the sleeve gastrectomy and the gastric bypass, are generally safe procedures with a favorable risk profile.
- Surgical complications that can occur include leak, bleeding, obstruction, fistula, ulcers, and thromboembolic disease, among others.
- Leaks after bariatric surgery benefit from early recognition, and are approached with operative, endoscopic, and radiologic modalities, depending on the clinical scenario.
- Metabolic complications depend on the surgical anatomy, and include nutritional deficiencies and dumping syndrome.

INTRODUCTION

Obesity is a serious and costly chronic disease that continues to increase in prevalence in the United States. It is defined as having a body mass index (BMI) of 30 kg/m^2 or more. From 2000 to 2018, the Centers for Disease Control and Prevention estimates that the prevalence of obesity increased from 30.5% to 42.4%.[1] Obesity-related conditions, such as type 2 diabetes, hypertension, stroke, and cardiovascular disease are leading causes of mortality, and severe obesity (defined as having a BMI of 40 kg/m^2 or more) is associated with a 50% to 100% increased risk of premature death.[2]

Bariatric surgery is an effective treatment of severe obesity, proven to have better durability than diet and medical therapy alone.[3,4] Weight loss is reported to range anywhere from 46% to 71% of a patient's extra weight, depending on the bariatric procedure, and most patients experience improvement or resolution of comorbidities, such as hypertension, hyperlipidemia, diabetes, and obstructive sleep apnea.[5,6]

General Surgery, Cedars Sinai Medical Center, 8635 West 3rd Street, Suite 650W, Los Angeles, CA 90048, USA
* Corresponding author.
E-mail address: Miguel.burch@cshs.org

Surg Clin N Am 101 (2021) 731–753
https://doi.org/10.1016/j.suc.2021.05.017
0039-6109/21/© 2021 Elsevier Inc. All rights reserved.

According to the American Society for Metabolic and Bariatric Surgery, in 2018, an estimated 252,000 total bariatric procedures were performed in the United States.[7] Practice patterns have changed over the years, with a decrease in use of the adjustable gastric band (AGB), and an increase of the sleeve gastrectomy, which accounted for approximately two-thirds of all bariatric procedures in 2018.[7] Multiple studies have shown that bariatric surgery has a good safety profile, with mortality estimated to be 0.3% to 0.6%, and complications ranging from 2% to 4%,[8,9] or similar to that of laparoscopic cholecystectomy or hysterectomy.

Early recognition and diagnosis of life-threatening processes in this specific cohort of patients is key in avoiding secondary morbidity and is often life-saving. When complications occur, referral to a bariatric surgeon or a bariatric center should be considered whenever possible, but general surgeons also encounter complications of bariatric surgery in the emergent setting. See **Fig. 1** for common bariatric operations.

This article is divided into two major sections: surgical postoperative complications and metabolic complications. Surgical complications are further organized into early and late.

POSTOPERATIVE SURGICAL COMPLICATIONS
Early Complications

Leak

Perhaps the most dreaded complication of bariatric surgery is a leak, or an anastomotic or staple line breakdown. Incidence of a leak after primary gastric bypass is estimated to be less than 1%, and 1% to 3% after sleeve gastrectomy.[10–12] Early

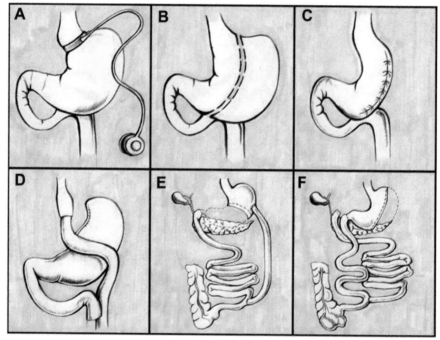

Fig. 1. Common bariatric operations. (*A*) Gastric banding. (*B*) Sleeve gastrectomy. (*C*) Gastric plication. (*D*) Gastric bypass. (*E*) Biliopancreatic diversion. (*F*) Biliopancreatic diversion with duodenal switch. (Campanile FC, Boru CE, Rizzello M, et al. Acute complications after laparoscopic bariatric procedures: update for the general surgeon. *Langenbecks Arch Surg.* 2013;398(5):669-686. https://doi.org/10.1007/s00423-013-1077-2.)

recognition and intervention for a leak in the postoperative period for this population is of utmost importance. Although patients may manifest with the typical signs, such as fevers, leukocytosis, hypotension, and tachypnea, postoperative tachycardia is one of the most important warning signals in the bariatric surgery cohort.[13,14] One study found that tachycardia greater than 100 beats per minute, in addition to systolic blood pressure less than 100 mm Hg, leukocytosis greater than 15,000/mm^3, age older than 48 years, and BMI greater than 48 kg/m^2 were all independent variables related to the presence of a leak.[13] Particularly concerning is tachycardia greater than 120 beats per minute, as this and tachypnea were two of the most sensitive indicators for a gastrointestinal leak.[15]

Patient symptoms may be nonspecific (pain, distention, and nausea) or may manifest as a sense of impending doom with anxiety or confrontational behavior. Physical examination, although important, may be less sensitive in these patients, and classic signs of guarding, rigidity, and peritoneal irritation may not be present. One study found that only one out of three patients with a leak after Roux-en-Y gastric bypass (RYGB) had severe abdominal pain or peritonitis.[15] Detection of subtle signs should prompt timely work-up. Sepsis, respiratory failure, and peritonitis are evidence of late stages of this deadly process.

If there is sufficient clinical suspicion for a leak, proceeding directly to the operating room is generally the safe option. If the patient is hemodynamically stable and the clinical picture is unclear, work-up should include a computed tomography (CT) scan with small volume (60–90 mL) water-soluble oral with or without intravenous contrast, or upper gastrointestinal series (UGI). CT scan has a higher sensitivity than UGI, and has the added advantage of detecting extraluminal fluid or air collections.[16] A pleural effusion can also be present on radiograph or CT imaging of the chest.

Sleeve gastrectomy. In a sleeve gastrectomy, most leaks occur proximally, close to the gastroesophageal junction and frequently present after hospital discharge.[11,12,17,18] To mitigate the risk of leak, surgeons have used various methods of staple line reinforcement including oversewing (which is also used for hemostasis), glue, or other tissue sealants. There is no current consensus on this practice or definitive evidence of reduction of leak rates.[12] In fact, one large database analysis suggested an increased risk of leak when staple line reinforcement was used.[19]

The priority in the acute setting is prompt and adequate drainage (either by surgical or radiologic means) and source control of intra-abdominal infection. In the acute setting (<72 postoperative hours), primary repair of the defect can be attempted. However, this may not be effective, which would make wide drainage a bigger imperative.[20] Leaks may also be associated with downstream stenosis or obstruction, which should be ruled out. Endoluminal stents have also been used in the management algorithms of sleeve leaks, with deployment of esophageal stents into the gastric lumen to exclude the leak. Many studies report success with this modality, but also mention complications, such as hemorrhage, migration, perforation, and stenosis.[21–23] Other endoscopic interventions, such as endoscopic suturing, double pigtail drainage, and endoluminal vacuum therapy are reported techniques that have demonstrated success.[24–26]

Another important consideration in the setting of a leak is establishing reliable feeding access, such as placement of feeding jejunostomy. This is especially relevant in patients who are likely to have a protracted course, such as those who cannot have closure of their defects and are relying on long-term stents. Chronic leaks are managed differently, depending on presentation (discussed later in the section on late complications).

Gastric bypass. In a gastric bypass, the most common site of a leak is the gastrojeju-nostomy, followed by the jejunojejunostomy; other possible sites include the gastric remnant, efferent Roux limb, and jejunum.[15,27] Because of multiple areas of concern, the preferred method of imaging is CT scan with limited volume of water-soluble contrast, with or without intravenous contrast. If a leak is strongly suspected even in the setting of negative imaging, or if a patient is unstable, re-exploration remains the definitive assessment. As with a leak after sleeve gastrectomy, surgical re-exploration has higher sensitivity, specificity, and accuracy than any other test, and the consequences of delayed operative intervention can compound morbidity.[20]

Leaks at the gastrojejunostomy are the most common, and such factors as anasto-motic tension and tissue ischemia can play a role. Surgical management is favored in the early postoperative setting, and if there is minimal contamination and tissue edema, direct repair or revision of the anastomosis can be attempted. If outside this time window, thorough operative washout, drainage of intra-abdominal collections, and placement of drains is performed.[28] In general, patients should be kept nil per os with broad-spectrum antibiotics.

For a leak from the remnant stomach, direct repair or a partial gastrectomy is per-formed with strong consideration for gastrostomy tube decompression. Leaks at the jejunojejunostomy typically require operative intervention for revision.[29] Stricture at this site can also be seen, and can lead to upstream dilation of the biliopancreatic limb, remnant stomach, or Roux limb.

Ensuring optimal nutrition is of critical importance and can include placement of a gastrostomy tube for early decompression and later feeding. If the remnant is not available or appropriate, then placement of a feeding jejunostomy tube in the common channel should be considered. If enteral nutrition is not possible, total parenteral nutri-tion is used.

Nonoperative treatment can be attempted if the patient is asymptomatic, clinically stable, and the leak appears small and contained (eg, a leak detected by a change in the surgical drain output character). In these cases, endoscopic stenting and/or percutaneous drains can also be used to control the intra-abdominal infection.[28,30] Nutritional support should be initiated, such as with total parenteral nutrition or enteral nutrition through a feeding tube.

Bleeding

Postoperative hemorrhage is intraluminal or intraperitoneal. Consistent with manage-ment of bleeding from other surgical procedures, patient stabilization, resuscitation, transfusion, and localization of the bleeding are tenets of management.

In the case of intraluminal bleeding, most occur within the first 30 days after sur-gery.[31] Endoscopy is diagnostic for proximal sources, such as the gastrojejunostomy in an RYGB. Endoscopic therapies, such as injection of epinephrine, probe cautery, or clipping, have been described.[32,33] Other anastomoses, such as the jejunojejunos-tomy or the ileoileal anastomosis in a biliopancreatic diversion (BPD)/duodenal switch (DS) are other potential sources for bleeding. It is possible for blood clots to become occlusive at various intraluminal points, such as the Roux limb, biliopancreatic limb, or jejunojejunostomy, thereby adding an obstructive element to this morbidity.[34]

CT scan with contrast can also help in the diagnosis especially if symptoms such as hematochezia or melena, suggesting intraluminal bleeding are absent. If the bleeding is intraperitoneal, operative exploration may be necessary. Staple lines should be examined at the time of re-exploration and clipped or oversewn; this is of particular importance with remnant stomach bleeding. Other possible sources, such as mesen-teric vessels, spleen and short gastrics, liver, omentum, and port sites, should all be checked.[31] Hematomas can be observed but if large, consideration should be given to exploration and evacuation.

Obstruction

Obstruction after bariatric surgery can happen from a variety of etiologies. In the acute postoperative and long-term periods, obstruction can be caused by internal hernia, small bowel obstruction, port site hernia, or anastomotic stenosis (discussed later in the section on late complications).

Delayed diagnosis of an internal hernia can have devastating consequences. These can occur after RYGBs and BPDs. In a gastric bypass, three potential locations for internal hernia are Petersen's space (the space between the mesocolon and Roux limb mesentery), the jejunojejunostomy mesentery defect, and transmesocolic space (if the Roux limb is retrocolic in nature) (**Fig. 2**). Patients can present with intermittent abdominal pain and inability to pass flatus; however, not all have nausea or vomiting caused by the altered anatomy and lack of a gastric reservoir. Obstruction in these patients can cause proximal dilation of the biliopancreatic limb and gastric remnant, eventually leading to increases in lipase and bilirubin. Because of the blind nature of the biliopancreatic limb, obstruction is a dangerous complication in RYGB patients and can result in blow-out of the gastric remnant.

If there are clinical signs of bowel ischemia, prompt surgical exploration should not be delayed. If there is diagnostic uncertainty and the patient is stable, cross-sectional

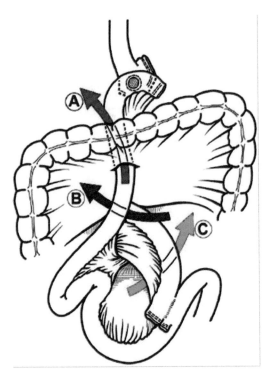

Fig. 2. Mesenteric defects. (A) Transverse mesocolic. (B) Petersen space. (C) Jejunojejunostomy mesentery. (*From:* Acquafresca PA, Palermo M, Rogula T, Duza GE, Serra E. Early surgical complications after gastric by-pass: a literature review. *Arq Bras Cir Dig ABCD Braz Arch Dig Surg.* 2015;28(1):74-80. https://doi.org/10.1590/S0102-67202015000100019.)

imaging is helpful. However, negative radiography should not delay surgical exploration if there is clinical suspicion. In one study, signs of small bowel obstruction were absent in 26.5% of patients with an internal hernia proven on surgical exploration.[35] Another ominous imaging finding is the mesenteric whirl sign, which suggests small bowel volvulus.

Closure of the mesenteric defects at the index bariatric operation is done to decrease the risk of an internal hernia.[36] However, even with initial closure, these mesenteric defects can reopen over time, especially in the setting of dramatic or rapid weight loss. One study reported internal hernia as a complication in 3.34% of the group that had no closure of defects at initial operation versus 1.15% when both defects were closed.[36]

Small bowel obstruction can also occur in the post-bariatric surgery patient. However, compared with non-bariatric patients, nasogastric decompression is usually ineffective in this population given lack of a gastric reservoir. Additionally, in the presence of an afferent biliopancreatic limb, there is no effective means of decompression for this portion of the bowel. If a transition point is distal to this, distention of this limb effectively constitutes a closed loop obstruction, and would therefore warrant prompt surgical intervention.

One other rare cause for small bowel obstruction that has been described after bariatric surgery is intussusception, with one series reporting an incidence of 0.4%.[37] The most common configuration is retrograde intussusception of the proximal common channel toward the jejunojejunostomy.[38] The cause of this phenomenon in bariatric patients is theorized to be peristaltic disturbances from ectopic pacemakers.[39] Treatment may involve reduction alone, reduction with resection of the affected segment, reduction with enteropexy, or resection en bloc (without reduction) and reconstruction.[37]

Port site and incisional hernias can also occur, with laparoscopic port sites greater than 10 mm at risk for possible bowel incarceration. Some case reports suggest that port sites smaller than 10 mm can also be at risk for herniation.[40] The incidence of this entity is hard to characterize, because many are asymptomatic, difficult to detect on physical examination, CT imaging is oftentimes helpful.[41] A systematic review found that BMI greater than 45 kg/m^2 had a significantly higher pooled incidence of trocar site hernia compared with studies with a mean patient BMI of less than 45 kg/m^2.[42] studies have reported an incidence of anywhere from 15.4% to 39.3%.[41,43,44] For the patient who develops acute-onset abdominal pain with intermittent obstructive symptoms, such as nausea and vomiting, consider a Richter hernia through a port site.[45]

Anastomotic stricture or stenosis in the acute postoperative period is typically caused by technical error. In a sleeve gastrectomy, narrowing or kinking in the creation of the sleeve can result in acute postoperative regurgitation, vomiting, dysphagia, and intolerance of oral intake. Various technical aspects of the operation can lead to this complication. Although there is no consensus on bougie size, most bariatric surgeons use a bougie to help size the sleeve stomach and to help avoid narrowing the angularis incisura.[46] Asymmetric stapling of the anterior and posterior walls of the stomach can lead to a twisted configuration that then results in a functional obstruction or kink. Finally, if oversewing of the staple line is used, care should be taken to avoid narrowing the lumen. An UGI is used to assess the morphology of the sleeve stomach; there may be smooth tapering to a narrowed segment seen. Endoscopy with balloon dilation or stenting can be used, depending on the timing after surgery.

Ulcers

Marginal ulcers can occur after RYGB in 0.35%, up to 25% of patients, depending on the mode of detection.[47–49] They can occur at any point after surgery, although the pathophysiology of ulcers presenting earlier (within weeks) of surgery is thought to be different than those that present in delayed fashion (>1 year). In general, they are thought to be caused by multiple factors: the jejunum lacks intrinsic ability to protect itself against acid, there may be a transient or subclinical ischemia of the anastomosis as it is healing, and baseline levels of acid production by the gastric pouch (and pouch size) may also play a role. Consideration should also be given to the possibility of a gastrogastric fistula. Several risk factors for marginal ulcers have been described, such as *Helicobacter pylori*, smoking, immunosuppression, use of nonsteroidal anti-inflammatory drugs, use of permanent sutures/foreign material, and size of gastric pouch.[49,50]

Patient presentation can range from asymptomatic, to abdominal pain, to perforation or massive bleeding. In one study, post-RYGB patients prospectively underwent endoscopy and 28% of those found to have a marginal ulcer were asymptomatic.[48] Approximately half describe epigastric burning, and about 15.1% experience bleeding as the main symptom; 1% to 2% present with perforation.[49,51]

If an ulcer is suspected based on a nonemergent clinical presentation, empiric treatment with a proton pump inhibitor (PPI) with an ulcer-coating medication is first-line. If there is diagnostic uncertainty, endoscopy may be performed, although CT and UGI may also be used. Endoscopy allows for direct visualization of the anastomosis, and subsequent endoscopy to check for healing is recommended. CT findings may only demonstrate some stranding in the area of the anastomosis.[52] UGI may also be performed, although barium contrast should be avoided if there is any concern for perforation. A marginal ulcer may appear as a focal outpouching close to the anastomosis, and there may be adjacent mucosal thickening.[53]

Treatment of marginal ulcers depends on the mode of presentation. Those that present with abdominal pain, nausea, and vomiting usually respond to PPI therapy, possibly with the addition of sucralfate.[54] Modifiable risk factors, such as smoking, alcohol consumption, and *H pylori* should also be addressed. In the case of a bleeding ulcer, PPI and endoscopic therapy is usually successful in most cases. During endoscopy, injection of epinephrine, cautery, or clipping is used.[34] Endoscopic suturing has also been described, but is limited to those that have the advanced resource and skill set.[55,56] In the event of bleeding that continues despite volume replacement and transfusion, or in the face of hemodynamic instability, surgical intervention is indicated. Oversewing of the ulcer or resection of the ulcer with revision of the gastrojejunostomy have been described.[57] Perforation requires surgical intervention, and such techniques as oversewing with or without omental patch are successful in most cases. Anastomotic revision has been described but its applicability may be limited by degree of contamination and edema, which significantly increases the risk of the complications.[58]

Ulcers that are recurrent or inadequately treated may manifest in delayed fashion as strictures or fistulae. Strictures may be treated endoscopically once the ulcer has healed, such as with dilation or stenting. In the setting of a recurrent ulcer, other contributing factors, such as enlarged gastric pouch, must be considered. An enlarged pouch has been shown to be directly related to risk of marginal ulcer.[54,59] Revision with pouch reduction may be necessary if marginal ulcer disease is refractory to maximum medical therapy. Another possibility for a recurrent ulcer refractory to maximum medical therapy (and in the absence of smoking, nonsteroidal anti-inflammatory drugs, and other risk factors) is a gastrogastric fistula. An UGI, endoscopy, or CT scan with oral contrast can be used to help rule out this possibility.

Thromboembolic disease

Thromboembolic events are a known complication after abdominal surgery, and bariatric surgery is no exception. Bariatric patients are at elevated risk for deep venous thrombosis (DVT) and pulmonary embolism (PE) given high BMI.[60,61] Studies estimate the prevalence of PE to be approximately 0.9%, and DVT 0.04% to 1.3%.[62,63] Rates of DVT/PE may also vary slightly by procedure, with rates of sleeve gastrectomy having a slightly lower rate of PE events than RYGB (0.1% vs 0.2%).[64]

PE accounts for a significant proportion of mortalities after elective bariatric surgery, with one study attributing 17% of the mortalities in their bariatric surgery cohort.[9] Moreover, based on an analysis of the Metabolic and Bariatric Surgery Accreditation and Quality Improvement Program database, improvements in venous thromboembolism rates would have the greatest effect on readmission and mortality.[65]

Some of the known risk factors for DVT/PE in this population includes age, operative length, prior history of DVT, transfusion, higher BMI, and open or revisional surgery.[63,64] Chemoprophylaxis, intermittent sequential compression devices, and early ambulation can all be used postoperatively to decrease the risk. However, there is no current consensus on the optimal dose or duration of thromboprophylaxis.[66–68] Some authors propose extended prophylaxis on discharge for high-risk patients, citing that most venous thromboembolism events happen after discharge[69]; high-risk characteristics include patients with a history of DVT, known hypercoagulable state, or limited ambulation (**Table 1**).[70]

Postoperative bariatric patients are also at increased risk for portomesenteric venous thrombosis. This is a rare entity that involves obstruction of the portal vein due to thrombus, possibly leading to bowel ischemia. One study reported an incidence of 1% after laparoscopic sleeve gastrectomy.[71] Patients can present with a range of symptoms, including abdominal pain, nausea, vomiting, fever, and back pain.

This complication was rarely seen before the widespread practice of the sleeve gastrectomy. It has been hypothesized that in a sleeve gastrectomy, there may be unintentional injury to the gastroepiploic or splenic veins that then leads to clot formation

Table 1
Risk factors for postdischarge VTE events

Risk Factor	Crude OR	Adjusted OR (95% CI)	Estimate	SEE
CHF	13.68	6.58 (1.95–22.20)	1.88	0.62
Paraplegia	9.20	5.71 (1.36–24.02)	1.74	0.73
Return to operating room	7.04	5.11 (3.25–8.04)	1.63	0.23
Dyspnea at rest	6.08	3.95 (1.57–9.95)	1.37	0.47
Nongastric band surgery	3.43	2.44 (1.55–3.85)	0.89	0.23
Age ≥60 y	2.03	1.96 (1.39–2.75)	0.67	0.17
Male	2.10	1.92 (1.44–2.57)	0.65	0.15
BMI ≥50 kg/m²	2.00	1.67 (1.26–2.23)	0.52	0.15
LOS ≥3 d	2.72	1.58 (1.16–2.14)	0.46	0.16
Operation time ≥3 h	2.45	1.57 (1.13–2.18)	0.45	0.17

Abbreviations: CHF, congestive heart failure; CI, confidence interval; LOS, length of stay; OR, odds ratio; SEE, standard error of estimate; VTE, venous thromboembolism.
From: Aminian A, Andalib A, Khorgami Z, et al. Who Should Get Extended Thromboprophylaxis After Bariatric Surgery?: A Risk Assessment Tool to Guide Indications for Post-discharge Pharmacoprophylaxis. *Ann Surg.* 2017;265(1):143-150. https://doi.org/10.1097/SLA.0000000000001686.

and propagation into the portal vein. Diagnosis includes contrasted CT scan or an MRI. Management for the patient with portomesenteric venous thrombosis without bowel ischemia is immediate therapeutic anticoagulation; patients with imaging or clinical findings suspicious for bowel ischemia should undergo prompt surgical exploration.

Wound infection

Obesity is a known risk factor for surgical site infection, as are multiple metabolic syndrome comorbidities, such as diabetes. In a large bariatric surgery database, wound infection (0.5%) was the second-most common 30-day complication behind bleeding.[65] Wound infection and abscess formation is decreased with the laparoscopic approach compared with open.[72] Superficial and deep superficial soft tissue infections were more common than deep-space abscesses.[73]

In a sleeve gastrectomy, the specimen retrieval port site is at higher risk, especially if there is rupture of the gastric specimen. Some surgeons support usage of a specimen retrieval bag, whereas other studies have found no difference with a non-endobag technique.[74,75] In a gastric bypass, the usage of the EEA stapler (Medtronic, Minneapolis, MN) has been shown to have a higher rate of infection, compared with use of the linear stapler.[76] The risk is decreased with sterile coverage of the circular site stapler for extraction, wound irrigation, loose skin approximation, usage of a Penrose, or wound packing.[77,78] A delayed infection of the subcutaneous port of an adjustable gastric band indicates erosion of the band until proven otherwise.

Late Complications

Delayed leak/fistula

Leaks that present in delayed fashion or become chronic fistulas may be more amenable to nonsurgical and/or endoscopic interventions. Late leaks that occur after sleeve gastrectomy have been described, and if the patient is stable and nontoxic, treatment can include radiologic drainage, endoscopic stenting, or intraluminal drainage, along with bowel rest and systemic antibiotics.[79] Other endoscopic techniques include over-the-scope clips, and endoluminal suturing.[80] Chronic leaks can also develop into fistulas, for which there are also advanced endoscopic management options, such as a septotomy, or endoluminal wound vacuum system.[79] Definitive surgical management for a chronic fistula is complex and should be delayed with nonsurgical means to allow for maturation of the fistulous tract, and nutritional optimization of the patient.[20] Correction of nutritional status is accomplished with a nasoenteric feeding tube, a jejunostomy tube, or a gastric tube in the remnant stomach. Optimization of nutrition is a cornerstone of therapy in a chronic inflammatory process such as a chronic leak/fistula.

Similar to the acute setting, the presence of a sleeve leak should also prompt workup to rule out a distal stricture. Conversion to an RYGB may be necessary.

Delayed leaks after RYGB can likewise be treated with radiologic and/or endoscopic means. In fact, multiple studies have quoted anywhere from 70% to 85% success rate with endoscopic stenting.[21,79] Other described techniques include endoscopic suturing or clipping. Surgical correction typically involves revision of the anastomosis, and as last resort, total gastrectomy with esophagojejunostomy.

Stricture/stenosis

Similar to the acute setting, late presentation of a sleeve gastrectomy stricture or stenosis includes vomiting and dysphagia. UGI is useful to localize the narrowing, and to characterize the length of the affected segment. Endoscopic stenting or balloon dilation can also be used in these scenarios, which is successful in 88% of cases.[81]

Some patients may require serial dilations to decrease the risk of perforation. If endoscopic measures fail, surgical options include longitudinal lateral gastrotomy with transverse closure (similar to a pyloroplasty), a seromyotomy, or conversion to an RYGB.

Stricture after a RYGB typically occurs at the gastrojejunostomy, with one study describing a gastrojejunostomy stenosis rate of 4.9%.[82] Endoscopy is diagnostic and therapeutic, and balloon dilation can be attempted as first-line therapy.[83] Patients may need multiple dilation sessions. Although eventual success rates are reported to be anywhere from 84.7% to 100%, there is a known risk of perforation, which would necessitate urgent surgical intervention.[79]

Gastrogastric fistula

A gastrogastric fistula is a rare complication after RYGB, and describes an abnormal connection between the gastric pouch and the remnant. Essentially, it is the re-establishment of continuity with the excluded stomach. Historically, this complication typically occurred because of failure to divide the stomach after stapling; more recently, etiologies include marginal ulcer and leak.[84,85] Additionally, because of the re-exposure of parietal cells in the remnant stomach to food, acid production is stimulated and the patient can also be at higher risk of ulcer formation. Because of this, patients diagnosed with a gastrogastric fistula should be place on PPI therapy.[86] Most patients present with pain (80%), followed by weight regain (73.3%).[84] Modes of diagnosis include endoscopy, UGI, or CT with oral contrast, with the most sensitive being UGI.[87,88] Treatment is almost always surgical, and includes either excision of fistula with a revision of the gastrojejunostomy, or excision of the fistula with remnant gastrectomy.[84,87] The gastric pouch should be appropriately resized in the process.

Gastroesophageal reflux disease

There is a complex relationship between obesity, gastroesophageal reflux disease (GERD), and bariatric surgery. Patients with increased BMI are at increased risk for GERD and related sequelae, such as erosive esophagitis and Barrett esophagus.[89] the sleeve gastrectomy is also thought to be associated with a risk of de novo GERD, or worsening of preexisting GERD symptoms. Reported incidence of de novo GERD after sleeve gastrectomy vary based on the published study, mainly because of different study definitions and method of diagnosis of GERD. Reports range anywhere from 11.7% up to 50%.[90,91] Part of the pathophysiology of worsened reflux after a sleeve gastrectomy is thought to be the high-pressures system of the sleeve stomach, and the increased intragastric pressure predisposing to reflux symptomatology. First-line treatment is similar to nonbariatric patients and includes PPIs. If GERD is refractory to medical therapy, consideration for conversion from a sleeve gastrectomy to RYGB is considered.

Complications after adjustable gastric banding

A particular set of complications is seen after gastric banding, which is a procedure that has generally fallen out of favor. Although the early postoperative morbidity profile is similar, if not better than the sleeve gastrectomy or the RYGB, there is a higher rate of long-term complications and reinterventions. Some studies have quoted up to a 28.4% long-term complication rate.[92,93] Minor device malfunctions, such as broken tubing, tubing disconnection, flipping of the access port, and fluid leak, can occur. More serious complications are discussed next.

Slipped band. The gastric band can become malpositioned and a portion of the stomach may slip above the band; this can be acute or chronic. Acute slippage can cause abdominal pain with nausea and vomiting, possibly with reflux. UGI is diagnostic, although an abdominal radiograph can also give information on the orientation of the gastric band. The first step in management should be deflation of the band by withdrawing all fluid from the subcutaneous port; this should be done in a timely manner to avoid development of gastric ischemia. If there is evidence of continued gastric obstruction or ischemia, rprompt emoval of the band is indicated.

Pouch dilation. A chronic malpositioned band or a band that was initially placed too low can predispose to dilation of the gastric pouch over time. Patients may complain of heartburn and vomiting, and loss of the sense of restriction. Pouch dilation is addressed with deflation of the band and serial imaging to see if the morphology of the pouch improves. Ultimately, surgical revision may be necessary to address an enlarged pouch.

Band erosion. Band erosion usually occurs later in the postoperative course. Removal is indicated in these cases because of risk of perforation or bleeding. Erosion may also present initially as a port site infection, so port site cellulitis or abscess should prompt further work-up to query the band itself. CT with oral contrast, UGI, or endoscopy are all used to assess for this problem. Surgical removal is necessary when an eroded band is identified. Of note, endoscopic removal of an eroded band is possible, but should be limited to cases where the gastric band buckle is intraluminal; otherwise adhesions to the buckle do not allow transoral removal.

Pseudoachalasia. Esophageal dysmotility has been reported as a late complication in gastric band patients.[94] Symptoms can include regurgitation, dysphagia, and emesis. It is hypothesized to occur because of weakening of the esophagus pushing against a relative obstruction. Over time, dilation of the esophagus can occur. Manometry is a highly sensitive test, and an esophagram can also be useful in assessing esophageal morphology. The first step in addressing the dysmotility is deflation of the band. If symptoms or dilation of the esophagus does not improve, the band should be removed, and the fibrotic capsule excised to completely relieve the obstruction.[95,96]

POSTOPERATIVE METABOLIC COMPLICATIONS
Nutritional Deficiencies

Changes in stomach capacity, decreased oral intake, hormonal changes, and altered absorption are all contributing reasons for bariatric patients being at increased risk of malnutrition and deficiencies in micronutrients and macronutrients. The risk of malnutrition with purely restrictive procedures, such as the adjustable gastric band (AGB) AGB, tends to be lower than the risk of malnutrition with surgeries that have a malabsorptive component (RYGB or BPD).[97] Consideration must be given to the patient's anatomy, such as the length of the common channel, where biliary and pancreatic secretions are mixed with enteric chyme for absorption. A common channel less than 120 cm from the ileocecal valve has been associated with severe malabsorption.[98] Prevention, and early recognition and treatment of nutrient deficiencies can help to avoid complications, some of which are irreversible (**Table 2**).

Water-soluble vitamins include thiamine/B_1, riboflavin/B_2, niacin/B_3, pantothenic acid/B_5, pyridoxine/B_6, biotin/B_7, folate/B_9, cyanocobalamin/B_{12}, and ascorbic acid/ vitamin C. Deficiencies in these vitamins tend to manifest sooner after bariatric surgery than fat-soluble vitamins, because the body has limited stores; one exception is vitamin B_{12}, where stores are usually sufficient for 3 to 5 years.[98]

Table 2
Nutritional deficiencies after bariatric surgery

Vitamin	Deficiency State	Symptoms	Dose[a]
Water-soluble vitamins			
Thiamine (vitamin B_1)	Beriberi	Neuropsychiatric: aggression, hallucinations, confusion, ataxia, nystagmus, paralysis of the motor nerves of the eye Neurologic or "dry" beriberi: convulsions, numbness, muscle weakness and/or pain of lower and upper extremities, brisk tendon reflexes High-output cardiac or "wet" beriberi: tachycardia or bradycardia, lactic acidosis, dyspnea, leg edema, right ventricular dilatation Gastroenterology: slow gastric emptying, nausea, vomiting, jejunal dilatation or megacolon, constipation	100 mg twice daily In patients with Wernicke encephalopathy or acute psychosis: 250 mg for 3–5 d, intramuscularly or intravenously
Riboflavin (vitamin B_2)	Ariboflavinosis	Anemia, dermatitis, stomatitis, glossitis	5–10 mg
Niacin (vitamin B_3)	Pellagra	Diarrhea, confusion, dermatitis, ataxia	100–500 mg thrice daily
Pantothenic acid (vitamin B_5)	Pantothenic acid deficiency	Depression, infections, orthostatic hypotension, paraesthesias, foot drop, gait disorder	2–4 g
Pyridoxine (vitamin B_6)	Pyridoxine deficiency	Dermatitis, neuropathy, confusion	30 mg
Folic acid (vitamin B_9)	Folate deficiency	Weakness, weight loss, anorexia	1–5 mg
Cobalamin (vitamin B_{12})	Pernicious anemia	Depression, malaise, ataxia, paraesthesias	0.5–2.0 mg orally: 1.000 μg intramuscularly monthly or 500 μg sublingually daily
Ascorbic acid (vitamin C)	Scurvy	Malaise, myalgias, gum disease, petechia	200 mg
Biotin (vitamin B_7)	Biotin deficiency	Loss of taste, seizures, hypotonia, ataxia, dermatitis, hair loss	20 mg
Fat-soluble vitamins			
Vitamin A	Vitamin A deficiency	Night blindness, itching, dry hair	10,000 IU

Vitamin D	Osteomalacia (in adults) Rickets (in children)	Arthralgias, depression, fasciculations, myalgias	Ergocalciferol 50,000 IU once weekly over 12 wk, then switch to daily cholecalciferol 1000–4000 IU
Vitamin E	Vitamin E deficiency	Anemia, ataxia, motor speech disorder, muscle weakness	800–1200 IU
Vitamin K	Vitamin K deficiency	Bleeding disorder	2.5–25.0 mg
Minerals			
Calcium	Osteoporosis	Usually absent	1.2–2.0 g
Iron	Iron deficiency anemia	Fatigue, shortness of breath, chest pain	Ferrous sulfate 325 mg or ferrous fumarate 200 mg plus vitamin C 125 mg up to 4 times daily
Trace elements			
Zinc	Hypozincemia	Skin lesions, nail dystrophy, alopecia, glossitis	Zinc sulfate 220 mg or zinc gluconate 30–50 mg every other day
Copper	Hypocupremia	Usually absent	Copper gluconate (2–4 mg) every other day
Selenium	Keshan disease	Dyspnea, fatigue, leg swelling	100 µg sodium selenite

[a] Supplements are administered once daily and orally unless stated otherwise.

From Bal BS, Finelli FC, Shope TR, Koch TR. Nutritional deficiencies after bariatric surgery. *Nat Rev Endocrinol.* 2012;8(9):544-556. https://doi.org/10.1038/nrendo.2012.48.

Thiamine has a short half-life (10–20 days). RYGB and BPD patients are at particular risk for thiamine deficiency given the bypass of the duodenum and jejunum, where absorption typically occurs. One study reported an incidence of 18.3% of thiamine deficiency in RYGB patients on follow-up.[99] However, Wernicke encephalopathy (a serious sequelae of thiamine deficiency) has been described after all types of bariatric surgery, including intragastric ballooning and sleeve gastrectomy.[100] Patients who suffer from poor oral intake, nausea, vomiting, and/or diarrhea should empirically be given intravenous or intramuscular thiamine, and it is crucial that this be done before dextrose administration. Wernicke encephalopathy is characterized by ophthalmoplegia, ataxia, and confusion. Wernicke-Korsakoff syndrome manifests as mental status changes and impairment of recent memory. These neurologic abnormalities and neuropsychiatric changes can be permanent, so prompt supplementation for at-risk patients is key.

Folate deficiency can result in neural tube defects, cardiovascular disease, and macrocytic anemia. Because of the susceptibility to this deficiency (along with B_{12}, iron, and calcium), bariatric patients who desire to become pregnant are recommended to undergo counseling before conception in addition to being tested for prenatal levels to ensure repletion of these important factors.[101,102] Currently, a minimum of 12 months between bariatric surgery and pregnancy is recommended to allow time for weight stabilization and nutritional monitoring.[102]

Vitamin B_{12} deficiency occurs in bariatric patients for multiple reasons including decreased ileal length, bacterial overgrowth, and decreases in the hydrochloric acid, pepsin, and intrinsic factor needed for its absorption. This deficiency may manifest in delayed fashion, because liver stores may be sufficient in the first few years. Symptoms include megaloblastic anemia, glossitis, neuropathy, paresthesias, autonomic dysfunction, and cognitive decline. The neuropathy may be permanent.

Fat-soluble vitamins include A, D, E, and K. RYGB and BPD patients are at risk, with the latter being at higher risk given their shorter ileal length, where absorption of fat-soluble vitamins occur. Vitamin A typically manifests after several months, because liver stores can last up to 1 year. Manifestations can include night blindness and decreased visual acuity, and the vision loss can be permanent if left untreated. Hypovitaminosis D can cause metabolic bone disease, leading to bone loss and predisposing to fractures. Also, low vitamin D causes compensatory activation of the parathyroid glands, which leads to increased resorption of calcium from bones; preoperative and postoperative parathyroid hormone testing may be necessary if low vitamin D levels are found to rule out secondary hyperparathyroidism.[97] Vitamins E and K are also micronutrients that require supplementation after bariatric surgery, but fortunately, clinically evident deficiencies are rarely seen in this population.

Essential minerals relevant to bariatric patients include calcium, iron, copper, selenium, and zinc. Calcium, in conjunction with vitamin D, are two of the most common micronutrient deficiencies in bariatric patients. Low iron levels are also common, because there is less exposure to hydrochloric acid and the primary absorption sites (duodenum and proximal jejunum) are bypassed. Zinc, copper, and selenium all function as coenzymes for essential enzymatic reactions, and can affect multiple body systems.

Dumping Syndrome

Dumping syndrome is characterized by nausea, abdominal pain, palpitations, and lightheadedness after ingestion of a high carbohydrate load meal. This phenomenon can occur after any type of gastric reconstructive surgery, such as after partial or total gastrectomy. Although this is more common after an RYGB or BPD, with reported incidence from 12% to 75%,[103–106] it can also occur after a sleeve gastrectomy.[105,107] There are two types of dumping syndrome: early and late.

Early dumping syndrome is thought to be a result of hyperosmolar chyme in the small bowel, which triggers the release of gastrointestinal hormones and the shift of fluids intraluminally due to the osmolar gradient. The chyme can also cause enteric distention. Symptoms typically occur in the first hour after meal ingestion and include abdominal pain, bloating, nausea, diarrhea, and borborygmi. vasomotor symptoms may also be present, such as flushing, palpitations, perspiration, tachycardia, and hypotension.

Late dumping syndrome, in contrast, typically manifests 1 to 3 hours after a meal and is mainly characterized by hypoglycemia and associated symptoms. Rapid gastric emptying leads to rapid absorption of glucose from the intestine, which then triggers insulin secretion; hypoglycemia results because of circulating levels of insulin and other gastrointestinal hormone imbalances.

Diagnosis is made based on symptom evaluation, with particular attention to the timing of meal ingestion, meal composition, and symptoms. Oral glucose tolerance test or radionuclide scintigraphy can also help aid in diagnosis.[103,104] First-line intervention is dietary change, by decreasing liquid intake and/or increasing solid food intake. Other recommendations include smaller, more frequent meals, and avoiding simple carbohydrates and lactose. If dietary changes fail, medications such as somatostatin analogues and anticholinergics are considered.[104] In medically refractory cases that cause lifestyle limitations, surgical intervention may be discussed.

Cholelithiasis

Patients after bariatric surgery are at higher risk of gallstone formation. This is especially true if there is rapid or excess weight loss.[108] Gallstone formation can occur in up to one-third of bariatric surgery patients.[109,110] Bariatric patients are often placed on ursodeoxycholic acid prophylaxis after their surgery to decrease the risk of gallstone formation.[111]

Although treatment of gallbladder disease in the bariatric patient is the same as for nonbariatric, there needs to be close evaluation of the common bile duct for choledocholithiasis, because RYGB anatomy precludes simple endoscopic access to the biliary tree. If choledocholithiasis is found, options include surgical common bile duct exploration; transgastric endoscopic retrograde cholangiopancreatography; percutaneous transhepatic access; or advanced endoscopic techniques, such as double-balloon endoscopic retrograde cholangiopancreatography.

Nephrolithiasis

Both obesity and bariatric surgery are risk factors for nephrolithiasis.[112] Malabsorptive procedures have a higher risk than purely restrictive procedures.[113] Pathophysiology includes several mechanisms, such as hyperoxaluria, hypocitraturia, and aciduria, which increase the risk of stone formation. most stones are composed of calcium oxalate.[113] Treatment of stones is the same as that of nonbariatric surgery patients; interventions for hyperoxaluria include low-fat, low-oxalate diet, and encouraging fluid intake.[114]

SUMMARY

There are surgical and metabolic complications that can occur after bariatric and metabolic procedures. The two most commonly performed operations are the sleeve gastrectomy and the gastric bypass. An understanding of the altered anatomy and physiology helps to guide management of morbidities. Leaks are a dreaded complication; early recognition and intervention is necessary for avoiding clinical deterioration. Obstruction can manifest in the form of internal hernias in RYGB patients, and a high degree of clinical suspicion is necessary because imaging may be negative or nondefinitive. Strictures and fistulae can also occur, and there is an increasing trend toward initial endoscopic management. Metabolic complications include nutritional deficiencies, especially in the setting of malabsorptive procedures, such as the RYGB and BPD. Patients should also be counseled on eating habits to avoid dumping syndrome.

CLINICS CARE POINTS

- Physical examination may be unreliable in postoperative bariatric surgery patients in detecting an acute intra-abdominal process.
- Postoperative tachycardia greater than 120 beats per minute is a leak until proven otherwise.
- Endoscopic stenting is considered to be part of the treatment algorithm in specific clinical scenarios for leaks and strictures; however, failure of endoscopic therapy necessitates surgical intervention.
- Nutritional access (nasojejunal tube, remnant gastrostomy tube, feeding jejunostomy tube) is an essential part of the management of leaks and fistulas.
- CT scans should be obtained when an acute intra-abdominal process is suspected in a stable RYGB patient, because it has advantages over UGI in assessing the remnant stomach and jejunojejunostomy.
- Diagnostic laparoscopy is the most reliable method of ruling out an internal hernia; negative radiologic imaging should not be considered definitive.
- Obstruction at the jejunojejunostomy in an RYGB patient is life-threatening, because it can lead to dilation of the biliopancreatic limb and remnant stomach, constituting a closed loop obstruction.
- Treatment of marginal ulcers depends on the clinical presentation. Patient counseling to avoid risk factors is important.
- Bariatric patients are at higher risk of DVT/PE; postoperative thromboprophylaxis should be used.
- Recurrent ulcers in an RYGB patient in the absence of other risk factors, such as smoking or nonsteroidal anti-inflammatory drug use, should prompt a work-up for a gastrogastric fistula.
- There is a high complication/reintervention rate after adjustable gastric banding; problems include pouch dilation, slipped band, band erosion, and pseudoachalasia.
- Post-bariatric surgery patients should be followed carefully for nutritional deficiencies; thiamine supplementation should be given empirically in the postoperative patient presenting with poor oral intake or dehydration.
- There are two forms of dumping syndrome: early and late. Dietary changes and medications are useful.

DISCLOSURE

The authors have nothing to disclose.

REFERENCES

1. CDC. Obesity is a common, serious, and costly disease. Centers for Disease Control and Prevention; 2020. Available at: https://www.cdc.gov/obesity/data/adult.html. Accessed December 11, 2020.
2. ASMBS. Obesity in America. American Society for Metabolic and Bariatric Surgery; 2018. Available at: https://asmbs.org/resources/obesity-in-america. Accessed December 11, 2020.
3. Schauer PR, Kashyap SR, Wolski K, et al. Bariatric surgery versus intensive medical therapy in obese patients with diabetes. N Engl J Med 2012;366(17): 1567–76.
4. Gloy VL, Briel M, Bhatt DL, et al. Bariatric surgery versus non-surgical treatment for obesity: a systematic review and meta-analysis of randomised controlled trials. BMJ 2013;347:f5934.
5. Chang S-H, Stoll CRT, Song J, et al. The effectiveness and risks of bariatric surgery: an updated systematic review and meta-analysis, 2003-2012. JAMA Surg 2014;149(3):275–87.
6. Buchwald H, Avidor Y, Braunwald E, et al. Bariatric surgery: a systematic review and meta-analysis. J Am Med Assoc 2004;292(14):1724–37.
7. ASMBS. Estimate of bariatric surgery numbers, 2011-2018. American Society for Metabolic and Bariatric Surgery; 2018. Available at: https://asmbs.org/resources/estimate-of-bariatric-surgery-numbers. Accessed December 11, 2020.
8. Ghiassi S, Morton JM. Safety and efficacy of bariatric and metabolic surgery. Curr Obes Rep 2020;9(2):159–64.
9. Smith MD, Patterson E, Wahed AS, et al. Thirty-day mortality after bariatric surgery: independently adjudicated causes of death in the longitudinal assessment of bariatric surgery. Obes Surg 2011;21(11):1687–92.
10. Podnos YD, Jimenez JC, Wilson SE, et al. Complications after laparoscopic gastric bypass: a review of 3464 cases. Arch Surg Chic Ill 1960 2003;138(9): 957–61.
11. Brethauer SA, Hammel JP, Schauer PR. Systematic review of sleeve gastrectomy as staging and primary bariatric procedure. Surg Obes Relat Dis Off J Am Soc Bariatr Surg 2009;5(4):469–75.
12. Rosenthal RJ, International Sleeve Gastrectomy Expert Panel, Diaz AA, et al. International Sleeve Gastrectomy Expert Panel Consensus Statement: best practice guidelines based on experience of >12,000 cases. Surg Obes Relat Dis Off J Am Soc Bariatr Surg 2012;8(1):8–19.
13. Arteaga-González I, Martín-Malagón A, Martín-Pérez J, et al. Usefulness of clinical signs and diagnostic tests for suspected leaks in bariatric surgery. Obes Surg 2015;25(9):1680–4.
14. Gagnière J, Slim K. Don't let obese patients be discharged with tachycardia after sleeve gastrectomy. Obes Surg 2012;22(9):1519–20.
15. Hamilton EC, Sims TL, Hamilton TT, et al. Clinical predictors of leak after laparoscopic Roux-en-Y gastric bypass for morbid obesity. Surg Endosc 2003;17(5): 679–84.
16. ASMBS Clinical Issues Committee. ASMBS guideline on the prevention and detection of gastrointestinal leak after gastric bypass including the role of imaging and surgical exploration. Surg Obes Relat Dis Off J Am Soc Bariatr Surg 2009;5(3):293–6.

17. Bashah M, Khidir N, El-Matbouly M. Management of leak after sleeve gastrectomy: outcomes of 73 cases, treatment algorithm and predictors of resolution. Obes Surg 2020;30(2):515–20.
18. Jurowich C, Thalheimer A, Seyfried F, et al. Gastric leakage after sleeve gastrectomy: clinical presentation and therapeutic options. Langenbecks Arch Surg 2011;396(7):981.
19. Berger ER, Clements RH, Morton JM, et al. The impact of different surgical techniques on outcomes in laparoscopic sleeve gastrectomies: the first report from the Metabolic and Bariatric Surgery Accreditation and Quality Improvement Program (MBSAQIP). Ann Surg 2016;264(3):464–73.
20. Kim J, Azagury D, Eisenberg D, et al. American Society for Metabolic and Bariatric Surgery Clinical Issues Committee. ASMBS position statement on prevention, detection, and treatment of gastrointestinal leak after gastric bypass and sleeve gastrectomy, including the roles of imaging, surgical exploration, and nonoperative management. Surg Obes Relat Dis Off J Am Soc Bariatr Surg 2015;11(4):739–48.
21. Murino A, Arvanitakis M, Le Moine O, et al. Effectiveness of endoscopic management using self-expandable metal stents in a large cohort of patients with post-bariatric leaks. Obes Surg 2015;25(9):1569–76.
22. Martin Del Campo SE, Mikami DJ, Needleman BJ, et al. Endoscopic stent placement for treatment of sleeve gastrectomy leak: a single institution experience with fully covered stents. Surg Obes Relat Dis Off J Am Soc Bariatr Surg 2018;14(4):453–61.
23. Simon F, Siciliano I, Gillet A, et al. Gastric leak after laparoscopic sleeve gastrectomy: early covered self-expandable stent reduces healing time. Obes Surg 2013;23(5):687–92.
24. Giuliani A, Romano L, Marchese M, et al. Gastric leak after laparoscopic sleeve gastrectomy: management with endoscopic double pigtail drainage. A systematic review. Surg Obes Relat Dis Off J Am Soc Bariatr Surg 2019;15(8):1414–9.
25. Fernandez AZ, Luthra AK, Evans JA. Endoscopic closure of persistent gastric leak and fistula following laparoscopic sleeve gastrectomy. Int J Surg Case Rep 2015;6C:186–7.
26. Leeds SG, Burdick JS. Management of gastric leaks after sleeve gastrectomy with endoluminal vacuum (E-Vac) therapy. Surg Obes Relat Dis Off J Am Soc Bariatr Surg 2016;12(7):1278–85.
27. Marshall JS, Srivastava A, Gupta SK, et al. Roux-en-Y gastric bypass leak complications. Arch Surg Chic Ill 1960 2003;138(5):520–3 [discussion 523-524].
28. Gonzalez R, Sarr MG, Smith CD, et al. Diagnosis and contemporary management of anastomotic leaks after gastric bypass for obesity. J Am Coll Surg 2007;204(1):47–55.
29. Lee S, Carmody B, Wolfe L, et al. Effect of location and speed of diagnosis on anastomotic leak outcomes in 3828 gastric bypass cases. J Gastrointest Surg 2007;11(6):708–13.
30. Ballesta C, Berindoague R, Cabrera M, et al. Management of anastomotic leaks after laparoscopic Roux-en-Y gastric bypass. Obes Surg 2008;18(6):623–30.
31. Rabl C, Peeva S, Prado K, et al. Early and late abdominal bleeding after Roux-en-Y gastric bypass: sources and tailored therapeutic strategies. Obes Surg 2011;21(4):413–20.
32. Fernández-Esparrach G, Bordas JM, Pellisé M, et al. Endoscopic management of early GI hemorrhage after laparoscopic gastric bypass. Gastrointest Endosc 2008;67(3):552–5.

33. Jamil LH, Krause KR, Chengelis DL, et al. Endoscopic management of early upper gastrointestinal hemorrhage following laparoscopic Roux-en-Y gastric bypass. Am J Gastroenterol 2008;103(1):86–91.

34. Spaw AT, Husted JD. Bleeding after laparoscopic gastric bypass: case report and literature review. Surg Obes Relat Dis Off J Am Soc Bariatr Surg 2005; 1(2):99–103.

35. Kawkabani Marchini A, Denys A, Paroz A, et al. The four different types of internal hernia occurring after laparascopic Roux-en-Y gastric bypass performed for morbid obesity: are there any multidetector computed tomography (MDCT) features permitting their distinction? Obes Surg 2011;21(4):506–16.

36. Blockhuys M, Gypen B, Heyman S, et al. Internal hernia after laparoscopic gastric bypass: effect of closure of the Petersen defect - single-center study. Obes Surg 2019;29(1):70–5.

37. Stephenson D, Moon RC, Teixeira AF, et al. Intussusception after Roux-en-Y gastric bypass. Surg Obes Relat Dis Off J Am Soc Bariatr Surg 2014;10(4): 666–70.

38. Bag H, Karaisli S, Celik SC, et al. A rare complication of bariatric surgery: retrograde intussusception. Obes Surg 2017;27(11):2996–8.

39. Mahmood A, Mahmood N, Robinson RB. Small bowel intussusception: a dangerous sequela of bariatric surgery. Radiol Case Rep 2007;2(1):10–2.

40. Bergemann JL, Hibbert ML, Harkins G, et al. Omental herniation through a 3-mm umbilical trocar site: unmasking a hidden umbilical hernia. J Laparoendosc Adv Surg Tech A 2001;11(3):171–3.

41. Ahlqvist S, Björk D, Weisby L, et al. Trocar site hernia after gastric bypass. Surg Technol Int 2017;30:170–4.

42. Karampinis I, Lion E, Grilli M, et al. Trocar site hernias in bariatric surgery-an underestimated issue: a qualitative systematic review and meta-analysis. Obes Surg 2019;29(3):1049–57.

43. Scozzari G, Zanini M, Cravero F, et al. High incidence of trocar site hernia after laparoscopic or robotic Roux-en-Y gastric bypass. Surg Endosc 2014;28(10): 2890–8.

44. Rebibo L, Dhahri A, Chivot C, et al. Trocar site hernia after laparoscopic sleeve gastrectomy using a specific open laparoscopy technique. Surg Obes Relat Dis Off J Am Soc Bariatr Surg 2015;11(4):791–6.

45. Cottam DR, Gorecki PJ, Curvelo M, et al. Preperitoneal herniation into a laparoscopic port site without a fascial defect. Obes Surg 2002;12(1):121–3.

46. Gagner M, Hutchinson C, Rosenthal R. Fifth International Consensus Conference: current status of sleeve gastrectomy. Surg Obes Relat Dis Off J Am Soc Bariatr Surg 2016;12(4):750–6.

47. Clapp B, Hahn J, Dodoo C, et al. Evaluation of the rate of marginal ulcer formation after bariatric surgery using the MBSAQIP database. Surg Endosc 2019; 33(6):1890–7.

48. Csendes A, Burgos AM, Altuve J, et al. Incidence of marginal ulcer 1 month and 1 to 2 years after gastric bypass: a prospective consecutive endoscopic evaluation of 442 patients with morbid obesity. Obes Surg 2009;19(2):135–8.

49. Coblijn UK, Goucham AB, Lagarde SM, et al. Development of ulcer disease after Roux-en-Y gastric bypass, incidence, risk factors, and patient presentation: a systematic review. Obes Surg 2014;24(2):299–309.

50. Di Palma A, Liu B, Maeda A, et al. Marginal ulceration following Roux-en-Y gastric bypass: risk factors for ulcer development, recurrence and need for

revisional surgery. Surg Endosc 2020. https://doi.org/10.1007/s00464-020-07650-0.

51. Coblijn UK, Lagarde SM, de Castro SMM, et al. Symptomatic marginal ulcer disease after Roux-en-Y gastric bypass: incidence, risk factors and management. Obes Surg 2015;25(5):805–11.

52. Adduci AJ, Phillips CH, Harvin H. Prospective diagnosis of marginal ulceration following Roux-en-Y gastric bypass with computed tomography. Radiol Case Rep 2016;10(2). https://doi.org/10.2484/rcr.v10i2.1063.

53. Carucci LR, Turner MA. Radiologic evaluation following Roux-en-Y gastric bypass surgery for morbid obesity. Eur J Radiol 2005;53(3):353–65.

54. Azagury DE, Abu Dayyeh BK, Greenwalt IT, et al. Marginal ulceration after Roux-en-Y gastric bypass surgery: characteristics, risk factors, treatment, and outcomes. Endoscopy 2011;43(11):950–4.

55. Barola S, Magnuson T, Schweitzer M, et al. Endoscopic suturing for massively bleeding marginal ulcer 10 days post Roux-en-Y gastric bypass. Obes Surg 2017;27(5):1394–6.

56. Barola S, Fayad L, Hill C, et al. Endoscopic management of recalcitrant marginal ulcers by covering the ulcer bed. Obes Surg 2018;28(8):2252–60.

57. Madan AK, DeArmond G, Ternovits CA, et al. Laparoscopic revision of the gastrojejunostomy for recurrent bleeding ulcers after past open revision gastric bypass. Obes Surg 2006;16(12):1662–8.

58. Moon RC, Teixeira AF, Goldbach M, et al. Management and treatment outcomes of marginal ulcers after Roux-en-Y gastric bypass at a single high volume bariatric center. Surg Obes Relat Dis Off J Am Soc Bariatr Surg 2014;10(2):229–34.

59. Edholm D, Ottosson J, Sundbom M. Importance of pouch size in laparoscopic Roux-en-Y gastric bypass: a cohort study of 14,168 patients. Surg Endosc 2016;30(5):2011–5.

60. Allman-Farinelli MA. Obesity and venous thrombosis: a review. Semin Thromb Hemost 2011;37(8):903–7.

61. Yang G, De Staercke C, Hooper WC. The effects of obesity on venous thromboembolism: a review. Open J Prev Med 2012;2(4):499–509.

62. Stein PD, Matta F. Pulmonary embolism and deep venous thrombosis following bariatric surgery. Obes Surg 2013;23(5):663–8.

63. Jamal MH, Corcelles R, Shimizu H, et al. Thromboembolic events in bariatric surgery: a large multi-institutional referral center experience. Surg Endosc 2015;29(2):376–80.

64. Gambhir S, Inaba CS, Alizadeh RF, et al. Venous thromboembolism risk for the contemporary bariatric surgeon. Surg Endosc 2020;34(8):3521–6.

65. Daigle CR, Brethauer SA, Tu C, et al. Which postoperative complications matter most after bariatric surgery? Prioritizing quality improvement efforts to improve national outcomes. Surg Obes Relat Dis Off J Am Soc Bariatr Surg 2018; 14(5):652–7.

66. Scholten DJ, Hoedema RM, Scholten SE. A comparison of two different prophylactic dose regimens of low molecular weight heparin in bariatric surgery. Obes Surg 2002;12(1):19–24.

67. Birkmeyer NJO, Finks JF, Carlin AM, et al. Comparative effectiveness of unfractionated and low-molecular-weight heparin for prevention of venous thromboembolism following bariatric surgery. Arch Surg Chic Ill 1960 2012;147(11):994–8.

68. Hamadi R, Marlow CF, Nassereddine S, et al. Bariatric venous thromboembolism prophylaxis: an update on the literature. Expert Rev Hematol 2019;12(9): 763–71.

69. Aminian A, Andalib A, Khorgami Z, et al. Who should get extended thromboprophylaxis after bariatric surgery? A risk assessment tool to guide indications for post-discharge pharmacoprophylaxis. Ann Surg 2017;265(1):143–50.
70. Mechanick JI, Youdim A, Jones DB, et al. Clinical practice guidelines for the perioperative nutritional, metabolic, and nonsurgical support of the bariatric surgery patient—2013 update: cosponsored by American Association of Clinical Endocrinologists, the Obesity Society, and American Society for Metabolic & Bariatric Surgery. Obes Silver Spring Md 2013;21(0 1):S1–27.
71. Salinas J, Barros D, Salgado N, et al. Portomesenteric vein thrombosis after laparoscopic sleeve gastrectomy. Surg Endosc 2014;28(4):1083–9.
72. Nguyen NT, Goldman C, Rosenquist CJ, et al. Laparoscopic versus open gastric bypass: a randomized study of outcomes, quality of life, and costs. Ann Surg 2001;234(3):279–89 [discussion 289-291].
73. Freeman JT, Anderson DJ, Hartwig MG, et al. Surgical site infections following bariatric surgery in community hospitals: a weighty concern? Obes Surg 2011;21(7):836–40.
74. Bou Nassif G, Scetbun E, Lecurieux-Lafayette C, et al. "Hand-over-hand grasping technique": a fast and safe procedure for specimen extraction in laparoscopic sleeve gastrectomy. Obes Surg 2017;27(5):1391.
75. Shoar S, Aboutaleb S, Karem M, et al. Comparison of two specimen retrieval techniques in laparoscopic sleeve gastrectomy: what is the role of endobag? Surg Endosc 2017;31(12):4883–7.
76. Shope TR, Cooney RN, McLeod J, et al. Early results after laparoscopic gastric bypass: EEA vs GIA stapled gastrojejunal anastomosis. Obes Surg 2003;13(3):355–9.
77. Zhang Y, Serrano OK, Scott Melvin W, et al. An intraoperative technique to reduce superficial surgical site infections in circular stapler-constructed laparoscopic Roux-en-Y gastric bypass. Surg Obes Relat Dis Off J Am Soc Bariatr Surg 2016;12(5):1008–13.
78. Alasfar F, Sabnis A, Liu R, et al. Reduction of circular stapler-related wound infection in patients undergoing laparoscopic Roux-en-Y gastric bypass, Cleveland Clinic technique. Obes Surg 2010;20(2):168–72.
79. Eisendrath P, Deviere J. Major complications of bariatric surgery: endoscopy as first-line treatment. Nat Rev Gastroenterol Hepatol 2015;12(12):701–10.
80. Nedelcu AM, Skalli M, Deneve E, et al. Surgical management of chronic fistula after sleeve gastrectomy. Surg Obes Relat Dis Off J Am Soc Bariatr Surg 2013;9(6):879–84.
81. Levy JL, Levine MS, Rubesin SE, et al. Stenosis of gastric sleeve after laparoscopic sleeve gastrectomy: clinical, radiographic and endoscopic findings. Br J Radiol 2018;91(1089):20170702.
82. Higa K, Ho T, Tercero F, et al. Laparoscopic Roux-en-Y gastric bypass: 10-year follow-up. Surg Obes Relat Dis Off J Am Soc Bariatr Surg 2011;7(4):516–25.
83. Huang CS, Forse RA, Jacobson BC, et al. Endoscopic findings and their clinical correlations in patients with symptoms after gastric bypass surgery. Gastrointest Endosc 2003;58(6):859–66.
84. Chahine E, Kassir R, Dirani M, et al. Surgical management of gastrogastric fistula after Roux-en-Y gastric bypass: 10-year experience. Obes Surg 2018;28(4):939–44.
85. Yao DC, Stellato TA, Schuster MM, et al. Gastrogastric fistula following Roux-en-Y bypass is attributed to both surgical technique and experience. Am J Surg 2010;199(3):382–5 [discussion 385-386].

86. Palermo M, Acquafresca PA, Rogula T, et al. Late surgical complications after gastric by-pass: a literature review. Arq Bras Cir Dig ABCD Braz Arch Dig Surg 2015;28(2):139–43.
87. Corcelles R, Jamal MH, Daigle CR, et al. Surgical management of gastrogastric fistula. Surg Obes Relat Dis Off J Am Soc Bariatr Surg 2015;11(6):1227–32.
88. Carrodeguas L, Szomstein S, Soto F, et al. Management of gastrogastric fistulas after divided Roux-en-Y gastric bypass surgery for morbid obesity: analysis of 1,292 consecutive patients and review of literature. Surg Obes Relat Dis Off J Am Soc Bariatr Surg 2005;1(5):467–74.
89. Hampel H, Abraham NS, El-Serag HB. Meta-analysis: obesity and the risk for gastroesophageal reflux disease and its complications. Ann Intern Med 2005; 143(3):199–211.
90. van Rutte PWJ, Smulders JF, de Zoete JP, et al. Outcome of sleeve gastrectomy as a primary bariatric procedure. Br J Surg 2014;101(6):661–8.
91. Mandeville Y, Van Looveren R, Vancoillie P-J, et al. Moderating the enthusiasm of sleeve gastrectomy: up to fifty percent of reflux symptoms after ten years in a consecutive series of one hundred laparoscopic sleeve gastrectomies. Obes Surg 2017;27(7):1797–803.
92. Mellert LT, Cheung M, Berbiglia L, et al. Reoperations for long-term complications following laparoscopic adjustable gastric banding: analysis of incidence and causality. Cureus 2020;12(5):e8127.
93. Tucker O, Sucandy I, Szomstein S, et al. Revisional surgery after failed laparoscopic adjustable gastric banding. Surg Obes Relat Dis Off J Am Soc Bariatr Surg 2008;4(6):740–7.
94. Khan A, Ren-Fielding C, Traube M. Potentially reversible pseudoachalasia after laparoscopic adjustable gastric banding. J Clin Gastroenterol 2011;45(9): 775–9.
95. Roman S, Kahrilas PJ. Pseudoachalasia and laparoscopic gastric banding. J Clin Gastroenterol 2011;45(9):745–7.
96. Suter M, Dorta G, Giusti V, et al. Gastric banding interferes with esophageal motility and gastroesophageal reflux. Arch Surg Chic Ill 1960 2005;140(7): 639–43.
97. Parrott J, Frank L, Rabena R, et al. American Society for Metabolic and Bariatric Surgery integrated health nutritional guidelines for the surgical weight loss patient 2016 update: micronutrients. Surg Obes Relat Dis Off J Am Soc Bariatr Surg 2017;13(5):727–41.
98. Bal BS, Finelli FC, Shope TR, et al. Nutritional deficiencies after bariatric surgery. Nat Rev Endocrinol 2012;8(9):544–56.
99. Clements RH, Katasani VG, Palepu R, et al. Incidence of vitamin deficiency after laparoscopic Roux-en-Y gastric bypass in a university hospital setting. Am Surg 2006;72(12):1196–202 [discussion 1203-1204].
100. Oudman E, Wijnia JW, van Dam M, et al. Preventing Wernicke encephalopathy after bariatric surgery. Obes Surg 2018;28(7):2060–8.
101. Fitzsimons KJ, Modder J, Greer IA. Obesity in pregnancy: risks and management. Obstet Med 2009;2(2):52–62.
102. Ciangura C, Coupaye M, Deruelle P, et al. Clinical practice guidelines for childbearing female candidates for bariatric surgery, pregnancy, and post-partum management after bariatric surgery. Obes Surg 2019;29(11):3722–34.
103. Tack J, Deloose E. Complications of bariatric surgery: dumping syndrome, reflux and vitamin deficiencies. Best Pract Res Clin Gastroenterol 2014;28(4): 741–9.

104. Berg P, McCallum R. Dumping syndrome: a review of the current concepts of pathophysiology, diagnosis, and treatment. Dig Dis Sci 2016;61(1):11–8.
105. Ahmad A, Kornrich DB, Krasner H, et al. Prevalence of dumping syndrome after laparoscopic sleeve gastrectomy and comparison with laparoscopic Roux-en-Y gastric bypass. Obes Surg 2019;29(5):1506–13.
106. Nielsen JB, Pedersen AM, Gribsholt SB, et al. Prevalence, severity, and predictors of symptoms of dumping and hypoglycemia after Roux-en-Y gastric bypass. Surg Obes Relat Dis Off J Am Soc Bariatr Surg 2016;12(8):1562–8.
107. Papamargaritis D, Koukoulis G, Sioka E, et al. Dumping symptoms and incidence of hypoglycaemia after provocation test at 6 and 12 months after laparoscopic sleeve gastrectomy. Obes Surg 2012;22(10):1600–6.
108. Li VKM, Pulido N, Fajnwaks P, et al. Predictors of gallstone formation after bariatric surgery: a multivariate analysis of risk factors comparing gastric bypass, gastric banding, and sleeve gastrectomy. Surg Endosc 2009;23(7):1640–4.
109. Shiffman ML, Sugerman HJ, Kellum JM, et al. Gallstone formation after rapid weight loss: a prospective study in patients undergoing gastric bypass surgery for treatment of morbid obesity. Am J Gastroenterol 1991;86(8):1000–5.
110. Guzmán HM, Sepúlveda M, Rosso N, et al. Incidence and risk factors for cholelithiasis after bariatric surgery. Obes Surg 2019;29(7):2110–4.
111. Talha A, Abdelbaki T, Farouk A, et al. Cholelithiasis after bariatric surgery, incidence, and prophylaxis: randomized controlled trial. Surg Endosc 2020;34(12):5331–7.
112. Semins MJ, Shore AD, Makary MA, et al. The association of increasing body mass index and kidney stone disease. J Urol 2010;183(2):571–5.
113. Lieske JC, Mehta RA, Milliner DS, et al. Kidney stones are common after bariatric surgery. Kidney Int 2015;87(4):839–45.
114. Bhatti UH, Duffy AJ, Roberts KE, et al. Nephrolithiasis after bariatric surgery: a review of pathophysiologic mechanisms and procedural risk. Int J Surg Lond Engl 2016;36(Pt D):618–23.

General Surgery
Management of Postoperative Complications Following Ventral Hernia Repair and Inguinal Hernia Repair

Yang Lu, MD[a], David C. Chen, MD[b], Ian T. MacQueen, MD[b],*

KEYWORDS

- Hernia repair • Wound complications • Ventral hernia repair complications
- Inguinal hernia repair complications • Hernia repair complications • Mesh infection

KEY POINTS

- Management of postoperative surgical site infection following hernia repair includes antibiotics, drainage of infected fluid collections, debridement of devitalized tissue, and mesh excision where appropriate.
- Management of recurrent inguinal hernia depends on the previous operation. After a failed anterior inguinal hernia repair, a posterior approach is recommended. Conversely, if recurrence occurs after a posterior repair, then an anterior repair should be attempted.
- Interventions for chronic postoperative inguinal pain should follow a "step-up approach" that includes watchful waiting, targeted pharmacologic agents, local anesthetic injections, radiofrequency ablation, and surgery (neurectomy, recurrent hernia repair, and mesh excision).

MANAGEMENT OF POSTOPERATIVE COMPLICATIONS FOLLOWING VENTRAL HERNIA REPAIR

Ventral hernia repair (VHR) is one of the most commonly performed general surgery operations worldwide. The variations of ventral hernia types and their surgical approaches make VHR a particularly challenging operation to standardize and to study. Although there is no universally accepted system of classification, approximately 75% of VHRs are performed for primary hernias such as epigastric, umbilical, and spigelian hernias, and approximately 25% of repairs are performed for incisional ventral

[a] Department of Surgery, David Geffen School of Medicine at UCLA, 10833 Le Conte Avenue, 72-227 CHS, Los Angeles, CA 90095, USA; [b] Department of Surgery, David Geffen School of Medicine, Lichtenstein Amid Hernia Clinic at UCLA, 1304 15th Street, Suite 102, Santa Monica, CA 90404, USA
* Corresponding author.
E-mail address: IMacqueen@mednet.ucla.edu

Surg Clin N Am 101 (2021) 755–766
https://doi.org/10.1016/j.suc.2021.05.018
0039-6109/21/© 2021 Elsevier Inc. All rights reserved.
surgical.theclinics.com

hernias.[1,2] In the United States, approximately 250,000 VHRs are performed annually, costing the health care system an estimated \$3 billion.[2-4] Furthermore, recurrence after primary VHR is common, exceeding 25% and particularly in those patients with body mass index greater than 35.[5] In the following section, we focus our review on the management of postoperative complications of VHR. These include the management of postoperative wound complications, hernia recurrence, postoperative pain, enterotomy, and seroma/hematoma formation.

Postoperative Wound Complications

Postoperative wound complications are common following VHRs, with rates ranging from 4% to 23%.[4,6,7] This wide range in reporting has led to focused efforts to improve standardization of post-VHR wound complications by assigning specific definitions, such as surgical site infection (SSI), surgical site occurrence (SSO), or surgical site occurrence requiring procedural intervention (SSOPI).[8] Well-published patient-level risk factors for SSO following VHR include morbid obesity, poor functional status, active smoking, malnutrition, diabetes, and chronic obstructive pulmonary disease.[7,9,10] However, aside from obesity, most other patient-related factors alone are not highly predictive of SSO. A recent propensity-matched cohort study even challenged the efficacy of modifying behavioral risk factors such as smoking, as there do not appear to be clinically significant differences in wound morbidity between active smokers and nonsmokers when examining short-term outcomes.[11] However, studies of longer-term outcomes and larger, more complex incisional hernia repairs, still emphasize the importance of smoking cessation in surgical preoptimization. Interestingly, although a history of past wound complications is not necessarily predictive of SSO in the future,[12] technical factors such open surgery, prolonged operative time, dirty infected wounds, contaminated wounds, and component separation are strongly associated with SSO.[7,9,10] Needless to say, wound complications following VHR are extremely important for hernia surgeons to diagnose and treat appropriately, as they are intimately related to hernia recurrence and need for reoperations.[4,6,7,13]

Diagnosis of post-VHR wound complications is largely based on clinical examination: erythema, induration, purulent exudate draining from incision, and positive wound culture obtained from the primary surgical site suggest SSI. Laboratory tests and imaging modalities such as computed tomography and ultrasonography may be useful in detecting deeper fluid collections. Treatment of wound infection following VHR is multifaceted and includes antibiotics, drainage of infected fluid collections, debridement of devitalized tissue, and mesh excision where appropriate. As the use of permanent mesh comprises more than 65% of all VHRs performed since 2010, the remainder of this section specifically discusses the treatment of mesh-related wound infections.[14,15]

Mesh-related postoperative wound infections

Mesh-related complications range from 5.6% to 10.0% and represent a particularly challenging subset of post-VHR wound morbidity, as they often require prolonged antibiotics and percutaneous drainage, and reoperations.[16-18] Furthermore, there are currently no standardized guidelines regarding mesh excision during reoperations. Most studies support that whenever feasible, implanted foreign material, including mesh, tacks, sutures, and scar tissue should be removed.[16-18] Exceptions may be made for partial excision of infected mesh if there is evidence of good incorporation of the remaining mesh to the native tissue.[18] Percutaneous drainage of peri-mesh collections in addition to antibiotics may be effective in select cases, and the type of bacterial pathogen did not predict efficacy of nonoperative management.[19] In situations in which there is failure of percutaneous drainage, an operative plan that includes surgical debridement of infected tissue, partial excision of mesh, drain placement, and negative pressure wound therapy may be considered. However, mesh infections with no incorporation of mesh into the surrounding tissues, should proceed with complete excision of the mesh and debridement of the surrounding tissues to healthy edges. Complete mesh excision to achieve "source control" carries higher risk of perioperative complications, such as enterotomy and fascial disruption, which leads to higher recurrence rates, whereas partial mesh excision leaves a foreign body behind, which serve as a nidus for subsequent and persistent wound infections.[20] A study by Kao and colleagues[21] examined the extent of mesh excision needed for effective control of post-herniorrhaphy mesh infections, and concluded that partial mesh excision is an acceptable technique in the setting of clean surgical wounds. However, this is associated with higher rates of wound complications and reoperations in clean-contaminated wounds and mesh-related infection and fistulas.[21] Thus, the ultimate decision when treating mesh infection should be made on an individualized basis with the patient understanding all possible treatment options.

Once mesh is excised, the patient is left with a recurrent ventral hernia, thus concomitant incisional hernia repair should be considered during the same operation as mesh excision. A recent study on concomitant incision hernia repair and mesh excision compared complete repair (fascial closure with mesh) versus partial repair (fascial closure without mesh or no fascial closure with mesh) and showed no difference in length of stay, SSIs, SSO, and readmission between the 2 groups within 30 days.[22] Surgeon judgment and experience plays into the decision to stage the operation versus attempting a repeat definitive repair, and is typically dependent on the burden of infection, ability to adequately achieve source control, quality of remaining tissue, size and complexity of the hernia, technical options for repair, and medical comorbidities. Other hernia repair strategies to consider when operating in a contaminated field is the use of biosynthetic absorbable mesh, which has been shown in a prospective longitudinal study to be efficacious with regard to long-term recurrence rates and quality-of-life outcomes.[23] Although controversy remains about appropriateness of placing a synthetic mesh in a contaminated field, a large retrospective study that examined the safety of macroporous permanent synthetic mesh placed in a retromuscular position during VHR reported a lower rate of postoperative SSI and hernia recurrence compared with biological or bioabsorbable meshes.[24]

Hernia Recurrence

Despite numerous techniques and types of mesh products a surgeon has in his or her arsenal to repair a ventral hernia, there remains a high recurrence rate. As we recall, approximately 25% of all VHRs are performed for incisional ventral hernias.[1,2] Moreover and unsurprisingly, incisional VHRs themselves carry a much higher risk of recurrence (60%–70%) than primary VHRs.[18] With each subsequent VHR, there is also a stepwise increase in long-term recurrence. These extremely high recurrence rates suggest a need for innovative strategies for VHR and incisional hernia prevention. Approximately 30% of patients who developed hernia recurrence had a preceding SSI.[16,25] In fact, an SSI doubled the chance of hernia recurrence and quadrupled the chance of reoperation.[16,25] Other patient-level risk factors include morbid obesity, diabetes, and active smoking.[26] Although most studies lack long-term outcomes to capture true recurrence rates, a 2012 prospective cohort study using the Danish Ventral Hernia Database estimated recurrence rates for umbilical and epigastric hernia repairs and incisional hernia repairs to be as high as 15% and 37%, respectively.[27]

Technical risk factors associated with higher recurrence rates include complex VHRs, contaminated fields, and repairs done without mesh.[16,25]

Techniques for preventing incisional hernias

Given the high prevalence, morbidity, and costs of ventral incisional hernias, the focus on hernia prevention is important and supported by high-level evidence. Adherence to surgical principles that decrease the incidence of incisional hernias after abdominal surgeries can reduce the overall VHR burden. In 2015, the European Hernia Society put forth guidelines to decrease the incidence of incisional hernias.[28]

A. Use a non-midline approach to a laparotomy whenever possible.
B. For elective midline incisions, perform a continuous suturing technique and avoid using rapidly absorbable sutures. Use a slowly absorbable monofilament suture in a single layer aponeurotic closure technique without separate closure of the peritoneum. A small bites technique with a suture to wound length ratio of at least 4:1 and the use of smaller (2–0) suture and (SH) needles is the current recommended method of fascial closure.
C. Prophylactic mesh augmentation appears effective and safe and can be suggested in high-risk settings like aortic aneurysm surgery and ostomy creation, and in obese patients.
D. For laparoscopic surgery, recommend closure of the fascial defect if trocars larger than or equal to 10 mm are used. For single incision laparoscopic surgery, meticulous closure of the fascial incision is suggested to avoid an increased risk of incisional hernias.

Laparoscopic versus open technique for incisional hernia repair

A 2011 Cochrane review of 10 randomized controlled trials comparing laparoscopic versus open hernia repairs reviewed 880 patients with primary ventral or incisional hernias.[29] Short-term evaluation (<2.5 years) of recurrence rate did not find differences between the 2 techniques. Although the risk of intraoperative enterotomy was slightly higher in laparoscopic hernia repair, there was reduced risk of wound infection (risk ratio = 0.26) and shortened hospital stay in most trials.[29] From 2009 to 2017 the percentage of minimally invasive inguinal hernia repairs increased from 23% to 38% and minimally invasive ventral hernias increased from 32% to 37%.[30] Laparoscopic VHR had total wound complication rates of approximately 1%, whereas open VHR had the highest total wound complication rates ranging from 5% to 6%.[30] Moreover, laparoscopic VHR is associated with shorter length of stay and decreased risk of SSI, but longer operating time compared with open repair.[31] In a thesis reviewing the Danish trials, Helgstrand and colleagues[27] found that large hernia defects and open repairs were independent predictors for 30-day complications after an incisional hernia repair. Open procedures and large hernia defects were independent risk factors for a later recurrence repair. Patients with large hernia defects (>15 cm) seem to benefit from an open mesh repair compared with laparoscopic repairs. Specifically, the open sublay mesh repair independently decreased the risk of recurrence repair compared with other open mesh repairs.[27]

Postoperative Pain after Laparoscopic Repair

Postoperative pain following laparoscopic repair is common but mostly resolves by 4 to 6 weeks. Persistent pain beyond 6 weeks ranges from 2% to 28% and can be attributed to nerve entrapment by a suture, tack, or mesh.[32] It is debatable whether absorbable tacks have been shown to cause any differences in pain than permanent tacks. Perioperative strategies to reduce postoperative pain include bilateral erector spinae blocks with 20 to 30 mL ropivacaine 0.5% at the level of the T7 transverse process undergoing laparoscopic VHR.[33] In addition, administration of a long-acting local anesthetic between the mesh and the peritoneum significantly reduces postoperative pain and narcotic use after laparoscopic VHR.[34] Last, mesh soaked with bupivacaine solution has been associated with reduced early postoperative pain.[35] Management of chronic postoperative pain after VHR includes analgesics, nonsteroidal anti-inflammatory medications, steroids, trigger point injection, nerve block, or excision of sutures or tacks.

Enterotomy

Iatrogenic enterotomy occurs in approximately 2% of patients undergoing laparoscopic VHR, making it a relatively uncommon but feared complication of laparoscopic VHR, half of which occur during lysis of adhesions.[36,37] When recognized intraoperatively, enterotomies with small defects should be primarily repaired or if a suture repair would cause luminal narrowing, then bowel resection should be considered. Inadvertent enterotomies present a challenge for the subsequent hernia repair, as it potentially contaminates the surgical field. Options includes aborting the hernia repair, converting to open approach and using a synthetic, biologic, or bioabsorbable mesh in the retrorectus or pre-peritoneal sublay position; or completing laparoscopic ventral hernia repair either using biologic or biosynthetic mesh intraperitoneally.[36,38] Unrecognized injuries from thermal injury or mesh fixation devices require re-exploration with intestinal repair, bowel resection, and either partial or complete mesh removal in some cases, and carry a significant risk of enterocutaneous fistula formation and mortality.[37]

Seromas/Hematomas

Seromas are common following open VHR because of the extensive dissection needed to create abdominal flaps large enough to accommodate mesh with sufficient fascia overlap to minimize recurrence. The incidence of postoperative seromas is highly variable from one series to another, although some report clinically significant seromas in up to 10% of patients.[39,40] Seromas form in the abdominal wall cavity left behind following a hernia repair and incidence of radiological seromas is present in almost all cases.[41] Although most seromas are asymptomatic, discovered incidentally, and usually resolve spontaneously, some require percutaneous drainage, sclerotherapy, or surgical excision. A review article in 2012 published by Morales-Conde[42] classified post-surgical seromas into 5 major subtypes based on clinical presentation and duration. Various groups have examined strategies to reduce postoperative seroma formation. A meta-analysis on postoperative seroma prevention reviewed techniques such as dissecting the abdomen in a place superficial to the Scarpa fascia; ligating blood vessels with sutures or clips; using quilting or progressive tension sutures; using fibrin, thrombin, or talc; and immobilizing the surgical site postoperatively.[43] The investigators concluded that surgical site compression did not prevent seroma accumulation. The use of sclerosants such as medical talc as prophylaxis was shown to increase the risk of seroma development in some studies.[44] However, higher-quality and longer-term outcome studies on the role of medical talc, fibrin glue, or negative pressure wound therapy for seroma prophylaxis need to be conducted to determine their true impact on SSOs. Once post-VHR seromas become encapsulated by chronic fibrous capsules, they may be managed with sclerotherapy (ie, talc or tetracycline antibiotics, and ethanol) or surgical excision to prevent re-accumulation.[45] Surgical excision may be performed via a mini-abdominoplasty incision, the fibrous capsule or pseudobursa excised, and closed with tension sutures to decrease the dead space, aided by suction drainage with a compressive dressing.[46] Finally, postoperative seromas need to be distinguished from hematomas, which are also common following VHR, but the latter appears more heterogeneous and higher attenuation on cross-sectional imaging. Most hematomas may be managed expectantly, whereas symptomatic, infected, and enlarging hematomas may require surgical evacuation.

POSTOPERATIVE COMPLICATIONS FOLLOWING INGUINAL HERNIA REPAIR

Like VHR, inguinal hernia repair (IHR) is one of the most commonly performed operations worldwide, with more than 20 million patients undergoing groin hernia repair annually.[47,48] The incidence of inguinal hernias increases with age, especially in the fifth to seventh decades of life.[49] Surgical repair in all cases has been the traditional management; however, recent literature has challenged this dogma. More evidence now supports watchful waiting for asymptomatic or minimally symptomatic inguinal hernias as a reasonable alternative in male patients older than 50.[50] This shift in thinking is in part due to the various postoperative complications that may follow this seemingly innocuous operation. In the following section, we focus our review on the management of postoperative complications specific to IHR, including the management of postoperative wound complications, chronic postoperative inguinal pain, sexual dysfunction or pain, and recurrence.

Postoperative Wound Complications

Superficial SSI rates following elective open IHR are generally low, with estimates between 3% and 5%.[51,52] The treatment is oral or intravenous antibiotics with high efficacy rates. The incidence of deep incisional SSI following IHR is similar between open versus laparoscopic IHR (0.1% and 0.2%, respectively).[51,52] Deep SSI should be suspected in any postoperative patient presenting with systemic symptoms, such as fevers, chills, or malaise. On examination, the surgical site may be erythematous, warm, and indurated. Sometimes a draining fistula in the groin region is noticed. Diagnosis is usually clinical, but imaging with computed tomography and ultrasonography can be useful for identifying deeper fluid collections, such as a postoperative fluid collection (seroma, hematoma, abscess), edema or stranding of the subcutaneous fat around the mesh, or other signs of tissue ischemia and necrosis. Treatment with antibiotics and percutaneous drainage can be effective in up to 76% of patients.[19] However, recurrent infection or lack of improvement of clinical course may warrant surgical drainage, debridement of devitalized tissue, and possible mesh excision similar to management of VHR mesh infections. Fluid cultures should be collected to guide antibiotic therapy. *Staphylococcus aureus* remains the most common organism; however, the type of bacteria does not necessarily predict mesh excision. Polytetrafluoroethylene mesh had a higher excision rate compared with both polypropylene and porcine dermal collagen meshes.[19] Last, neither fluid collection size nor location predicts mesh excision.[19]

Chronic Postoperative Inguinal Pain

An increasingly recognized complication following IHR is chronic postoperative inguinal pain (CPIP), defined as inguinal pain that persists more 6 months after a patient's index operation. Incidence ranges between 8% and 16% and significantly impacts activities of daily living in 0.5% and 6.0% of patients.[53–55] Neuropathic causes of CPIP can be attributed to scarring of or injury to the sensory nerves, including the iliohypogastric, ilioinguinal, and genital branch of the genitofemoral nerve during an open repair, and the genitofemoral trunk, lateral femoral cutaneous, and femoral nerve during a laparoscopic repair. Perioperatively, the important role of identification and pragmatic resection of nerves has been investigated to minimize the occurrence of chronic pain.[56,57]

The diagnosis and management of CPIP starts with a thorough history and physical examination to understand the precise location and determine the underlying etiology of pain. A "pain map" of the groin, abdomen, thigh, and genitals is useful in delineating the extent of neuralgia. Dermatomal sensory mapping can be done using a surgical marker with pluses indicating pain, zeros indicating no pain, and minuses referring to numbness.[58] The pain map ensures consistency between examinations and clues the surgeon into which nerves might be involved in chronic pain pathogenesis.

For CPIP, interventions should follow a "step-up approach" that includes watchful waiting, pharmacologic treatments, local anesthetic injections, sensory stimulation, radiofrequency or pharmacologic ablations, and surgery (mesh removal, reoperation for recurrence, and/or neurectomy).[59,60]

Watchful waiting: First-line management of chronic pain following IHR is to examine the patient and explain the condition. Because pain typically declines with time after surgery, a watchful strategy can be trialed in the beginning; however, with caution against modifying lifestyle to sedentary activities, as chronic pain can severely impair quality of life. Basic analgesics can be used during this period of watchful waiting. If there are no improvements in the condition after a few months, then systematic pharmacologic interventions in collaboration with pain specialists should be trialed. This includes a combination of nonsteroidal anti-inflammatory drugs, gabapentinoids, tricyclic antidepressants, and selective serotonin reuptake inhibitors or serotonin-norepinephrine reuptake inhibitors. Topical administration of analgesics has also been studied, specifically lidocaine and capsaicin transdermal patches, but these have not shown to provide lasting benefit.

Local anesthetic injections are useful for both pain relief and for diagnostic purposes to identify which nerves are involved in CPIP. Tailored injections demonstrated some efficacy, indicating that the peripheral nerves were involved in the chronic pain, but without lasting effect in most studies. A study using repeated injections of lidocaine, steroids, and hyaluronic acid to treat chronic pain demonstrated a 22% efficacy rate compared with the 71% success rate for the neurectomy group.[61] The injections were safe with rare minor complications and minimally invasive, thus the investigators concluded that it should be considered to use injections before surgery with neurectomy.

Radiofrequency can be used to block the nerve through temperature-moderated tissue ablation and can be performed at the peripheral nerve level or at the proximal nerve root level.[62–66] Pulsed radiofrequency at the dorsal root ganglia with heating to temperature of 40 to 42°C resulted in pain relief for up to 20 weeks. Thermocoagulation of nerves at a higher intensity of 70 to 90°C provided pain relief lasting 12 months.[62–66]

If nonoperative treatments do not ameliorate CPIP, then a combined surgical neurectomy with or without mesh excision should be considered depending on the symptomatology and mechanism of injury.[67–69] Neurectomy can be performed via an anterior open approach or via a posterior minimally invasive technique. Surgical strategy will be determined by the initial technique for IHR and the likelihood of accessing the nerve at its site of injury. Following anterior approaches, an anterior approach with neurectomy and mesh removal is typically recommended. Conversely, following posterior approaches, such as totally extraperitoneal (TEP) or transabdominal preperitoneal (TAPP), a posterior approach is recommended with exploration of the field and removal of tacks and mesh, and a laparoscopic or robotic-assisted neurectomy. An added justification for neurectomy to be performed during the same operation is to avoid need for a subsequent surgical procedure in a reoperative surgical field following mesh removal, as it may be incredibly difficult. Thus, when performing mesh removal after a previous Lichtenstein repair, it is recommended to remove any of the anterior inguinal nerves likely to be involved. Selective neurectomy may be safely used if there are no suggested neuropathic symptoms in the distribution of a nerve and there is no risk to the nerve from reoperation. In recognizing the difficulty and potential dangers of operating in a scarred surgical field, a laparoscopic retroperitoneal triple neurectomy can be considered in select patients to conduct neurectomy proximal to the nerves following preperitoneal or intraperitoneal approaches.[70,71]

Sexual Dysfunction or Pain

Sexual dysfunction and sexual pain are common following IHR. A systematic review with a median follow-up of 10.5 months found that open IHR was associated with sexual dysfunction and persistent sexual pain in 4% and 12% of patients, respectively.[72] In male patients, testicular complications range from 0.3% to 7.2%.[72,73] Interference with blood supply to the testicle, dissection of indirect hernia from the cord structures may lead to testicular pain, ischemic orchitis, and testicular atrophy. The same processes may also result from mesh migration, causing extrinsic compression of cord structures or fibrotic reaction that leads to ischemia. Injury of the vas deferens may lead to ejaculatory issues. Another study of 176 men undergoing unilateral IHR reported that TEP resulted in higher quality of life and sexual function scores than open (Lichtenstein) repair at 7 and 30 days, but these differences were not replicated at 90 days.[74]

Hernia Recurrence

Despite numerous technological advancements made in IHR since its conception, recurrence is still reported in 0.5% to 15% of patients depending on the type of repair performed, patient comorbidities, and duration of time from the index repair.[75–77] The lowest rates of hernia recurrence (1%–2%) are reported after tension-free mesh repairs, such as open modified Lichtenstein, TEP, and TAPP, with the exception being the Shouldice tissue repair performed at high-volume centers.[78–80] On the other hand, recurrence rates are reported as high 15% after other types of primary tissue repairs.[78–80] Management of recurrent hernia depends on the preceding operation. In general, after an anterior repair, a posterior approach is recommended. Conversely, if recurrence occurs after a posterior repair, an anterior repair typically should be attempted. After a failed anterior and posterior approach, then referral should be considered to a specialist hernia surgeon to determine the best option for remediation.[57]

SUMMARY

VHRs and IHRs are commonly performed general surgery procedures, with postoperative complications ranging from wound morbidities, hernia recurrence, chronic pain, and mesh-related issues. Management is highly variable given the wide heterogeneity of hernia types and their unique surgical approaches. Thus, treatment decisions should be made on an individualized basis based on surgeon experience and with the patient understanding all possible options.

DISCLOSURE

The authors have nothing to disclose.

REFERENCES

1. Muysoms FE, Miserez M, Berrevoet F, et al. Classification of primary and incisional abdominal wall hernias. Hernia 2009;13(4):407–14.
2. Poulose BK, Shelton J, Phillips S, et al. Epidemiology and cost of ventral hernia repair: making the case for hernia research. Hernia 2012;16:179–83.
3. Bower C, Roth JS. Economics of abdominal wall reconstruction. Surg Clin North Am 2013;93:1241–53.
4. Ventral Hernia Working Group, Breuing K, Butler CE, et al. Incisional ventral hernias: review of the literature and recommendations regarding the grading and technique of repair. Surgery 2010;148(3):544–58.
5. Desai KA, Razavi SA, Hart AM, et al. The effect of BMI on outcomes following complex abdominal wall reconstructions. Ann Plast Surg 2016;76:S295–7.
6. Baucom RB, Ousley J, Oyefule OO, et al. Evaluation of long-term surgical site occurrences in ventral hernia repair: implications of preoperative site independent MRSA infection. Hernia 2016;20(5):701–10.
7. Fischer JP, Wink JD, Nelson JA, et al. Wound risk assessment in ventral hernia repair: generation and internal validation of risk stratification system using the ACS-NSQIP. Hernia 2015;19(1):103–11.
8. Haskins IN, Horne CM, Krpata DM, et al. A call for standardization of wound events reporting following ventral hernia repair. Hernia 2018;22:729–36.
9. Levi B, Zhang P, Lisiecki J, et al. Use of morphometric assessment of body composition to quantify risk of surgical-site infection in patients undergoing component separation ventral hernia repair. Plast Reconstr Surg 2014;133(4):559e–66e.
10. Finan KR, Vick CC, Kiefe CI, et al. Predictors of wound infection in ventral hernia repair. Am J Surg 2005;190(5):676.
11. Petro CC, Haskins IN, Tastaldi L, et al. Does active smoking really matter before ventral hernia repair? An AHSQC analysis. Surgery 2019;165(2):406–11.
12. Blatnik JA, Krpata DM, Novitsky YW, et al. Does a history of wound infection predict postoperative surgical site infection after ventral hernia repair? Am J Surg 2012;203(3):370–4.
13. Luijendijk RW, Hop WC, van den Tol MP, et al. A comparison of suture repair with mesh repair for incisional hernia. N Engl J Med 2000;343(6):392–8.
14. Flum DR, Horvath KKT. "Have outcomes of incisional hernia repair improved with time?" A population-based analysis. Ann Surg 2003;237:129–35.
15. Poulose BK. So what's the chance of this mesh causing me a problem in the long run? Ann Surg 2018;267:e66.
16. Kokotovic D, Bisgaard T, Helgstrand F. Long-term recurrence and complications associated with elective incisional hernia repair. JAMA 2016;316:1575–82.
17. Cobb WS, Carbonell AM, Kalbaugh CL, et al. Infection risk of open placement of intraperitoneal composite mesh. Am Surg 2009;75:762–8.
18. Holihan JL, Alawadi Z, Martindale RG, et al. Adverse events after ventral hernia repair: the vicious cycle of complications. J Am Coll Surg 2015;221:478–85.
19. Kuo YC, Mondschein JI, Soulen MC, et al. Drainage of collections associated with hernia mesh: is it worthwhile? J Vasc Interv Radiol 2010;21(3):362.
20. Szczerba SR, Dumanian GA. Definitive surgical treatment of infected or exposed ventral hernia mesh. Ann Surg 2003;237:437–41.
21. Kao AM, Arnold MR, Augenstein VA, et al. Prevention and treatment strategies for mesh infection in abdominal wall reconstruction. Plast Reconstr Surg 2018;142(3 Suppl):149S.

22. Devin CL, Olson MA, Tastaldi L, et al. Surgical management of infected abdominal wall mesh: an analysis using the American Hernia Society Quality Collaborative. Hernia 2021. https://doi.org/10.1007/s10029-020-02355-8.

23. Rosen MJ, Bauer JJ, Harmaty M, et al. Multicenter, prospective, longitudinal study of the recurrence, surgical site infection, and quality of life after contaminated ventral hernia repair using biosynthetic absorbable mesh: the COBRA study. Ann Surg 2017;265(1):205–11.

24. Warren J, Desai SS, Boswell ND, et al. Safety and efficacy of synthetic mesh for ventral hernia repair in a contaminated field. J Am Coll Surg 2020;230(4):405–13.

25. Burger JW, Luijendijk RW, Hop WC, et al. Long-term follow-up of a randomized controlled trial of suture versus mesh repair of incisional hernia. Ann Surg 2004;240(4):578–83.

26. Donovan K, Denham M, Kuchta K, et al. Predictors for recurrence after open umbilical hernia repair in 979 patients. Surgery 2019;166(4):615–22.

27. Helgstrand F, Rosenberg J, Kehlet H, et al. Reoperation versus clinical recurrence rate after ventral hernia repair. Ann Surg 2012;256(6):955–8.

28. Muysoms FE, Antoniou SA, Bury K, et al, European Hernia Society. European Hernia Society guidelines on the closure of abdominal wall incisions. Hernia 2015; 19(1):1–24.

29. Sauerland S, Walgenbach M, Habermalz B, et al. Laparoscopic versus open surgical techniques for ventral or incisional hernia repair. Cochrane Database Syst Rev 2011;(3):CD007781.

30. Madion M, Goldblatt MI, Gould JC, et al. Ten-year trends in minimally invasive hernia repair: a NSQIP database review. Surg Endosc 2021. [E-pub ahead of print].

31. Kaoutzanis C, Leichtle SW, Mouawad NJ, et al. Postoperative surgical site infections after ventral/incisional hernia repair: a comparison of open and laparoscopic outcomes. Surg Endosc 2013;27:2221e2230.

32. Earle D, Roth JS, Saber A, et al, SAGES Guidelines Committee. SAGES guidelines for laparoscopic ventral hernia repair. Surg Endosc 2016;30(8):3163–83.

33. Chin KJ, Adhikary S, Sarwani N, et al. The analgesic efficacy of pre-operative bilateral erector spinae plane (ESP) blocks in patients having ventral hernia repair. Anaesthesia 2017;72(4):452–60.

34. Gough AE, Chang S, Reddy S, et al. Periprosthetic anesthetic for postoperative pain after laparoscopic ventral hernia repair: a randomized clinical trial. JAMA Surg 2015;150(9):835–40.

35. Chawla T, Shahzad N, Ahmad K, et al. Post-operative pain after laparoscopic ventral hernia repair, the impact of mesh soakage with bupivacaine solution versus normal saline solution: a randomised controlled trial (HAPPIEST Trial). J Minim Access Surg 2020;16(4):328–34.

36. Krpata DM, Prabhu AS, Tastaldi L, et al. Impact of inadvertent enterotomy on short-term outcomes after ventral hernia repair: an AHSQC analysis. Surgery 2018;164(2):327–32.

37. LeBlanc KA, Elieson MJ, Corder JM 3rd. Enterotomy and mortality rates of laparoscopic incisional and ventral hernia repair: a review of the literature. JSLS 2007; 11(4):408–14.

38. Sharma A, Khullar R, Soni V, et al. Iatrogenic enterotomy in laparoscopic ventral/incisional hernia repair: a single center experience of 2,346 patients over 17 years. Hernia 2013;17(5):581–7.

39. Tonolini M, Ippolito S. Multidetector CT of expected findings and early postoperative complications after current techniques for ventral hernia repair. Insights Imaging 2016;7:541–51.

40. Lacour M, Ridereau Zins C, Casa C, et al. CT findings of complications after abdominal wall repair with prosthetic mesh. Diagn Interv Imaging 2017;98: 517–28.

41. Susmallian S, Gewurtz G, Ezri T, et al. Seroma after laparoscopic repair of hernia with PTFE patch: is it really a complication? Hernia 2001;5:139–41.

42. Morales-Conde S. A new classification for seroma after laparoscopic ventral hernia repair. Hernia 2012;16:261–7.

43. Janis JE, Khansa L, Khansa I. Strategies for postoperative seroma prevention: a systematic review. Plast Reconstr Surg 2016;138(1):240–52.

44. Parameswaran R, Hornby ST, Kingsnorth AN. Medical talc increases the incidence of seroma formation following onlay repair of major abdominal wall hernias. Hernia 2013;17:459–63.

45. Sood A, Kotamarti VS, Therattil PJ, et al. Sclerotherapy for the management of seromas: a systematic review. Eplasty 2017;17:e25.

46. Vidal P, Berner JE, Will PA. Managing complications in abdominoplasty: a literature review. Arch Plast Surg 2017;44(5):457–68.

47. Rutkow IM. Demographic and socioeconomic aspects of hernia repair in the United States in 2003. Surg Clin North Am 2003;83:1045–51.

48. Kingsnorth A, LeBlanc K. Hernias: inguinal and incisional. Lancet 2003;362: 1561–71.

49. Ruhl CE, Everhart JE. Risk factors for inguinal hernia among adults in the US population. Am J Epidemiol 2007;165:1154–61.

50. de Goede B, Wijsmuller AR, van Ramshorst GH, et al, INCA Trialists' Collaboration. Watchful waiting versus surgery of mildly symptomatic or asymptomatic inguinal hernia in men aged 50 years and older: a randomized controlled trial. Ann Surg 2018;267(1):42–9.

51. Moon V, Chaudry GA, Choy C, et al. Mesh infection in the era of laparoscopy. J Laparoendosc Adv Surg Tech A 2004;14(6):349.

52. Falagas ME, Kasiakou SK. Mesh-related infections after hernia repair surgery. Clin Microbiol Infect 2005;11(1):3.

53. Aasvang EK, Gmaehle E, Hansen JB, et al. Predictive risk factors for persistent postherniotomy pain. Anesthesiology 2010;112(4):957–69.

54. Andresen K, Burcharth J, Fonnes S, et al. Chronic pain after inguinal hernia repair with the ONSTEP versus the Lichtenstein technique, results of a double-blinded multicenter randomized clinical trial. Langenbecks Arch Surg 2017;402(2):213–8.

55. Ergonenc T, Beyaz SG, Ozocak H, et al. Persistent postherniorrhaphy pain following inguinal hernia repair: A cross-sectional study of prevalence, pain characteristics, and effects on quality of life. Int J Surg 2017;46:126–32.

56. Graham DS, MacQueen IT, Chen DC. Inguinal neuroanatomy: implications for prevention of chronic postinguinal hernia pain. Int J Abdom Wall Hernia 2018; 1:1–8.

57. HerniaSurge Group. International guidelines for groin hernia management. Hernia 2018;22(1):1–165.

58. Bjurström MF, Álvarez R, Nicol AL, et al. Quantitative validation of sensory mapping in persistent postherniorrhaphy inguinal pain patients undergoing triple neurectomy. Hernia 2017;21(2):207–14.

59. Werner MU. Management of persistent postsurgical inguinal pain. Langenbecks Arch Surg 2014;399(5):559–69.

60. Bjurstrom MF, Nicol AL, Amid PK, et al. Pain control following inguinal herniorrhaphy: current perspectives. J Pain Res 2014;7:277–90.

61. Verhagen T, Loos MJA, Scheltinga MRM, et al. The Groin-Pain trial: a randomized controlled trial of injection therapy versus neurectomy for postherniorraphy inguinal neuralgia. Ann Surg 2017;26.
62. Rozen D, Ahn J. Pulsed radiofrequency for the treatment of ilioinguinal neuralgia after inguinal herniorrhaphy. Mt Sinai J Med 2006;73:716–8.
63. Rozen D, Parvez U. Pulsed radiofrequency of lumbar nerve roots for treatment of chronic inguinal herniorraphy pain. Pain Physician 2006;9:153–6.
64. Cohen SP, Foster A. Pulsed radiofrequency as a treatment for groin pain and orchialgia. Urology 2003;61:645.
65. Mitra R, Zeighami A, Mackey S. Pulsed radiofrequency for the treatment of chronic ilioinguinal neuropathy. Hernia 2007;11:369–71.
66. Werner MU, Bischoff JM, Rathmell JP, et al. Pulsed radiofrequency in the treatment of persistent pain after inguinal herniotomy: a systematic review. Reg Anesth Pain Med 2012;37:340–3.
67. Amid PK. A 1-stage surgical treatment for postherniorrhaphy neuropathic pain: triple neurectomy and proximal end implantation without mobilization of the cord. Arch Surg 2002;137(1):100–4.
68. Amid PK. Causes, prevention, and surgical treatment of postherniorrhaphy neuropathic inguinodynia: triple neurectomy with proximal end implantation. Hernia 2004;8(4):343–9.
69. Amid PK, Chen DC. Surgical treatment of chronic groin and testicular pain after laparoscopic and open preperitoneal inguinal hernia repair. J Am Coll Surg 2011; 213(4):531–6.
70. Moore AM, Bjurstrom MF, Hiatt JR, et al. Efficacy of retroperitoneal triple neurectomy for refractory neuropathic inguinodynia. Am J Surg 2016;212(6):1126–32.
71. Chen DC, Hiatt JR, Amid PK. Operative management of refractory neuropathic inguinodynia by a laparoscopic retroperitoneal approach. JAMA Surg 2013; 148(10):962–7.
72. Ssentongo AE, Kwon EG, Zhou S, et al. Pain and dysfunction with sexual activity after inguinal hernia repair: systematic review and meta-analysis. J Am Coll Surg 2020;230(2):237.
73. Hawn MT, Itani KM, Giobbie-Hurder A, et al. Patient-reported outcomes after inguinal herniorrhaphy. Surgery 2006;140(2):198.
74. Isil RG, Avlanmis O. Effects of totally extraperitoneal and lichtenstein hernia repair on men's sexual function and quality of life. Surg Endosc 2020;34(3):1103.
75. Maneck M, Köckerling F, Fahlenbrach C, et al. Hospital volume and outcome in inguinal hernia repair: analysis of routine data of 133,449 patients. Hernia 2020;24(4):747–57.
76. Nordin P, Van Der Linden W. Volume of procedures and risk of recurrence after repair of groin hernia: national register study. BMJ 2008;336:934–7.
77. Köckerling F, Bittner R, Kraft B, et al. Does surgeon volume matter in the outcome of endoscopic inguinal hernia repair? Surg Endosc 2016;31:573–85.
78. Köckerling F, Jacob D, Wiegank W, et al. Endoscopic repair of primary versus recurrent male unilateral inguinal hernias: are there differences in the outcome? Surg Endosc 2016;30:1146–55.
79. Köckerling F, Koch A, Lorenz R, et al. Open repair of primary versus recurrent male unilateral inguinal hernias: perioperative complications and 1-year follow-up. World J Surg 2016;40:813–25.
80. Miserez M, Peeters E, Aufenacker T, et al. Update with level 1 studies of the European Hernia Society guidelines on the treatment of inguinal hernia in adult patients. Hernia 2014;18:151–63.

Endocrine Surgery
Management of Postoperative Complications Following Endocrine Surgery of the Neck

Oliver J. Fackelmayer, MD, James X. Wu, MD,
Michael W. Yeh, MD*

KEYWORDS

- Endocrine surgery • Neck hematoma • Thyroidectomy • Parathyroidectomy
- Lymph node dissection • Hypoparathyroidism • Hypocalcemia
- Recurrent laryngeal nerve injury

KEY POINTS

- Neck hematomas can threaten the airway and require prompt management with bedside decompression and return to the operating room.
- Neck wound infection/abscess is rare but should be managed with washout, drainage, and antibiotics.
- Lymph leak can occur after lymph node dissection, and management ranges from surgical drain placement to interventional lymphangioembolization depending on the output volume and duration of leak.
- Postthyroidectomy hypoparathyroidism can result in symptomatic hypocalcemia. Devitalized parathyroid glands should be autotransplanted. The authors administer prophylactic supplementation with calcium ± calcitriol based on the postoperative parathyroid hormone level.
- Recurrent laryngeal nerve injury ranges from mild transient unilateral neuropraxia with temporary voice changes to bilateral vocal cord paralysis requiring tracheostomy. Management is complex and multidisciplinary.

INTRODUCTION

Cervical endocrine operations commonly include parathyroidectomy, thyroid lobectomy, thyroidectomy, central neck dissection, and selective or modified radical neck dissection. Being the inlet to the human body, the neck comprises a dense collection of vital structures contained in a small, roughly cylindrical volume. It is an unforgiving

All authors report no commercial or financial disclosures or conflicts of interest.
No funding sources to declare.
Section of Endocrine Surgery, UCLA David Geffen School of Medicine, UCLA Endocrine Center, 100 Medical Plaza Driveway, Suite 310, Los Angeles, CA 90095, USA
* Corresponding author.
E-mail address: MYeh@mednet.ucla.edu

Surg Clin N Am 101 (2021) 767–784
https://doi.org/10.1016/j.suc.2021.05.019
0039-6109/21/© 2021 Elsevier Inc. All rights reserved.

surgical.theclinics.com

place in which to operate. The vital structures at risk include the recurrent laryngeal nerves (RLN) to the intrinsic muscles of the larynx, additional cranial nerves, parathyroid glands essential for calcium homeostasis, aerodigestive structures, and great vessels. The limited space of the neck also makes relatively small-volume bleeding and fluid collections potentially hazardous, as they can lead precipitously to airway compromise. Here, the authors discuss complications of neck surgery, including cervical hematoma and other fluid collections, hypocalcemia from hypoparathyroidism, and nerve injuries, along with the prevention, mitigation, and management (summarized in **Table 1**).

NECK HEMATOMA

Neck hematoma is a feared and potentially lethal complication of cervical endocrine surgery. It is defined as the postoperative collection of blood in the operative bed. Because of the small volume and noncompliance of the neck as a body compartment, hematomas can threaten the airway through extrinsic compression as well as venous congestion resulting in laryngeal edema.

In study of 3660 patients undergoing thyroid surgery, 76 (2.1%) required reoperation for a compressive hematoma.[1]

The risk of postoperative hematoma is dependent on the operation performed: lowest for focused parathyroidectomy followed by thyroid lobectomy and highest for total thyroidectomy with central neck dissection (**Fig. 1**).[2] In a study of 30,000 thyroid operations, the rate of postoperative bleeding following thyroidectomy was

Table 1
Complication prevention, mitigation, and management overview

Complication	Prevention	Mitigation	Management
Cervical hematoma	Technical hemostasis Perioperative management of antiplatelets & anticoagulants	Observation period after surgery	Reoperation
Seroma/chyle leak	Avoidance of injury to thoracic duct Ligation of major lymphatics	Drain placement at initial operation	Aspiration Reoperation with drain placement Lymphangiography and embolization Surgical ligation of thoracic duct
Surgical site infection	Aseptic technique	Antibiotics	Antibiotics Wound care
Hypocalcemia	Minimize extent of surgery Preservation of parathyroid glands Autotransplantation of parathyroid glands	Routine postoperative calcium supplementation PTH-based calcitriol supplementation	Calcium/calcitriol supplementation rhPTH HCTZ
Recurrent laryngeal nerve injury	Minimize extent of surgery	Neuromonitoring Staged operation Nerve repair or transposition	Swallow evaluation Laryngoscopy Cord medialization

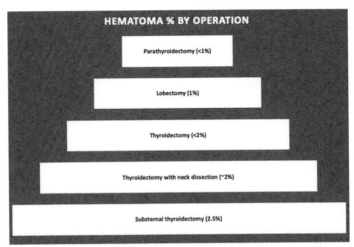

HEMATOMA % BY OPERATION

Parathyroidectomy (<1%)

Lobectomy (1%)

Thyroidectomy (<2%)

Thyroidectomy with neck dissection (~2%)

Substernal thyroidectomy (2.5%)

Fig. 1. Risk of bleeding by operation.[1] *Data from* Dehal A, Abbas A, Hussain F, et al. Risk factors for neck hematoma after thyroid or parathyroid surgery: ten-year analysis of the nationwide inpatient sample database. Perm J 2015;19(1):22-8.

double that of unilateral lobectomies, 2% versus 1%.[3] Older age and male sex have also been shown to be independent risk factors for postoperative bleeding.

A study based on the American College of Surgeons–National Surgical Quality Improvement Program (ACS-NSQIP) database showed a 1.3% rate of hematoma in more than 14,000 patients who underwent thyroidectomy at 98 hospitals. Although hospital performance varied for other thyroidectomy-specific complications, no variance was found in the rate of hematoma, suggesting that no surgeon or hospital, regardless of expertise, is immune to this stubborn complication.[4]

Prevention

The prevention of postoperative neck hematoma rests on careful technical hemostasis. Critical bleeding points that should be routinely checked before closing the neck include the superior pole pedicle, inferior thyroid artery and its branches, ligament of Berry, inferior pole veins, and the cut surface of the thyroid isthmus during lobectomy. In the authors' practice, they commonly perform suture ligation of the ligament of Berry using 5-0 monofilament suture for hemostasis medial to the RLN terminus. Similarly, the application of small titanium clips to the branches of the inferior thyroid artery near the nerve can be helpful in an area where the avoidance of energy-based hemostasis is desirable. Tiny bleeders lying very close to the nerve may respond to digital compression. An intraoperative Valsalva maneuver, performed by the anesthesiologist by sustaining an airway pressure above 25 mm Hg for several seconds, may assist in revealing areas of bleeding, especially from inferior pole veins, which may be avulsed during delivery of a substernal goiter. It is the authors' practice to routinely place thrombin-soaked gelatin foam into the field at the conclusion of hemostasis. The strap muscles should be closed loosely, in a manner permitting the anterior egress of blood such that any bleeding would be more likely to manifest clinically rather than being trapped in a small deep space adjacent to the airway.

The use of electrosurgery devices in thyroid surgery has become widespread. Ultrasonic and bipolar sealing devices have been associated with reduced operative time as well as reduced blood loss as compared with conventional techniques. The choice of electrosurgery device, bipolar sealer versus ultrasonic coagulation, had no impact on rates of postoperative hematoma, cost, or operative times.[5] New analyses indicate these devices are associated with a statistically significant reduced risk of postoperative neck hematoma.[6,7]

Preoperative management of anticoagulants and antiplatelet agents
The risk of neck hematoma may be increased in those who are chronically anticoagulated or maintained on antiplatelet medications. In a single-institution study of 4500 patients, the overall observed postoperative hematoma rate was low at 0.5% but significantly increased for patients on antiplatelet therapy (2.2%) and anticoagulation therapy (10.7%).[8]

Aspirin and clopidogrel should be held for 1 week before operation whenever possible. In patients receiving dual antiplatelet therapy after percutaneous coronary intervention, surgery should be delayed 6 months regardless of stent type, and then surgery should be performed while the patient is off antiplatelet medications.[9] A small number of patients with severe coronary disease will require the continuation of aspirin throughout the perioperative period with a small but significant increased absolute risk of 0.8%.[10,11] The optimal perioperative management of patients undergoing cervical endocrine surgery who chronically take anticoagulants or antiplatelet drugs rests on proper comparative assessment of the bleeding risk and the thromboembolic risk. Because these risks vary according to the procedure performed and the indication for anticoagulation, no specific guidelines exist regarding the timing of either preoperative drug cessation or postoperative resumption. A suggested framework of drug cessation and resumption is presented in **Table 2**. Drug cessation may be timed to allow 5 half-lives of elimination to occur preoperatively for anticoagulants and to allow the genesis of a sufficient number of functional platelets for antiplatelet drugs. Bridge therapy with enoxaparin after cessation of warfarin should only be considered in patients at very high risk for thromboembolic events, such as those with a mechanical mitral valve. Antiplatelet medications are generally restarted 3 to 5 days following surgery. Warfarin, because of its delayed onset of action, can be resumed without a bridge the day following surgery. Novel oral anticoagulants can generally be resumed 2 to 3 days following surgery.[12]

Table 2 Anticoagulant and antiplatelet characteristics			
Medication	Mechanism of Action	Half-Life (h)	When to Stop
Warfarin (Coumadin)	Vitamin K antagonist	20–60	5 d (average 4 d for international normalized ratio <1.5)
Low-molecular-weight heparin (enoxaparin)	Antithrombin III mediated selective inhibition of factor Xa	2	24 h
Dabigatran (Pradaxa)	Direct thrombin inhibition	8–15	24–48 h
Rivaroxaban (Xarelto)	Direct factor Xa inhibition	5–13	24–48 h
Apixaban (Eliquis)	Direct factor Xa inhibition	12	24–48 h
Aspirin	Cyclooxygenase inhibition	3–10	7 d
Clopidogrel (Plavix)	Adenosine diphosphate receptor antagonist, irreversible	8	5–7 d

Postoperative hemorrhagic events are both more frequent and more lethal than thromboembolic events in chronically anticoagulated patients undergoing elective surgery.[13] As such, the authors err on the side of resuming anticoagulant and antiplatelet drugs later during the postoperative period in situations of ambiguity. The authors have not experienced any thromboembolic events using this strategy.

Mitigation

Postoperative observation

Given the statistical inevitability of a small number of neck hematomas following cervical endocrine surgery, every surgeon performing these procedures must establish a team-based detection and mitigation strategy to prevent progression of these events to lethality. The mainstay of mitigation is the inclusion of a postoperative observation period. Most hematomas manifest within the first few hours after surgery (**Fig. 2**), with the frequency of events falling off steeply after 6 hours. In the authors' practice, they discharge patients 4 hours after parathyroidectomy, 6 hours after thyroid lobectomy or total thyroidectomy with low bleeding risk (as assessed by the individual surgeon), and 23 hours after total thyroidectomy with moderate to high bleeding risk or when neck dissection is performed.[14] Other factors, such as the patient's ability to communicate, adequacy of social supports, and distance between the patient's home and the hospital, are also considered. The authors favor monitoring patients in "open" observation units where beds are separated by curtains or glass walls, permitting a maximum number of "eyes" on each patient to increase the likelihood of early hematoma detection.

Management

Most hematomas present as a firm and visible bulge in the anterior neck, often associated with ecchymosis (**Fig. 3**). In rare circumstances, a small, asymptomatic, nonexpanding or obviously superficial hematoma can be managed with manual compression by the surgeon and observation in a closely monitored setting provided there is immediate access to an operating room. An expanding cervical hematoma with symptoms of respiratory distress indicates impending airway compression and will progress to respiratory failure.

The first priority is to secure the patient's airway. If the patient is awake, alert, and breathing normally, management may take place after efficient transport to an operating room under the immediate supervision of both a surgeon and an

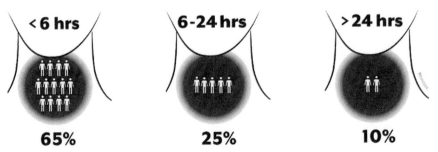

Onset of Post-Operative Hematoma

< 6 hrs	6-24 hrs	> 24 hrs
65%	**25%**	**10%**

Fig. 2. Timing of hematomas requiring intervention.[14]

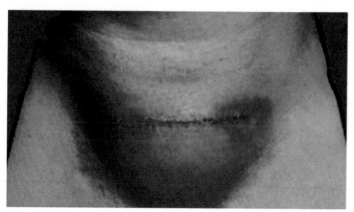

Fig. 3. Cervical hematoma. (Image credit Masha Livhits, MD; UCLA David Geffen School of Medicine)

anesthesiologist. If the patient is in respiratory distress, the surgeon should call for help from nursing and anesthesia staff and then perform immediate bedside decompression of the neck with either a scalpel or scissors. This should be done in a way that opens not only the skin but also any other intervening layers between the skin and airway that have been closed, such as the platysma and sometimes even the strap muscle layer, as these may impede the egress of hematoma contents.

Bedside decompression usually relieves respiratory distress, permitting patient transport to the operating room where intubation and hematoma exploration can be performed. Patients who remain in respiratory distress after bedside decompression should be intubated to secure the airway. This is an uncommon scenario that may signal the presence of a residual, deep, undrained fluid collection that is compressing the trachea.

Definitive management consists of hematoma exploration under general anesthesia. After the evacuation of clot, irrigation with water and dilute hydrogen peroxide helps to destain the tissues, facilitating visual identification of bleeding points. Hemostasis should proceed methodically, as described above. An obvious culprit vessel (or vessels) is often, but not always, found.

SEROMA FORMATION AND CHYLE LEAK

Other postoperative fluid collections include seromas and chyle (lymphatic) leaks. Seromas are usually small and self-limited in their course; some may require simple aspiration. Injury to the thoracic duct during left lateral neck dissection, or large lymphatic channels on either side, can result in chyle leaks at a rate of approximately 0.9% of thyroidectomy with cervical lymph node dissection.[15]

Prevention

Knowledge of the relevant anatomy may help the surgeon identify the thoracic duct or lymphatic channels for early ligation and to avoid inadvertent injury. Operations in the left lateral neck are at much higher risk of lymph leak given the anatomic path of the thoracic duct (**Fig. 4**). In the authors' practice, they observe the risk of major lymph leak on the right side is far lower, and major injury is unlikely unless an anomalous right sided thoracic duct is present.

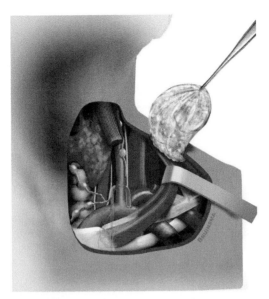

Fig. 4. Thoracic duct anatomy.

Surgeons should not attempt to dissect the very delicate thoracic duct or lymphatic channels, as the dissection may lead to injury. Some surgeons routinely tie all inferior attachments of the lateral neck lymph nodes from phrenic nerve to internal jugular vein before division. Any visible lymphatic channels that require division in the course of neck dissection should be clipped, tied, or sealed with an electrosurgical device.

Mitigation

After division of the inferior border of the specimen in a lateral neck dissection, a chyle leak may manifest as pooling of clear or milky fluid. If recognized during operation, careful and complete suture ligation or clipping is required. If attempts to close the leak are unsuccessful, then the area can also be injected with fibrin glue and/or the potential space can be obliterated with a rotational muscle flap.

If not recognized and successfully managed at the initial operation, a chyle leak will present with either high-volume drain output (sometimes exceeding 500 cc per day) or an enlarging ballotable fluid collection in the absence of a drain.

Management

A large undrained chyle leak should be drained immediately upon discovery, either operatively or with the placement of a percutaneous drain. Failure to establish drainage may result in an organized (fibrotic) lymph collection, which causes significant patient discomfort and takes months to resolve. A small undrained chyle leak may be adequately managed by vertical positioning (encouraging the patient to stand, sit upright, or sleep with head elevated) and weighted compression of the supraclavicular fossa (the authors often ask their patients to place a bag of rice over the area). High-volume drain output is first managed with a low-fat diet and maintenance of bulb suction. If the leak fails to resolve, the bulb should be converted to gravity drainage to reduce potentiation of the leak. In the case of a persistent high-volume chyle leak, the authors do not attempt reoperation with the goal of ligating lymphatic channels, as these are exceedingly difficulty to identify in an inflamed/scarred reoperative field. In this scenario, the authors consider thoracic duct ligation (**Fig. 5**) or

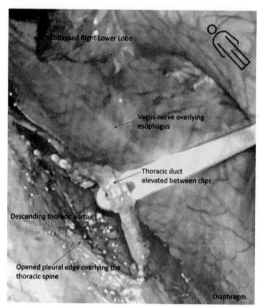

Fig. 5. Thoracoscopic ligation of the thoracic duct in the right hemithorax just cephalad to the diaphragm. (Image credit Fredric Pieracci, MD; Denver Health Medical Center)

embolization. An interventional approach, such as lymphangiography with emboliza-tion, is an excellent option but only available in specialized centers with appropriately skilled interventionalists (**Fig. 6**).

SURGICAL SITE INFECTION
Prevention

Wound infection for cervical operations is uncommon. Prevention includes maximal sterile technique with appropriate skin preparation. These operations are considered clean cases and do not mandate routine antibiotic prophylaxis. Risk factors for wound infection include lymph node dissection (odds ratio [OR] 3.2) and drain placement (OR 1.8).[16]

Mitigation

The surgeon may elect to administer antibiotics if the technical factors above or clin-ical risk factors are present.

Management

As with any superficial surgical site infection, the surgeon may elect to open the wound to allow drainage and healing by secondary intention. Cosmetic outcomes in this sce-nario remain excellent. A short course of antibiotics targeting gram-positive organisms is often warranted, especially in the presence of any cellulitis, with close follow-up of the wound.

HYPOCALCEMIA

Hypocalcemia following thyroidectomy is common and underreported.[1] Transient postoperative hypocalcemia with low parathyroid hormone (PTH) level lasting less than 6 months occurs in approximately 25% of patients, whereas permanent

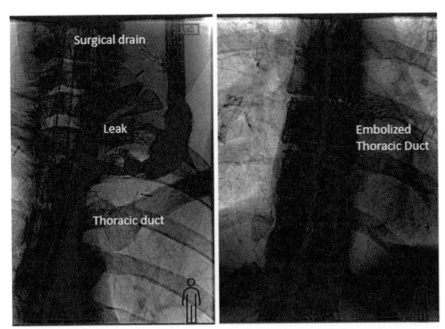

Fig. 6. Lymphangiography showing cervical thoracic duct injury with leak in the region of a surgical drain (*left*) and embolization of the thoracic duct (*right*). (Image credit Edward W. Lee, MD; PhD, Dept. Of Radiological Sciences, UCLA David Geffen School of Medicine)

hypoparathyroidism occurs in less than 3% of patients. Severe postoperative hypocalcemia requiring the administration of intravenous calcium, emergent emergency room or office visit, or hospital readmission occurs in 5% of patients.[17] Risk factors for transient hypoparathyroidism include preoperative vitamin D deficiency, parathyroid autotransplantation, and longer operative time, and the extent of central neck dissection (**Table 3**). Risk factors for permanent hypoparathyroidism include a diagnosis of Graves disease and reoperation for bleeding. Age also influences the rate of postoperative hypoparathyroidism. Among Medicare patients who underwent surgery for thyroid cancer, hypoparathyroidism occurred in 5.1% of those aged less than 65 years, and 13.6% in those aged greater than 65 years.[18]

Prevention

Prevention of postoperative hypocalcemia rests on the technical preservation of parathyroid tissue. If appropriate, lobectomy rather than total thyroidectomy is preferred to spare manipulation of 2 parathyroid glands. Bilateral central neck dissection is associated with a nonlinear increase in the rate of permanent hypoparathyroidism and should be avoided if possible.[19]

Parathyroid autotransplantation

Intraoperatively, all efforts should be made to protect and preserve the parathyroid glands in situ on their native vascular pedicle. Should a parathyroid be devascularized, or removed, it should be autotransplanted (**Fig. 7**). One should treat every parathyroid gland identified as the only remaining gland, making every effort to prevent permanent hypoparathyroidism. After thyroidectomy, one should inspect the specimen for any inadvertently removed parathyroid glands, which should then be autotransplanted.

Table 3
Rates of hypoparathyroidism following thyroidectomy with and without unilateral versus bilateral central neck dissection[19]

	Total Thyroidectomy		
	Without Central Neck Dissection	Unilateral Central Neck Dissection	Bilateral Central Neck Dissection
Transient (%)	27.7	36.1	51.9
Permanent (%)	6.3	7.0	16.2

Although preservation of parathyroid glands in situ is desirable, parathyroid autotransplantation should be performed when the adequacy of the vascular supply is in question. Parathyroid autotransplantation increases the rate of temporary hypoparathyroidism but does not increase the rate of permanent hypoparathyroidism.[20,21] Routine autotransplantation of one or more parathyroid glands as a strategy to reduce the rate of permanent hypoparathyroidism did not alter the outcome.[22] With appropriate technique, autotransplanted parathyroid glands almost always regain function by the sixth postoperative week.[23]

Mitigation

Postoperative calcium supplementation following thyroid surgery
Prophylactic calcium supplementation after total thyroidectomy can reduce the incidence of symptomatic postoperative hypocalcemia because of hypoparathyroidism. Several protocols have been described in the literature.[24–26] In the authors' practice, all patients are given scheduled calcium supplementation following total or completion thyroidectomy (**Fig. 8**).[25] A PTH level is obtained 1 hour after the operation, and

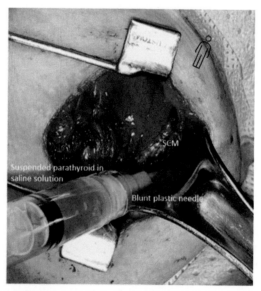

Fig. 7. Autotransplantation via injection of morcellated parathyroid tissue resuspended in cold buffered saline solution into the sternocleidomastoid muscle using a blunt tip applicator.

supplementation is adjusted to (1) augment the dose of calcium and (2) add calcitriol as needed per the algorithm. The authors' protocol has virtually eliminated hypocalcemic symptoms during hospitalization, the need for intravenous calcium postoperatively, and readmissions related to hypocalcemia, without causing any instances of hypercalcemia. Furthermore, virtually any hypocalcemic event can be managed over the phone in a recently discharged patient who has calcitriol immediately at hand.

Postoperative calcium supplementation following parathyroid surgery
Prevention of postoperative hypocalcemia after parathyroidectomy is similarly managed with a protocol for prophylactic calcium and vitamin D supplementation. In the authors' practice, they tailor the regimen to each patient's highest preoperative calcium level (**Table 4**).

Hungry bone syndrome
Hungry bone syndrome is a phenomenon whereby rapid deposition of serum calcium into "hungry" demineralized bones causes profound, prolonged hypocalcemia after parathyroidectomy. Patients with end-stage renal disease, severe osteoporosis, or prolonged, untreated hyperthyroidism (severe Graves disease undergoing total thyroidectomy) are at risk for hungry bone syndrome. Other risk factors include volume of adenoma resected, preoperative blood urea nitrogen concentration, preoperative alkaline phosphatase level, and younger age.[27] Treatment requires aggressive supplementation of calcium supplementation. Although the oral route is the first choice, intravenous calcium is frequently required in patients who have undergone subtotal parathyroidectomy for renal hyperparathyroidism. These patients often benefit from dialysis with a high calcium bath. Calcitriol may be given to increase oral calcium absorption. Hypomagnesemia can contribute to refractory hypocalcemia and should be corrected. Hypophosphatemia, however, should be tolerated, as supplementation of phosphorus can bind calcium, thus worsening hypocalcemia. Patients with renal hyperparathyroidism may benefit from preoperative calcitriol loading for 3 to 5 days

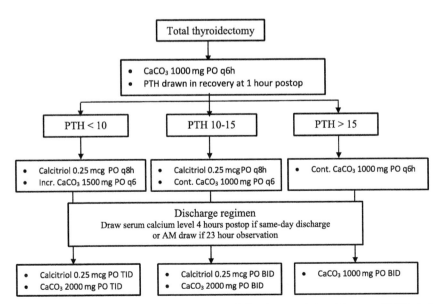

Fig. 8. Protocolized postoperative management following total thyroidectomy.[25] BID, twice a day; Incr., increased; PO, orally; postop., postoperatively; TID, 3 times a day.

Table 4			
Postparathyroidectomy supplementation			
	Highest Preoperative Serum Calcium		
	<11.5	11.5–12.5	>12.5
Calcium carbonate dose	1000 mg	2000 mg	2000 mg
Dosing interval	bid	bid	tid

All patients receive 2000 units cholecalciferol daily.

before surgery; this mitigates postoperative hypocalcemia and may shorten the length of hospitalization.[28]

Management

Permanent hypoparathyroidism is managed with calcium supplementation and calcitriol to maintain normal serum calcium levels. Unfortunately, lack of PTH action on the kidney causes urinary losses of supplemented calcium with resultant hypercalciuria, nephrolithiasis, and nephrocalcinosis.[29] Adding hydrochlorothiazide in this situation can decrease the urine calcium with the advantageous result of increasing serum calcium. Long-term follow-up showed patients with permanent hypoparathyroidism have 2- to 17-fold greater rates of chronic kidney disease stage 3 or worse relative to age-appropriate norms.[30] Severe cases may require recombinant PTH. Recombinant human parathyroid hormone (rhPTH) can reduce the need for large doses of calcium and calcitriol, especially if patients develop hypercalciuria. Natpara is an 84-amino-acid rhPTH recalled in the United States by the Food and Drug Administration in 2019 and is currently available only under a Special Use Program.[31] Teriparatide (Forteo) is a 34-amino-acid rhPTH identical to the N-terminal portion of the native protein. A more stable and longer-acting prodrug formulation (TranCon PTH) is in phase 2 clinical trials.[32] Institution of rhPTH therapies has been limited by the high cost, required administration via subcutaneous injection, and need for additional long-term efficacy and safety data.

RECURRENT LARYNGEAL NERVE INJURY

Injury to the RLN is the most dreaded complication of thyroid and parathyroid surgery, causing significant morbidity, reduced quality of life, and litigation.[33] The severity of RLN injury can range from mild neuropraxia with temporary voice changes to severe permanent hoarseness from vocal cord paralysis. The glottic gap that results from vocal cord paresis also increases the risk of aspiration. Bilateral RLN injury can result in significant airway compromise, often requiring tracheostomy.

Prevention

A unilateral operation where appropriate, such as lobectomy or focused parathyroidectomy, only places one of the RLNs at risk. In the operating room, knowledge of anatomy of the RLN is crucial, as it allows early identification and protection of the nerve (**Table 5**).[34] The RLN will bifurcate in approximately 36% of cases, occurring at a median distance of 18 mm on the right and 13 mm on the left from the cricothyroid (**Fig. 9**). The anterior division carries motor fibers to all of the intrinsic muscles of the larynx except the cricothyroid and the posterior crico-arytenoid muscles. The posterior division innervates the posterior crico-arytenoid muscle, responsible for abducting the vocal cords. It is also important to recognize when there is the possibility of a non-

Table 5
Relationship of the left and right recurrent laryngeal nerves to the inferior thyroid artery[34]

Recurrent Laryngeal Nerve	Relationship to Inferior Thyroid Artery (%)		
	Anterior	Posterior	Between Branches
Left	17.2	62.6	20.2
Right	37.1	37.0	29.0

RLN, which always occurs on the right and in patients with an anomalous course of right subclavian artery posterior to the esophagus.[35] Neuromonitoring is an adjunct tool to be used at the discretion of the operating surgeon. A special endotracheal tube monitors the muscular contractions of the intrinsic muscles of the larynx; thus, a paralytic must not be used. The data do not support use of neuromonitoring to prevent injury to the RLN.[36] Despite that fact, a study based on the ACS-NSQIP database found that surgeons at best performing hospitals for RLN injury were more likely to use intraoperative nerve monitoring and energy devices with nerve injuries reported in 755 out of 13,144 operations (5.7% overall, 4.2% lobectomy, 6.6% total thyroidectomy).[4]

Mitigation

For patients undergoing reoperation or who have large or symptomatic thyroid cancer, it is prudent to evaluate vocal cord motion before surgery. Risk factors for vocal cord palsy include older age, nodule size ≥ 3.5 cm, presence of voice symptoms, and prior neck surgery. In a review of more than 6000 patients, 41 patients were identified as having a vocal cord palsy, and all 41 of them had at least 1 risk factor, that is, no vocal

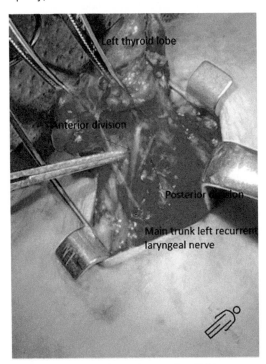

Fig. 9. Branching of the RLN into anterior and posterior divisions.

cord palsies existed without any risk factors.[37] Vocal cord motion can be evaluated via flexible laryngoscopy or laryngeal ultrasound. If disease is adherent to the RLN, every effort should be made to preserve the functioning nerve.

Management

If using intraoperative nerve monitoring, surgeons may recognize a recurrent nerve injury when stimulation of the nerve no longer produces a signal. The surgeon should be familiar with how to troubleshoot the nerve monitor to rule out technical errors or displacement of endotracheal tube. The surgeon can verify whether the nerve is being adequately stimulated by placing a finger on the posterior cricoid plate to palpate a laryngeal twitch when stimulating the distal RLN. When a nerve injury is suspected but the nerve is grossly intact, it should not be manipulated and given a chance to recover postoperatively. It is prudent to then stage the operation and avoid dissection of the contralateral nerve until a later date, when the injured nerve has a chance to recover. This practice is in line with the 2020 American Association of Endocrine Surgeons guidelines, recommendation 43 and 44.[38]

If the RLN is inadvertently transected or intentionally sacrificed, injury identified intraoperatively can be managed by primary anastomosis with nerve wrap or conduit, interposition graft with a segment of ansa cervicalis, or anastomosis directly to the ansa cervicalis (**Fig. 10**). Regardless of choice of technique, the resulting anastomosis should be tension free. Reanastomosis will not restore nerve function but will maintain muscular tone and result in better voice outcomes. If the nerve was cauterized, the ends should be trimmed to healthy tissue before anastomosis. Postoperatively, patients with RLN injury are at increased aspiration risk and should undergo swallow evaluation. Patients who continue to aspirate with oral intake can be evaluated for vocal cord injection to medialize the paralyzed vocal cord.

If bilateral RLN injury is suspected, it is acceptable to trial extubating the patient. If there is sufficient space between the paralyzed vocal cords, patients with bilateral injury may avoid tracheostomy. The anesthesia team should be aware of the possibility of airway compromise and should be ready to reintubate the patient at the first sign of respiratory distress. The surgical team should also be ready to secure a surgical airway if needed, and instruments should be kept sterile. Do *not* leave the operating room with a patient having stridorous respirations. If the patient has stridor and/or dyspnea, reintubate and perform a tracheostomy. If the patient is breathing comfortably, they should be closely monitored for 72 hours, as postoperative laryngeal edema could still threaten the airway. Steroids, supplemental oxygen, and Heliox can be used as a bridge to intubation from above or establishing a surgical airway.[39] Heliox is a gaseous mixture of helium and oxygen with resultant decreased airway resistance and easier ventilation in patients with difficulty breathing.

External branch of superior laryngeal nerve

Although overshadowed by fear of injury to the RLN, injury to the external branch of the superior laryngeal nerve is a source of morbidity from thyroid surgery (**Table 6**).[40,41] It innervates the cricothyroid muscle; injury compromises higher pitched phonation, singing, and voice projection. Careful visual inspection or testing with a nerve monitor, if available, should be performed before ligation of superior pole vessels to avoid injury to this nerve.

SUMMARY

The neck contains many densely arranged critical structures. Significant and permanent morbidity can result from surgical complications following endocrine surgery.

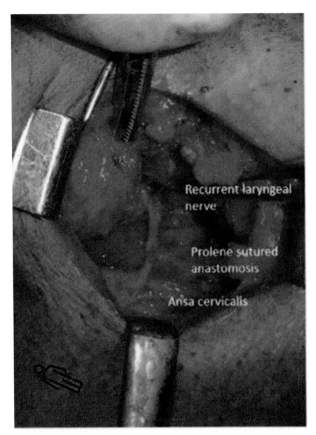

Fig. 10. RLN to ansa cervicalis anastomosis.

Table 6
The Cernea classification describes the variation of the external branch of the superior laryngeal nerve as it passes deep to the superior thyroid artery[40]

	Distance from Superior Thyroid Pole	Percent of Nerves[41]
Type I	>1 cm above	7.3
Type IIa	<1 cm but above	42.7
Type IIb	Below	48.3

Fortunately, the overall rate of complications remains low, especially when surgery is performed by high-volume surgeons. The authors hope increased awareness of potential complications of endocrine operations of the neck as well as the prevention, mitigation, and management thereof can minimize morbidity and improve patient care.

CLINICS CARE POINTS

- Understanding the potential complications of cervical endocrine operations allows for prompt recognition and management.
- Patients should be assessed in the immediate postoperative period for stridor, dysphonia, dysphagia, neck swelling, perioral or digital paresthesia, and nerve deficits.
- Guidelines put forth by the AAES (38) provide a helpful framework for performing safe cervical endocrine operations but should be tailored to the specific practice setting, resources, and expertise of the surgeon.
- Cervical endocrine operations should be performed by high-volume surgeons when possible.

DISCLOSURE

The authors have nothing to disclose.

REFERENCES

1. Bergenfelz A, Jansson S, Kristoffersson A, et al. Complications to thyroid surgery: results as reported in a database from a multicenter audit comprising 3,660 patients. Langenbecks Arch Surg 2008;393(5):667–73.
2. Dehal A, Abbas A, Hussain F, et al. Risk factors for neck hematoma after thyroid or parathyroid surgery: ten-year analysis of the nationwide inpatient sample database. Perm J 2015;19(1):22–8.
3. Promberger R, Ott J, Kober F, et al. Risk factors for postoperative bleeding after thyroid surgery. Br J Surg 2012;99(3):373–9.
4. Liu JB, Sosa JA, Grogan RH, et al. Variation of thyroidectomy-specific outcomes among hospitals and their association with risk adjustment and hospital performance. JAMA Surg 2018;153(1):e174593.
5. Rahbari R, Mathur A, Kitano M, et al. Prospective randomized trial of ligasure versus harmonic hemostasis technique in thyroidectomy. Ann Surg Oncol 2011; 18(4):1023–7.
6. Moran K, Grigorian A, Elfenbein D, et al. Energy vessel sealant devices are associated with decreased risk of neck hematoma after thyroid surgery. Updates Surg 2020;72(4):1135–41.
7. Mahoney RC, Vossler JD, Woodruff SL, et al. Predictors and consequences of hematoma after thyroidectomy: an American College of Surgeons National Surgical Quality Improvement Program database analysis. J Surg Res 2020;260:481–7.
8. Oltmann SC, Alhefdhi AY, Rajaei MH, et al. Antiplatelet and anticoagulant medications significantly increase the risk of postoperative hematoma: review of over 4500 thyroid and parathyroid procedures. Ann Surg Oncol 2016;23(9): 2874–82.
9. Bittl JA, Baber U, Bradley SM, et al. Duration of dual antiplatelet therapy: a systematic review for the 2016 ACC/AHA guideline focused update on duration of dual antiplatelet therapy in patients with coronary artery disease: a report of

the American College of Cardiology/American Heart Association Task Force on Clinical Practice Guidelines. J Am Coll Cardiol 2016;68(10):1116–39.

10. Graham MM, Sessler DI, Parlow JL, et al. Aspirin in patients with previous percutaneous coronary intervention undergoing noncardiac surgery. Ann Intern Med 2018;168(4):237–44.

11. Devereaux PJ, Mrkobrada M, Sessler DI, et al. Aspirin in patients undergoing noncardiac surgery. N Engl J Med 2014;370(16):1494–503.

12. Hornor MA, Duane TM, Ehlers AP, et al. American College of Surgeons' Guidelines for the perioperative management of antithrombotic medication. J Am Coll Surg 2018;227(5):521–36.e1.

13. Kearon C, Hirsh J. Management of anticoagulation before and after elective surgery. N Engl J Med 1997;336(21):1506–11.

14. Terris DJ, Snyder S, Carneiro-Pla D, et al. American Thyroid Association statement on outpatient thyroidectomy. Thyroid 2013;23(10):1193–202.

15. Park I, Her N, Choe JH, et al. Management of chyle leakage after thyroidectomy, cervical lymph node dissection, in patients with thyroid cancer. Head Neck 2018; 40(1):7–15.

16. Salem FA, Almquist M, Nordenström E, et al. A nested case-control study on the risk of surgical site infection after thyroid surgery. World J Surg 2018;42(8): 2454–61.

17. Kazaure HS, Zambeli-Ljepovic A, Oyekunle T, et al. Severe hypocalcemia after thyroidectomy: an analysis of 7366 patients. Ann Surg 2019. https://doi.org/10. 1097/SLA.0000000000003725.

18. Papaleontiou M, Hughes DT, Guo C, et al. Population-based assessment of complications following surgery for thyroid cancer. J Clin Endocrinol Metab 2017; 102(7):2543–51.

19. Giordano D, Valcavi R, Thompson GB, et al. Complications of central neck dissection in patients with papillary thyroid carcinoma: results of a study on 1087 patients and review of the literature. Thyroid Sep 2012;22(9):911–7.

20. Wang B, Zhu CR, Liu H, et al. The effectiveness of parathyroid gland autotransplantation in preserving parathyroid function during thyroid surgery for thyroid neoplasms: a meta-analysis. PLoS One 2019;14(8):e0221173.

21. Iorio O, Petrozza V, De Gori A, et al. Parathyroid autotransplantation during thyroid surgery. Where we are? A systematic review on indications and results. J Invest Surg 2019;32(7):594–601.

22. Lo CY. Parathyroid autotransplantation during thyroidectomy. ANZ J Surg 2002; 72(12):902–7.

23. Olson JA, DeBenedetti MK, Baumann DS, et al. Parathyroid autotransplantation during thyroidectomy. Results of long-term follow-up. Ann Surg 1996;223(5): 472–8 [discussion 478-80].

24. Albuja-Cruz MB, Pozdeyev N, Robbins S, et al. A "safe and effective" protocol for management of post-thyroidectomy hypocalcemia. Am J Surg 2015;210(6): 1162–8 [discussion 1168-9].

25. Wiseman JE, Mossanen M, Ituarte PH, et al. An algorithm informed by the parathyroid hormone level reduces hypocalcemic complications of thyroidectomy. World J Surg 2010;34(3):532–7.

26. Mazotas IG, Yen TWF, Park J, et al. A postoperative parathyroid hormone-based algorithm to reduce symptomatic hypocalcemia following completion/total thyroidectomy: a retrospective analysis of 591 patients. Surgery 2018;164(4): 746–53.

27. Kritmetapak K, Kongpetch S, Chotmongkol W, et al. Incidence of and risk factors for post-parathyroidectomy hungry bone syndrome in patients with secondary hyperparathyroidism. Ren Fail 2020;42(1):1118–26.

28. Witteveen JE, van Thiel S, Romijn JA, et al. Hungry bone syndrome: still a challenge in the post-operative management of primary hyperparathyroidism: a systematic review of the literature. Eur J Endocrinol 2013;168(3):R45–53.

29. Mannstadt M, Bilezikian JP, Thakker RV, et al. Hypoparathyroidism. Nat Rev Dis Primers 2017;3:17080.

30. Mitchell DM, Regan S, Cooley MR, et al. Long-term follow-up of patients with hypoparathyroidism. J Clin Endocrinol Metab 2012;97(12):4507–14.

31. Available at: https://www.fda.gov/safety/recalls-market-withdrawals-safety-alerts/ takeda-issues-us-recall-natpar-parathyroid-hormone-injection-due-potential- rubber-particulate. Accessed February 8, 2021.

32. Available at: https://clinicaltrials.gov/ct2/show/NCT04009291. Accessed February 8, 2021.

33. Swonke ML, Shakibai N, Chaaban MR. Medical malpractice trends in thyroidectomies among general surgeons and otolaryngologists. OTO Open 2020;4(2). 2473974X20921141.

34. Shindo ML, Wu JC, Park EE. Surgical anatomy of the recurrent laryngeal nerve revisited. Otolaryngol Head Neck Surg 2005;133(4):514–9.

35. Yeh MW, Carter JN, Sidhu SB, et al. A case of sibling rivalry? J Am Coll Surg 2006; 202(5):846–7.

36. Barczyński M, Konturek A, Cichoń S. Randomized clinical trial of visualization versus neuromonitoring of recurrent laryngeal nerves during thyroidectomy. Br J Surg Mar 2009;96(3):240–6.

37. Maher DI, Goare S, Forrest E, et al. Routine preoperative laryngoscopy for thyroid surgery is not necessary without risk factors. Thyroid 2019;29(11):1646–52.

38. Patel KN, Yip L, Lubitz CC, et al. Executive summary of the American Association of Endocrine Surgeons guidelines for the definitive surgical management of thyroid disease in adults. Ann Surg 2020;271(3):399–410.

39. Slinger C, Slinger R, Vyas A, et al. Heliox for inducible laryngeal obstruction (vocal cord dysfunction): a systematic literature review. Laryngoscope Investig Otolaryngol 2019;4(2):255–8.

40. Cernea CR, Ferraz AR, Nishio S, et al. Surgical anatomy of the external branch of the superior laryngeal nerve. Head Neck 1992;14(5):380–3.

41. Pagedar NA, Freeman JL. Identification of the external branch of the superior laryngeal nerve during thyroidectomy. Arch Otolaryngol Head Neck Surg 2009; 135(4):360–2.

Management of Postoperative Complications Following Endovascular Aortic Aneurysm Repair

Mohammad Qrareya, MD[a], Bara Zuhaili, MD[b],*

KEYWORDS

- Aortic aneurysms • Ruptured aneurysm • Endovascular aneurysm repair (EVAR)
- Thoracic endovascular aortic repair (TEVAR) • Endoleak • Post-EVAR complications
- Spinal cord ischemia • LSA coverage

Endovascular repair of aortic aneurysm (EVAR) is a well-established minimally invasive method used to treat both thoracic and abdominal aortic pathologic conditions. Currently, EVAR accounts for almost 50% of all aortic aneurysm repairs performed in patients with aortic pathologic conditions in the United States.[1] Cumulative data show that the safety profile of EVAR is improving, and it is comparable to open surgical repair with lower perioperative morbidity and hospital length of stay.[2] However, many complications and challenges have arisen with more utilization of EVAR. Complications related to EVAR can be categorized as device related or systemic. Device-related complications include endoleaks, endograft migration, endograft infection, limb kinking or occlusion, and endograft collapse. Systemic complications include organ ischemia, postimplantation syndrome, and cerebrovascular events.

DEVICE RELATED COMPLICATION
Endoleaks

Endoleaks are the most common complications associated with EVAR. Approximately 15% to 30% of patients with EVAR and 4.5% to 15% of patients with thoracic endovascular aortic repair (TEVAR) have endoleaks within the first 30 days postoperatively.[3,4]

In endoleak, the aneurysmal sac is not fully isolated from systemic circulation, leading to continuous blood flow that pressurizes the residual sac,[1] which could result in

[a] Cardiovascular Surgery Department, Mayo Clinic, 1216 2nd Street Northeast, Rochester, MN 55902, USA; [b] Michigan Vascular Center, Michigan State University, 5020 West Bristol Road, Flint, MI 48507, USA
* Corresponding author.
E-mail address: bzuhaili@michiganvascular.com

Surg Clin N Am 101 (2021) 785–798
https://doi.org/10.1016/j.suc.2021.05.020
0039-6109/21/© 2021 Elsevier Inc. All rights reserved.

surgical.theclinics.com

aneurysmal expansion and possible rupture if left untreated. Five subtypes of endo-leaks have been described.[5]

Type I endoleaks

Type I endoleak develops at the attachment points between the graft and the aortic wall, where the graft fails to achieve circumferential sealing.[6] Type Ia occurs at the proximal attachment point, whereas type Ib occurs at the distal attachment point. The overall incidence of type I endoleak is around 7%, with almost equal incidence between type Ia (3.3%) and Ib (3.7%),[7–9] whereas the incidence of type I endoleak after EVAR is around 3.3% at completion of surgery.[10]

Several anatomic configurations may predispose patients to develop endoleaks. Patients with short, angulated, and/or large-diameter necks are at increased risk of developing type I endoleaks. The risk is higher if there is concomitant circumferential thrombus or calcification.[6] Type I endoleak can be detected as early as the completion arteriography at the end of the case. It can also be detected at the postoperative imaging follow-up. If type I endoleak is detected on computed tomography angiography (CTA), the authors recommend observation for 1 year before intervening unless rapid expansion is noted.

The most common method for type Ia treatment is the aortic cuff extension,[1] especially in cases of mal-deployed or undersized grafts. Another option is a balloon angioplasty via a large-caliber balloon to achieve optimal distention of the endograft at the proximal attachment point. If that does not rectify it, endovascular repair with reballooning graft attachments sites with expandable metal stents can be applied to secure the attachments point.

New techniques, such as EndoAnchors (Medtronic Inc., Minneapolis, MN, USA), whereby helical screws provide transmural fixation for the graft to the aorta, are showing promising results.[11] The Nellix endovascular aneurysm sealing system (Endologix, Irvine, CA, USA) was also used successfully for type Ia endoleak management.[12]

If endoleak persists despite endovascular attempts, open conversion is the next option for suitable surgical patients.[6]

Compared with type Ia endoleaks, type Ib endoleaks are easier to manage.[6] Various options are available, including iliac extender limbs, bare metal stents, coil embolization of the internal iliac arteries, and/or covered stents (**Fig. 1**). In cases whereby coverage of an internal iliac artery (IIA) is necessary, the artery should be embolized before addressing the attachment site leak to avoid subsequent type II endoleaks.[6] Flow to at least one of the internal iliac arteries should be preserved when possible to avoid intractable buttock claudication, sexual dysfunction, and/or the rare incident of rectal ischemia, and bowel ischemia.[6] In the rare cases when the aforementioned techniques are unsuccessful, embolization of the endoleak can be performed with an NBCA glue.[6] Despite these advances in endovascular techniques, some cases with persistent endoleaks may require open surgical repair for definitive treatment.

Type II endoleak

Type II endoleak is the most common type of endoleak, with an estimated 8% to 10% incidence in EVAR patients.[13,14] Type II endoleaks most commonly occur during the first 6 months after surgery.[14] Type II endoleak will show on CTA as a retrograde blood flow through collateral arteries, mainly the inferior mesenteric artery (IMA) and lumbar arteries. Other vasculatures may be present as the source of retrograde flow, such as the accessory renal artery, the sacral arteries, and the hypogastric artery.[14]

There is no consensus on the management strategy of type II endoleaks.[6,14] There is no significant difference in aneurysmal rupture rate or aneurysmal-associated

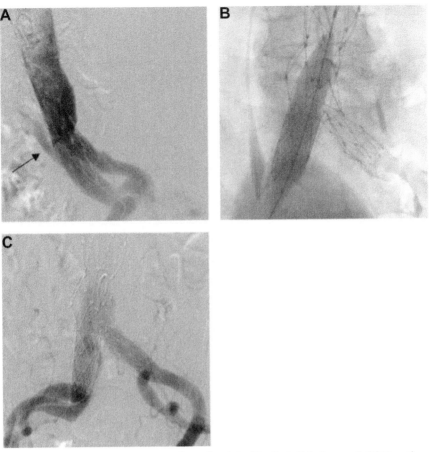

Fig. 1. (*A*) A type Ib endoleak arising from the right iliac limb (*black arrow*). (*B*) Type Ib endoleak seen at the right distal limb of the endograft was treated by an expandable balloon stent. (*C*) The complete resolution of type Ib endoleak was achieved by Palmaz stent deployment within the endograft's right distal limb. (Reprinted from "Management of Endoleaks following Endovascular Aneurysm Repair." by White et al, 2009, Seminars in interventional radiology, 26 (1), 33-38. Copyright (2009) by Thieme Medical Publishers.)

mortality after EVAR between patients with and without type II endoleak.[13,15] In addition, there is a high rate of spontaneous resolution over time[6,14,16] (**Fig. 2**). Thus, many investigators advocate for more conservative approach.[7,17]

Others suggest a more aggressive approach with aortic side branches embolization preoperatively or intraoperatively.[18] This approach can be associated with coil migration, longer procedure times, prolonged fluoroscopy exposure, and higher costs.

The most commonly accepted criteria to intervene on type II endoleaks are sac diameter expansion is greater than 10 mm and/or persistent leaks lasting more than 6 months.[6,13,14] Techniques for type IIa endoleaks management include percutaneous transarterial embolization[19] (**Fig. 3**), translumbar direct sac embolization[20] (**Fig. 4**), and laparoscopic or open ligation of the feeding artery.[6] Angiography is the first step to delineate the extent of collateralization and vessel structure and tortuosity. The decision for either technique is decided accordingly.

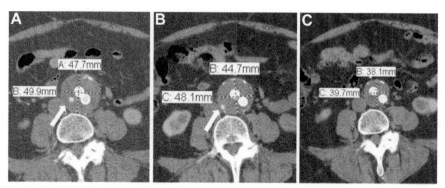

Fig. 2. Abdominal aortic aneurysm shrinking after EVAR despite type II persistence. (*A*) At 1 year. (*B*) Sac shrinking with type II endoleak persistence (*arrow*). (*C*) Endoleak resolution and aneurysm continues to shrink at year 3. (Reprinted from "Type II endoleaks" by Avgerinos et al, 2014, Journal of Vascular Surgery, 60 (5), 1386-1391. Copyright (2014) by Elsevier.)

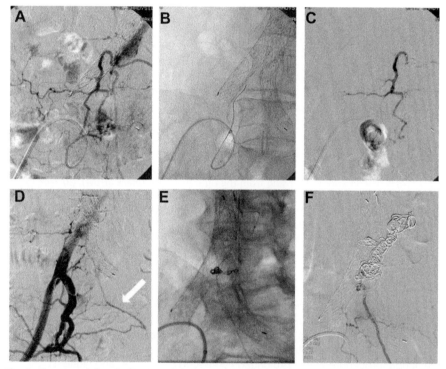

Fig. 3. Transarterial embolization. (*A*) The endoleak is imaged through A 5F selective catheter advanced through a 6F sheath placed in the IIA. (*B*) A microcatheter is guided over a microwire toward the lumbar artery origin. (*C*) Endoleak is sealed by using microcoils. (*D*) Endoleak persists on 6 months' follow-up surveillance, with additional feeders identified (*arrow*) with continuous expansion in abdominal aortic aneurysm (AAA) sac. (*E*) Access to AAA sac is achieved by using a microcatheter. (*F*) Nidus and feeder branches are coiled, and endoleak resolves. (Reprinted from "Type II endoleaks" by Avgerinos et al, 2014, Journal of Vascular Surgery, 60 (5), 1386-1391. Copyright (2014) by Elsevier.)

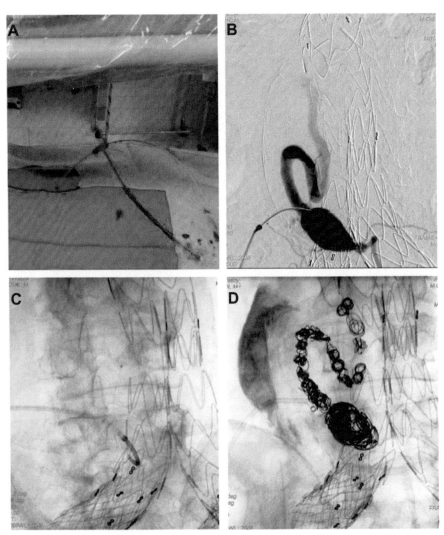

Fig. 4. Translumbar embolization. (*A*) Access has been established to the AAA sac through the left paraspinal approach by using a 6F 30-cm sheath while the patient is in a prone position. (*B*) Endoleak is delineated through a sacogram. (*C*) Embolization is guided through a 5F catheter. (*D*) Multiple coils are used for nidus embolization. (Reprinted from "Type II endoleaks" by Avgerinos et al, 2014, Journal of Vascular Surgery, 60 (5), 1386-1391. Copyright (2014) by Elsevier.)

Type III endoleak

Type III endoleak emerges when the endograft fails to maintain structural integrity. This happens because of dehiscence of modular graft components (type IIIa) or as a result of tears in the endograft fabric (type IIIb).[21] The incidence of type III endoleaks ranges between 3% and 4.5%, with type IIIa accounting for most cases.[21] Type IIIb is a rare complication.[21] Type III endoleaks' diagnosis is often challenging. Management of type III endoleak aims to retain the graft's structural integrity while maintaining full isolation of aneurysmal sac from the systemic circulation.[1,22] Most type III endoleaks can be managed with an endovascular approach by deploying a modular endograft with angioplasty to achieve optimal sealing (**Fig. 5**).[21,22] Risk of recurrence after repair can be as high as 25%, and hence, close surveillance after repair is required.[21]

Other techniques, such as Aorto Uni-iliac endograft with femoral-femoral crossover bypass graft, can also be performed.[6]

Type IV endoleaks

Type IV endoleak is extremely rare.[23] It is not an actual leak, and rather, it is a fluid or blood filtration through the graft porosity.[6] Most investigators report spontaneous resolution of type IV once the patient's coagulation status is restored to baseline. With rapid improvement in graft fabric materials, type IV endoleaks have been largely eliminated.[6]

Type V endoleaks

Type V endoleak, also known as endotension, refers to enlarging the aneurysmal sac without evidence of perigraft blood flow by using conventional imaging modalities.[6,24] The cause of endotension is not fully understood. Several theories have been proposed to explain the mechanism behind it, such as pulse-wave transmission to the aneurysmal sac from the adjacent stent graft or the presence of undetectable endoleaks.[24] Type V endoleak management remains controversial because of the poor understanding of its cause. Observation can be considered in some instances; however, no specific criteria are set to determine which patients are candidates for conservative management.[6] Other investigators advocate for open conversion as a mainstream approach. Less-invasive options have also been applied in a small series of cases with good outcomes, such as the deployment of proximal and distal extension cuffs,[25] aspiration or laparoscopic fenestration of the aneurysmal sac, and relining of the graft with conversion from polytetrafluoroethylene endograft to a less porous one like polyester.[6]

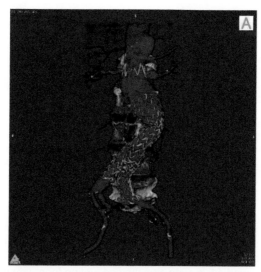

Fig. 5. Three-dimensional reconstruction of abdominal aorta shows complete separation of the stent-graft main body segment. (Reprinted from "An Uncommon Case of Type III Endoleak Treated with a Custom-made Thoracic Stent Graft" by Massara et al, 2016, Annals of Vascular Surgery, 35 (2), 206.e1-206.e3. Copyright (2016) by Elsevier.)

Endograft Migration

Device migration is a common complication.[6] It is more common after EVAR (1%–10%) compared with TEVAR 1% to 2.8%. It is defined as the displacement of the stent by more than 5 to 10 mm from its original location (**Fig. 6**).[6] Factors contributing to stent migration include aortic wall degeneration, undersize or oversize graft, continuous dilation of the aneurysm neck, and aortic tortuosity.[6] Management for endograft migration is the same as type I endoleak. Additional options include using endostaples to fixate the graft to the aortic wall.[26]

Endograft Collapse

Endograft collapse is a rare complication of TEVAR.[6] It is more common following traumatic aortic injuries or spontaneous aortic dissection,[27] but there are also a few reported cases of endograft collapse following an EVAR of abdominal aorta.[28] The underlying cause of graft collapse can be classified into device-related factors and anatomic factors. Device-related factors include low radial force devices, endograft oversizing, material fatigue, and bird-beak phenomena.[1,29] Anatomic factors include a narrow aortic diameter, tight aortic arch, and young healthy aorta.[29] Management of graft collapse following TEVAR includes redo TEVAR and open surgical repair.[29]

The goal of endovascular repair is to increase the radial force at the collapsed portion and enhance the opposition to the aortic wall through either the deployment of a large balloon-expandable stent or placement of additional endograft.[29] Although proximal extension is not always necessary, it can be done if there is a sufficient landing zone.[30] If the landing zone is not sufficient, coverage of the left subclavian artery (LSA) can be done with or without carotid-subclavian bypass, depending on the overall hemodynamics of the patient. If the landing zone is still not sufficient despite covering the LSA, open conversion is mandated rather than graft extension through the left common carotid artery (LCCA).[30] Coverage of the LCCA is strongly

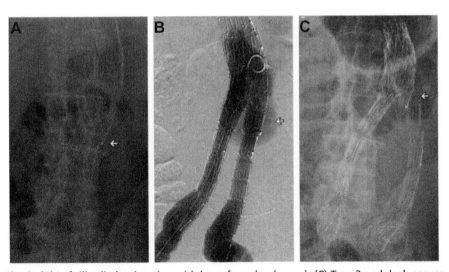

Fig. 6. (A) Left iliac limb migration with loss of overlap (*arrow*). (B) Type 3 endoleak ensues (*arrow*) (C) and eventual limb dislocation (*arrow*). (Reprinted from "Endovascular aneurysm repair (EVAR) follow-up imaging: the assessment and treatment of common postoperative complications" by Ilyas et al, 2015, Clinical Radiology, 70 (2), 183-196. Copyright (2015) by Elsevier.)

discouraged unless the patient is in severe extremis. Open conversion remains an option if the endovascular option has failed or if there is concern for collapse recurrence.[29]

Endograft Occlusion or Limb Kinking

Endograft occlusion and limb kinking (**Fig. 7**) is a time-sensitive complication, as it often leads to acute lower-limb ischemia.[1] It can also lead to the development of type I or type III endoleaks in addition to endograft migration.[1] Risk factors include aortic neck angulation, narrow diameter of the distal aorta, and continuous decrease in the residual aneurysm sac overtime.[31] The management goal in endograft occlusion or kinking is to preserve blood flow to the distal parts of circulation. Open thrombectomy via ipsilateral groin cutdown is usually the first step. Once thrombectomy is done, the underlying cause for the thrombosis or kinking should be rectified. Usually this can be achieved with stents to reinforce the endograft or an additional endograft limbs within the defected graft itself. Cross-femoral bypass can be used as a last resort.

Endograft Infection

Aortic graft infection (AGI) following abdominal EVAR or TEVAR is a rare but life-threatening complication.[1] Less than 1% of patients develop AGI, but the 5-year mortality is as high as 80% in TEVAR group and 50% in EVAR group.[32] Several factors can increase the risk of graft infection. These factors include emergent repair, septic

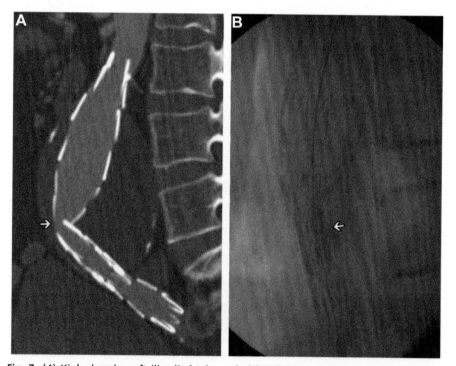

Fig. 7. (A) Kinked endograft iliac limbs (arrow). (B) Relining overlapped segment with a bridging stent graft (arrow). (Reprinted from "Endovascular aneurysm repair (EVAR) follow-up imaging: the assessment and treatment of common postoperative complications" by Ilyas et al, 2015, Clinical Radiology, 70 (2), 183-196. Copyright (2015) by Elsevier.)

process requiring hospitalization, suprarenal clamping, open repair, procedure location (operating room vs radiology suite), contaminated index procedure, use of femoral incision, immunosuppression, and hospital-acquired infections.[32,33]

Early-stage infection tends to present with abdominal pain, abdominal distention, bleeding with anastomotic disruption, surgical site infection, superficial soft tissue infection, and/or fluid collection around the endograft.[34]

Late AGI appearing several months after surgery usually presents with nonspecific signs and symptoms, such as fever, malaise, and/or abdominal pain. Gastrointestinal bleeding, hemoptysis, and/or anemia may develop because of the formation of aortoenteric or aortobronchial fistula.[35]

The first step in managing AGI is initiating of empiric broad-spectrum intravenous antibiotics, and overall medical optimization until a decision is made for the next step.[32] The next step is determined by the patient hemodynamics and baseline health status. If the patient is hemodynamically stable and healthy at baseline, the definitive treatment is debridement of the necrotic tissue, removal of all graft materials, repair of any existing fistula track, and reconstruction of circulation with appropriate conduit.[32,35,36] The conduit can be either rifampin-soaked ePTFE/polyester, cryopreserved segment, or harvested veins from femoral-popliteal distribution (NAIS [Neoaortoiliac System] procedure).[32] Within those conduit options, the NAIS procedure has the highest morbidity and is only tolerated by a minority of patients with AGI.[32,35]

In less stable or less healthy patients, the next step would be local debridement of the infection site, oversewing of the aorta stump, and extra-anatomic reconstruction, such as axillary-bifemoral bypass.[35] In the thoracic aorta, extra-anatomic bypass is more challenging because of the complex anatomy and the need for thoracotomy and possible left heart bypass.[32,35]

In extreme cases of patients with prohibitive risk of surgery, temporizing measures can be taken. Examples of those measures are endovascular stent graft to cover the origin of the aortoenteric fistula and percutaneous drainage of the infected aneurysmal sac.[35,36] The outcome of those temporizing measures is extremely poor, and thus, they are reserved for patients who cannot survive operative intervention for AGI.[35]

SYSTEMIC COMPLICATIONS
Ischemia

Organ ischemia following the EVAR and TEVAR procedure is a common complication. Kidneys, pelvis, abdominal muscles, bowel, and lower-extremities ischemia incidence is estimated to be 9% after EVAR.[1] Spinal cord, left upper-extremity ischemia, and subclavian steal syndrome are more commonly associated with TEVAR with an incidence rate ranging between 5% and 37.5%.[37–39]

Ischemia results from arterial microembolism thrombosis, arterial dissection, obstruction owing to graft malpositioning, or coverage of native arteries because of graft correct positioning (ie, IMA).[1]

In kidneys, a short aneurysm neck increases the risk of inadvertent coverage of renal arteries' origin.[1] In this case, the renal artery or arteries will not be visualized on completion arteriography and renal artery or arteries stenting can be attempted.[1] However, in the case of failed stenting or continuous deterioration of renal function, surgical bypass is required to preserve kidney function.[1]

In cases of bowel ischemia, the colon can be affected following EVAR because of inferior mesenteric artery (IMA) origin coverage by the endograft. The affected territory is the left colon in this case. In contrast to IMA involvement, the superior mesenteric artery (SMA) is less commonly affected, and the cause of SMA involvement is thromboembolic rather than inadvertent coverage of SMA origin. The affected territories in SMA involvement include small bowel and right colon. Bowel ischemia is rarely seen after TEVAR.[1] It typically occurs when the distal tip of the endograft covers the celiac artery origin with possible subsequent small-bowel ischemia.[1] Patients tend to develop bloody diarrhea and abdominal pain postoperatively. The risk increases in cases of prior IIA embolization or known occlusion. Low threshold for lower endoscopy is crucial for early diagnosis. Mild colonic ischemia with no transmural necrosis can be managed through intravenous hydration and bowel rest. In the case of transmural necrosis with or without organ failure or sepsis, explanatory laparotomy with possible colectomy should be done.

Pelvic ischemia has also been reported following EVAR of the abdominal aorta.[1] Pelvic ischemia is more prevalent when bilateral IIA embolization is required because of the complex anatomy or to exclude IIA aneurysm. Clinically, patients with IIA embolization may experience buttock claudication, erectile dysfunction, skin hypoperfusion, and/or rectal ischemia.[40,41] Patients tend to improve over time without intervention[1]; however, if ischemia persists, surgical revascularization of IIA should be considered. Some measures can also be done intraoperatively to preserve blood flow into IIA territories, such as placement of parallel endograft, iliac branch devise, operator modification of existing endograft, and bell-bottom technique.[1,42]

Spinal cord ischemia (SCI) following EVAR of the abdominal aorta is an infrequent complication with only a few cases reported in the literature.[1] SCI is mostly associated with TEVAR with almost 12% of patients developing SCI.[43] Risk factors for developing SCI include age greater than 70 years, perioperative hypotension (mean arterial pressure <70 mm Hg), renal insufficiency, coverage of left subclavian artery (LSA) without revascularization, previous abdominal aortic aneurysm repair, use of 3 or more stent grafts, emergency surgery, iliac artery injury, postoperative increased cerebrospinal fluid pressure, and prolong duration of the procedure.[44,45] Symptoms of SCI develop rapidly within 12 hours postoperatively and may lead to paraplegia.[46] Spinal cord drainage is recommended to reduce the risk of SCI if extensive coverage of the thoracic aorta is planned (>200 mm), or previous AAA repair. cerebrospinal fluid drainage is recommended for at least 48 to 72 hours after TEVAR and should be monitored and adjusted aggressively in intensive care unit settings.[47]

Cerebrovascular Events

The incidence of cerebrovascular events following TEVAR is equitable to open surgery, with middle cerebral artery strokes as the most common and posterior circulations as the least common.[1] Risk factors that may predispose TEVAR patients for stroke include history of stroke, mobile atheroma in the aortic arch, proximal landing zone, placement of proximal cuff, emergency procedure, and LSA coverage.[48,49]

Potential sequela for LSA coverage includes but not limited to left arm ischemia, SCI, and stroke.[49] Debate is still equivocal on the importance of LSA revascularization before its intended coverage in TEVAR.[49] The Society for Vascular Surgery and the European Society for Vascular Surgery currently recommend LSA revascularization in patients who need elective TEVAR whereby proximal sealing is required and in patients with anatomic configuration that compromises perfusion to critical organs.[47,50] In the case of urgent TEVAR with proximal sealing, LSA revascularization is considered according to each case factor, including anatomy, availability of surgical service, and urgency.[50] A meta-analysis concluded that LSA revascularization did not show a superiority in preventing stroke and SCI, whereas it significantly reduced left arm ischemia.[44]

Postimplantation Syndrome

It is estimated that 13% to 60% of patients experience acute inflammatory response following an EVAR procedure.[1] This syndrome is characterized by fever, elevated inflammatory biomarkers like C-reactive protein (CRP), and leukocytosis.[51] The cause behind postimplantation syndrome has not entirely been delineated. There is no definite management for postimplantation syndrome besides aspirin and close follow-up.

The POMEVAR trial suggested methylprednisolone administration preoperatively.[51] Results showed a lower concentration of inflammatory markers in the treatment group. Clinically, it was associated with pronounced reduction in systemic inflammatory response syndrome and faster recovery after EVAR.[51] Larger studies are needed to confirm those findings and elaborate any side effects of such intervention on the long-term outcome.

CONCLUDING POINTS

1. EVAR/TEVAR are becoming standard of care with lower perioperative mortality and morbidity.
2. Safety profile for EVAR and TEVAR is well documented.
3. Complications following EVAR and TEVAR can be classified into graft-related complications and systemic complications.
4. Graft complications include endoleaks, graft infection, migration, collusion, kinking, and collapse.
5. Systemic complications include ischemia, cerebrovascular events, and postimplantation syndrome.
6. The management of EVAR and TEVAR complications is individualized via either minimally invasive or open surgical conversion according to patients' presence and baseline characteristics.
7. Further studies are warranted to delineate the best preventive/therapeutic approach for drastic complications, particularly SCI.

DISCLOSURE

The authors have nothing to disclose.

REFERENCES

1. Daye D, Walker TG. Complications of endovascular aneurysm repair of the thoracic and abdominal aorta: evaluation and management. Cardiovasc Diagn Ther 2018;8(Suppl 1):S138–56.
2. Propper BW, Abularrage CJ. Long-term safety and efficacy of endovascular abdominal aortic aneurysm repair. Vasc Health Risk Manag 2013;9:135–41.
3. Hirsch AT, Haskal ZJ, Hertzer NR, et al. ACC/AHA 2005 practice guidelines for the management of patients with peripheral arterial disease (lower extremity, renal, mesenteric, and abdominal aortic): a collaborative report from the American Association for Vascular Surgery/Society for Vascular Surgery, Society for Cardiovascular Angiography and Interventions, Society for Vascular Medicine and Biology, Society of Interventional Radiology, and the ACC/AHA Task Force on Practice Guidelines (Writing Committee to Develop Guidelines for the Management of Patients With Peripheral Arterial Disease): endorsed by the American Association of Cardiovascular and Pulmonary Rehabilitation; National Heart, Lung, and Blood Institute; Society for Vascular Nursing; TransAtlantic Inter-

Society Consensus; and Vascular Disease Foundation. Circulation 2006;113(11): e463–654.

4. Makaroun MS, Dillavou ED, Wheatley GH, et al. Five-year results of endovascular treatment with the Gore TAG device compared with open repair of thoracic aortic aneurysms. J Vasc Surg 2008;47(5):912–8.

5. Moll FL, Powell JT, Fraedrich G, et al. Management of abdominal aortic aneurysms clinical practice guidelines of the European Society for Vascular Surgery. Eur J Vasc Endovasc Surg 2011;41(Suppl 1):S1–58.

6. Chen J, Stavropoulos SW. Management of endoleaks. Semin Intervent Radiol 2015;32(3):259–64.

7. Buth J, Harris PL, van Marrewijk C, et al. The significance and management of different types of endoleaks. Semin Vasc Surg 2003;16(2):95–102.

8. Buth J, Laheij RJ. Early complications and endoleaks after endovascular abdominal aortic aneurysm repair: report of a multicenter study. J Vasc Surg 2000;31(1 Pt 1):134–46.

9. Mohan IV, Laheij RJ, Harris PL, et al. Risk factors for endoleak and the evidence for stent-graft oversizing in patients undergoing endovascular aneurysm repair. Eur J Vasc Endovasc Surg 2001;21(4):344–9.

10. Tan TW, Eslami M, Rybin D, et al. Outcomes of patients with type I endoleak at completion of endovascular abdominal aneurysm repair. J Vasc Surg 2016; 63(6):1420–7.

11. Giudice R, Borghese O, Sbenaglia G, et al. The use of EndoAnchors in endovascular repair of abdominal aortic aneurysms with challenging proximal neck: single-centre experience. JRSM Cardiovasc Dis 2019;8. 2048004019845508.

12. Hughes CO, de Bruin JL, Karthikesalingam A, et al. Management of a type Ia endoleak with the Nellix endovascular aneurysm sealing system. J Endovasc Ther 2015;22(3):309–11.

13. Sidloff DA, Stather PW, Choke E, et al. Type II endoleak after endovascular aneurysm repair. Br J Surg 2013;100(10):1262–70.

14. Avgerinos ED, Chaer RA, Makaroun MS. Type II endoleaks. J Vasc Surg 2014; 60(5):1386–91.

15. van Marrewijk C, Buth J, Harris PL, et al. Significance of endoleaks after endovascular repair of abdominal aortic aneurysms: the EUROSTAR experience. J Vasc Surg 2002;35(3):461–73.

16. Silverberg D, Baril DT, Ellozy SH, et al. An 8-year experience with type II endoleaks: natural history suggests selective intervention is a safe approach. J Vasc Surg 2006;44(3):453–9.

17. Sidloff DA, Gokani V, Stather PW, et al. Type II endoleak: conservative management is a safe strategy. Eur J Vasc Endovasc Surg 2014;48(4):391–9.

18. Ward TJ, Cohen S, Fischman AM, et al. Preoperative inferior mesenteric artery embolization before endovascular aneurysm repair: decreased incidence of type II endoleak and aneurysm sac enlargement with 24-month follow-up. J Vasc Interv Radiol 2013;24(1):49–55.

19. Bail DH, Walker T, Giehl J. Vascular endostapling systems for vascular endografts (T)EVAR–systematic review–current state. Vasc Endovascular Surg 2013;47(4): 261–6.

20. Bonvini R, Alerci M, Antonucci F, et al. Preoperative embolization of collateral side branches: a valid means to reduce type II endoleaks after endovascular AAA repair. J Endovasc Ther 2003;10(2):227–32.

21. Maleux G, Poorteman L, Laenen A, et al. Incidence, etiology, and management of type III endoleak after endovascular aortic repair. J Vasc Surg 2017;66(4): 1056–64.

22. Parmer SS, Carpenter JP, Stavropoulos SW, et al. Endoleaks after endovascular repair of thoracic aortic aneurysms. J Vasc Surg 2006;44(3):447–52.

23. Wachal K, Szmyt K, Oszkinis G. Diagnosis and treatment of a patient with type IV endoleak as a late complication after endovascular aneurysm repair. Wideochir Inne Tech Maloinwazyjne 2014;9(4):667–70.

24. Toya N, Fujita T, Kanaoka Y, et al. Endotension following endovascular aneurysm repair. Vasc Med 2008;13(4):305–11.

25. Kougias P, Lin PH, Dardik A, et al. Successful treatment of endotension and aneurysm sac enlargement with endovascular stent graft reinforcement. J Vasc Surg 2007;46(1):124–7.

26. Deaton DH. Improving proximal fixation and seal with the HeliFx Aortic EndoAnchor. Semin Vasc Surg 2012;25(4):187–92.

27. Muhs BE, Balm R, White GH, et al. Anatomic factors associated with acute endograft collapse after Gore TAG treatment of thoracic aortic dissection or traumatic rupture. J Vasc Surg 2007;45(4):655–61.

28. Mohapatra A, Magnetta MJ, Snatchko ME, et al. Acute aortic occlusion secondary to aortic endograft migration and collapse. J Vasc Surg Cases Innov Tech 2017;3(3):183–4.

29. Tadros RO, Lipsitz EC, Chaer RA, et al. A multicenter experience of the management of collapsed thoracic endografts. J Vasc Surg 2011;53(5):1217–22.

30. Steinbauer MG, Stehr A, Pfister K, et al. Endovascular repair of proximal endograft collapse after treatment for thoracic aortic disease. J Vasc Surg 2006;43(3): 609–12.

31. Fransen GA, Desgranges P, Laheij RJ, et al. Frequency, predictive factors, and consequences of stent-graft kink following endovascular AAA repair. J Endovasc Ther 2003;10(5):913–8.

32. Smeds MR, Duncan AA, Harlander-Locke MP, et al. Treatment and outcomes of aortic endograft infection. J Vasc Surg 2016;63(2):332–40.

33. Shiraev T, Barrett S, Heywood S, et al. Incidence, management, and outcomes of aortic graft infection. Ann Vasc Surg 2019;59:73–83.

34. Kilic A, Arnaoutakis DJ, Reifsnyder T, et al. Management of infected vascular grafts. Vasc Med 2016;21(1):53–60.

35. Sorber R, Osgood MJ, Abularrage CJ, et al. Treatment of aortic graft infection in the endovascular era. Curr Infect Dis Rep 2017;19(11):40.

36. Murphy EH, Szeto WY, Herdrich BJ, et al. The management of endograft infections following endovascular thoracic and abdominal aneurysm repair. J Vasc Surg 2013;58(5):1179–85.

37. Si Y, Fu W, Liu Z, et al. Coverage of the left subclavian artery without revascularization during thoracic endovascular repair is feasible: a prospective study. Ann Vasc Surg 2014;28(4):850–9.

38. Weigang E, Parker JA, Czerny M, et al. Should intentional endovascular stent-graft coverage of the left subclavian artery be preceded by prophylactic revascularisation? Eur J Cardiothorac Surg 2011;40(4):858–68.

39. Klocker J, Koell A, Erlmeier M, et al. Ischemia and functional status of the left arm and quality of life after left subclavian artery coverage during stent grafting of thoracic aortic diseases. J Vasc Surg 2014;60(1):64–9.

40. Arko FR, Lee WA, Hill BB, et al. Hypogastric artery bypass to preserve pelvic circulation: improved outcome after endovascular abdominal aortic aneurysm repair. J Vasc Surg 2004;39(2):404–8.

41. Bratby MJ, Munneke GM, Belli AM, et al. How safe is bilateral internal iliac artery embolization prior to EVAR? Cardiovasc Intervent Radiol 2008;31(2):246–53.

42. Farivar BS, Kalsi R, Drucker CB, et al. Implications of concomitant hypogastric artery embolization with endovascular repair of infrarenal abdominal aortic aneurysms. J Vasc Surg 2017;66(1):95–101.

43. Setacci F, Sirignano P, De Donato G, et al. Endovascular thoracic aortic repair and risk of spinal cord ischemia: the role of previous or concomitant treatment for aortic aneurysm. J Cardiovasc Surg (Torino) 2010;51(2):169–76.

44. Sobocinski J, Patterson BO, Karthikesalingam A, et al. The effect of left subclavian artery coverage in thoracic endovascular aortic repair. Ann Thorac Surg 2016;101(2):810–7.

45. Awad H, Ramadan ME, El Sayed HF, et al. Spinal cord injury after thoracic endovascular aortic aneurysm repair. Can J Anaesth 2017;64(12):1218–35.

46. Alvarez-Tostado JA, Moise MA, Bena JF, et al. The brachial artery: a critical access for endovascular procedures. J Vasc Surg 2009;49(2):378–85 [discussion 385].

47. Riambau V, Bockler D, Brunkwall J, et al. Editor's choice - management of descending thoracic aorta diseases: clinical practice guidelines of the European Society for Vascular Surgery (ESVS). Eur J Vasc Endovasc Surg 2017;53(1):4–52.

48. Gutsche JT, Cheung AT, McGarvey ML, et al. Risk factors for perioperative stroke after thoracic endovascular aortic repair. Ann Thorac Surg 2007;84(4):1195–200 [discussion 1200].

49. Sepehripour AH, Ahmed K, Vecht JA, et al. Management of the left subclavian artery during endovascular stent grafting for traumatic aortic injury - a systematic review. Eur J Vasc Endovasc Surg 2011;41(6):758–69.

50. Matsumura JS, Lee WA, Mitchell RS, et al. The Society for Vascular Surgery Practice Guidelines: management of the left subclavian artery with thoracic endovascular aortic repair. J Vasc Surg 2009;50(5):1155–8.

51. de la Motte L, Kehlet H, Vogt K, et al. Preoperative methylprednisolone enhances recovery after endovascular aortic repair: a randomized, double-blind, placebo-controlled clinical trial. Ann Surg 2014;260(3):540–8 [discussion 548-9].

Management of Postoperative Complications Following Common Pediatric Operations

Danny Lascano, MD[a,b], Lorraine I. Kelley-Quon, MD, MSHS[a,b,c],*

KEYWORDS

• Pediatric • Child • Surgery • Postoperative • Complications

KEY POINTS

- The general surgical principles of source control with broad-spectrum antibiotics, drainage, and bowel rest can be successfully used to manage most complications after appendectomy in children.
- Nonoperative management of uncomplicated appendicitis fails in approximately 30% of children.
- Jugular vein route is a superior access point with fewer complications at time of insertion (compared with subclavian approach) and fewer long-term complications (compared with femoral approach).
- Hypertrophic pyloric stenosis is not a surgical emergency, and infants should be appropriately resuscitated to avoid complications related to severe alkalosis.
- Family education and daily attention to gastrostomy tube care will minimize long-term complications associated with leakage and infection.
- Recurrence after inguinal herniorrhaphy is rare in children, with higher rates reported in preterm infants or infants with respiratory comorbidities.

INTRODUCTION

Approximately 3.9 million surgical interventions are performed in children annually in the United States.[1] The most common surgeries performed on children include appendectomy, central venous access (CVA) placement, pyloromyotomy, gastrostomy,

[a] Division of Pediatric Surgery, Children's Hospital Los Angeles, 4650 Sunset Boulevard, Mailstop #100, Los Angeles, CA 90027, USA; [b] Department of Surgery, Keck School of Medicine of the University of Southern California, Los Angeles, CA, USA; [c] Department of Preventive Medicine, University of Southern California, Los Angeles, CA, USA
* Corresponding author. Division of Pediatric Surgery, Children's Hospital Los Angeles, 4650 Sunset Boulevard, Mailstop #100, Los Angeles, CA 90027.
E-mail address: lkquon@chla.usc.edu

Surg Clin N Am 101 (2021) 799–812
https://doi.org/10.1016/j.suc.2021.05.021
0039-6109/21/© 2021 Elsevier Inc. All rights reserved.

and herniorrhaphy.[2] The current review presents common postoperative complications occurring in children after these operations and the most up-to-date management algorithms for care.

APPENDECTOMY
Patient Evaluation Overview

In the United States, 55,000 to 90,000 appendectomies are performed on children each year, making it the most common pediatric surgery performed.[2,3] The lifetime incidence of appendicitis in children is 9%, with the peak cases reported in children 10 to 14 years old.[4] Pediatric appendicitis is categorized in 3 states defined by intraoperative or imaging findings that dictate management and risk of complications:

1. Uncomplicated appendicitis: not gangrenous, and no abscess on imaging
2. Complicated appendicitis: perforated, gangrenous, or suppurative
3. Complicated appendicitis with abscess[5]

Presentation and clinical suspicion for perforation vary by age, as younger children more commonly present with complicated appendicitis.[6] The current standard surgical care for children with uncomplicated appendicitis is laparoscopic appendectomy.[7] Overall, laparoscopic procedures have decreased rates of postoperative small-bowel obstruction in children with uncomplicated appendicitis to approximately 1%.[8]

Treatment for children with complicated appendicitis includes primary appendectomy, delayed or interval appendectomy with intravenous/oral antibiotics, or antibiotics alone without appendectomy.[5] Upfront laparoscopic appendectomy for complicated appendicitis has equivalent outcomes to traditional nonoperative management while improving quality of life.[9,10] For children with complicated appendicitis with a well-formed abscess, treatment typically involves drainage of the abscess, usually by interventional radiology or a laparoscopic washout and drain placement, and a course of antibiotics with or without interval appendectomy in 6 to 12 weeks.[11,12] In practice, most children receive up to 2 weeks of antibiotics, either intravenously or intravenously and followed by oral antibiotics.[13] If an abscess is not drainable and the child is doing well, children may be treated with just antibiotics with plans for interval appendectomy in 6 to 8 weeks. In some cases, providers may forego interval appendectomy, as only 8% of children with perforated appendicitis managed nonoperatively present with recurrent appendicitis.[14] Alternatively, some advocate for an interval appendectomy given the small but nonzero risk of malignancy.[15]

Complications After Appendectomy

Complications after appendectomy are uncommon in children and include wound infection (1.5%–2.7%), intraabdominal abscess (3.1%–3.6%), ileus (1.3%–2.3%), and wound hematoma (3.3%).[16,17] The low rates of complications can largely be attributed to the fact that most children undergoing appendectomy are otherwise healthy, and most receive laparoscopic surgery.[5,18] The general surgical principles of source control with broad-spectrum antibiotics, drainage, and bowel rest in the setting of ileus can be successfully used to manage most complications after appendectomy for appendicitis.[12,19] Unique to children, abscesses after surgical treatment of perforated appendicitis may present as failure to thrive and weight loss. Image-guided drainage of fluid collections greater than 3 to 5 cm is typically successful.[15] When abscesses are unable to be drained, an attempt of antibiotics alone has some success.[20] For children discharged on an oral course of antibiotics, it is important to ascertain compliance, as patients may not tolerate antibiotics because of side-effect profile or medication taste (eg, metronidazole).[21] On the other hand, some oral antibiotics require access to a compounding pharmacy because they are unavailable as liquid formulations and/or to adjust for a child's weight-based dose.[22]

Nonoperative Management of Uncomplicated Appendicitis

Currently, nonoperative management of uncomplicated appendicitis is increasing in prevalence, particularly during the severe acute respiratory syndrome coronavirus 2 pandemic.[23] Recent multi-institution studies of found that 67.1% of children receiving antibiotics alone as part of a nonoperative protocol avoided surgery within the first year and reported fewer disability days.[24,25] With the increasing prevalence of nonoperative management of uncomplicated appendicitis, surgeons must recognize that clinical signs of fever, persistent abdominal pain, and inability to tolerate oral intake indicate failure of nonoperative management, and appendectomy is needed for definitive treatment.

CENTRAL VENOUS ACCESS
Patient Evaluation Overview

CVA is the second most common pediatric surgery performed.[2] Indications for CVA in children include failure to obtain peripheral access or need for long-term central access. The type of access is determined by the child's needs with nontunneled CVA devices and umbilical CVA devices in neonates for 7 to 10 days, PICCs (peripherally inserted central catheters) for short- to medium-term use (4 weeks to 6 months), and tunneled and implantable catheters for long-term use (months to years).[26–28] The number of lumens should be kept to a minimum, as more lumens are associated with higher catheter-related bloodstream infections.[29] Access points for CVA include the external jugular vein, internal jugular vein, brachiocephalic vein, facial vein, femoral vein, and subclavian vein.[30] Devices used include traditional cuffed central venous catheters, such as Broviac or Hickman catheters, as well as a totally implantable reservoir with a subcutaneous port either in titanium or in plastic used for children who need intermittent therapies, such as chemotherapy.

Acute Complications of Central Venous Access

Complications of CVA include the pneumothorax, arterial puncture, bleeding, arrhythmias, nerve injuries, and catheter malposition (**Table 1**).[26,31] In children, jugular vein route is a superior access point with fewer complications at time of insertion (compared with subclavian approach) and fewer long-term complications (compared with the femoral approach).[32] CVA placement in children differs from adults in that appropriate initial placement may also be complicated by small-caliber catheters and the short distance between access points and the superior vena cava–right atrial junction. Small-caliber catheters are prone to kinking off at internal jugular and subclavian access sites and can be minimized by moving a child's head and testing patency in different positions before completion of placement. In addition, a catheter that is too long may lead to arrhythmias when abutting the right atrium. This complication may be appreciated during initial placement if premature ventricular contractions are present. Prompt intraoperative retraction of the catheter avoids sustained arrythmias and rare complications, such as cardiac perforation and tamponade.[30]

Conversely, a catheter that is too far above the superior vena cava–right atrial junction may flip retrograde into the subclavian, brachiocephalic, or jugular veins, leading to suboptimal infusion or the dangerous cerebral infusion of medications.[33] Optimal

Table 1
Complications of central venous access

Complications	Preventive Measures	Treatments
Infected catheter and port	Avoid multiple lumens, cuffed CVA for long-term use, avoid soiled or exposed areas (eg, overlapping diaper placement)	Antibiotics and/or removal
Pneumothorax	Use ultrasound and/or fluoroscopy for placement	Chest tube, aspiration of air
Arterial puncture	Use ultrasound and/or fluoroscopy for placement, use micropuncture kit before inserting final catheter and dilating to final size	Compressions, if large, may need exploration and primary repair or ligation
Arrhythmias, cardiac perforation, tamponade	Chest radiograph or fluoroscopy to assess final location confirming tip at atrial-caval junction	Reposition the catheter tip
Nerve injuries	Use ultrasound and/or fluoroscopy for placement	If caused by hematoma, consider evacuating, physical therapy, neurology consult
Thrombosis	Subclavian = jugular > femoral, when not accessed, keep heparinized in a weight-based amount	Treat with anticoagulation, hematology consult, consider catheter removal
Pulled/damaged catheter	Securing the catheter with a cuffed catheter, sutures, repair the catheter	Use a commercial repair kit, can use the same tract/catheter and via a wire insert new catheter or reinsert at another site
Hematoma	Use ultrasound and/or fluoroscopy for placement	Compression, if causing collateral issues may consider drainage
Catheter fracture, distal embolization, catheter adherent to vessel wall	Remove catheter before 6 mo if possible	Transverse snare, venotomy, and open removal of fragment, fluoroscopy, leave the catheter in place if risk outweighs benefit
Malposition of the catheter with growth	Remove catheter before 6 mo if possible, evaluate with chest radiograph to make sure it remains in adequate position as child grows	Removal and/or replacement

catheter placement often requires repeated use of intraoperative fluoroscopy and ultrasound throughout the procedure to ensure proper placement and functioning. Finally, although femoral and saphenous vein access is possible in low-birth-weight neonates and infants, it is typically avoided because of the increased risk of mechanical complications, such as thrombosis and central line infections, owing to overlapping diaper placement.[34,35]

Long-Term Complications of Central Venous Access

Long-term complications of single and repetitive CVA procedures include loss of access, venous insufficiency, central venous stenosis, deep venous thrombosis, adherence of catheter to veins, catheter fracture, malposition of the catheter with growth, and line infection leading to bacteremia.[30] For external leakage from a damaged catheter, it is prudent to avoid removing the catheter. The catheter should be repaired using an appropriate repair kit, such as the Broviac or Hickman repair kits, which should be tailored to the manufacturer of the catheter. In addition, heparin should be injected and left in the catheter upon completion in a weight-adjusted dose, and the repair site should be splinted so that the child destabilizes the repair.[36] The catheter can be used 4 hours after the glue sets. If, after repair, the catheter becomes occluded, tissue plasminogen activator in a weight-adjusted dose can be carefully administered and left in the catheter for 4 hours. If the catheter remains occluded after repair, replacement may be required.[36] If this initial repair or replacement cannot be performed because of lack of a trained physician, advanced provider, nursing staff, or technician or because of lack of equipment, it may be prudent to have the patient transferred to a facility to perform the repair.[37]

Breakage or fracture of a catheter because of tight adherence of the catheter to the wall of the vein or mechanical breakage or fracture from a product defect can occur, particularly with CVAs that are in place for longer than 6 months.[38] Options to retrieve a catheter that cannot be removed manually include radiological intervention using a guidewire/transverse snare to remove the fragment, venotomy and open removal of the adhered fragment, or leaving the catheter in place if the risk of the invasiveness of surgery outweighs the risk of embolic events from the catheter fragment.[39,40] The loss of CVA and central venous stenosis is common for children with chronic illnesses, such as short gut syndrome.[37] An ultrasound duplex to assess vessel patency may help with preoperative planning, although an intraoperative venogram may be more sensitive and specific and can allow intervention to open up any occluded or stenotic vessels.[41] In cases where traditional vascular access options do not exist, endovascular approaches can be obtained.[42,43]

PYLOROMYOTOMY
Patient Evaluation Overview

Hypertrophic pyloric stenosis typically occurs between 2 and 12 weeks of life and is a common cause of nonbloody, nonbilious projectile emesis in infants, impacting one out of every 400 infants.[44] Infants typically present volume-depleted, with concomitant hypochloremic, hypokalemic metabolic alkalosis. Infants should be resuscitated with 0.45% saline with 5% dextrose with or without potassium (depending on whether the infant has voided) at a rate of 1.5× fluid maintenance rate, which can be reduced to 1× maintenance when serum bicarbonate is less than 25 mmol/L.[45,46] Generally ,a chloride greater than 100 mEq/dL, bicarbonate less than 28 mEq/dL, and urine output greater than 1 mL/kg/h are adequate thresholds for surgery.[46] After appropriate resuscitation, surgery is accomplished by either a laparoscopic or an open pyloromyotomy, with the central goal of performing an extramucosal longitudinal incision that splits the pylorus open, allowing gastric contents to pass.

Inadequate Preoperative Resuscitation

It is important for surgeons and families to recognize that hypertrophic pyloric stenosis is not a surgical emergency. Careful preoperative volume and electrolyte management is key to avoiding metabolic and respiratory postoperative complications. Even an infant presenting with normal electrolytes warrants further volume resuscitation, as infants will become quickly hypotensive on induction of anesthesia if intravascularly depleted. If electrolytes are left uncorrected, this can lead to life-threatening postoperative apnea, as any uncorrected metabolic alkalosis can be associated with significant compensatory hypoventilation.[47]

Technical Complications

Overall complications for pyloromyotomy are between 3% and 10% and are outlined in **Table 2**.[46,48] Wound infections are the most common complication, with no difference seen with usage of prophylactic antibiotics.[48,49] Infection or dehiscence requiring reoperation is rare and is seen more commonly in cases of open pyloromyotomies.[50] Incisional hernias may also be seen at more than twice the rate in open cases than laparoscopic cases.[51] An incomplete pyloromyotomy, often presenting as persistent emesis for several days after surgery, requires reoperation and is typically due to

Table 2
Complications of pyloromyotomy

Complications	Preventive Measures	Treatments
Aspiration of gastric contents on induction of anesthesia	Passage of a Replogle tube into the stomach 3 times or more with suctioning while awake before induction	Supportive care for aspiration
Intraoperative hypotension	Ensure adequate resuscitation and euvolemia with urine output urine output >1 mL/kg/h can add potassium to fluid once voiding	Volume boluses of 20 mL/kg 0.9% NaCl as needed
Incomplete pyloromyotomy	"Shoe-shine maneuver," visualize bulging mucosa through pyloromyotomy and transverse gastric fibers in proximal pyloromyotomy edge, insufflate stomach to observe passage of gas to duodenum	Reoperation and complete pyloromyotomy
Postoperative apnea	Resuscitate child with 0.45% NaCl with 5% dextrose aiming for chloride >100 mEq/dL, bicarbonate <28 mEq/dL	Continuous postoperative monitoring
Wound complications	Laparoscopic pyloromyotomy	Consider antibiotics for infection, local wound care
Full-thickness defect of duodenum	"Shoe-shine maneuver," visualize bulging mucosa through pyloromyotomy, insufflate stomach to check for bubbles in pyloromyotomy	Repair with closure of the full-thickness defect and perform pyloromyotomy on the opposed side of perforation

insufficient extension on the gastric side of the pyloromyotomy.[52,53] Mucosal perforation occurs rarely[52,54] and is preferentially repaired with the closure of the full-thickness defect and pyloromyotomy on the opposite side of the perforation or primary repair of the mucosa.[54] Performance of a "shoe-shine" maneuver to confirm the independent movement of the edges of the cut pylorus and visual confirmation of bulging of the mucosa through the pyloromyotomy can be performed to decrease the likelihood of both incomplete pyloromyotomy and mucosal perforation.[48,55]

GASTROSTOMY
Patient Evaluation Overview

Gastrostomy tube placement may be necessary to establish durable enteral access for children for a wide range of indications.[56] Techniques include open, laparoscopic, percutaneous endoscopic gastrostomy (PEG) tube placement, and laparoscopic-assisted PEG by either a surgeon, gastroenterologist, or interventional radiologist.[57,58] Approaches to enteral access depend on a child's weight, age, and size, as well as the surgeon's experience. Care should be taken to select the appropriate tube for the child's nutritional needs and home environment, as larger-caliber tubes are required to accommodate pureed diets; low-profile tubes may be needed to prevent patient-initiated dislodgement, and single-unit gastrojejunostomy tubes are not approved for use in small infants and children because of risk of intestinal perforation.

Surgical Complications of Gastrostomy Placement

Common complications related to gastrostomy tube placement are shown in **Table 3**.[59,60] Major complications in PEGs can be reduced by using a laparoscopic-assisted approach to visualize adjacent organs, although cost and need for a surgeon have precluded widespread adoption. Key steps to minimize complication risk with PEG placement include transillumination of the abdominal wall, aspiration of air with simultaneous visualization with endoscopy, and optimizing gastric insufflation to avoid bringing the colon adjacent to the needle puncture. Buried bumper syndrome, in which the PEG gastric bumper erodes into the gastric wall and lodges itself between the gastric wall and skin, can be avoided by minimizing tension on the bumper at the time of placement and proper education of family for home care.[61]

For many parents of children who receive a gastrostomy, accidental dislodgement is a concern after surgery.[62] Early dislodgement after surgery warrants evaluation in the emergency room, but after 6 weeks, families may be advised to use a Foley catheter to maintain the tract and to go to their clinicians' office for replacement. In general, surgical tubes may be exchanged 3 to 6 week postoperatively, whereas for PEGs, many recommend 6 to 8 weeks.[63] In the case of early inadvertent tube dislodging, an attempt can be made to reinsert with a gastrostomy tube study to confirm placement. At times, if the tract has closed, the Seldinger technique with radiological imaging can be used to go through the closed lumen and reinsert the tube. If there is any difficulty, the child should go to the operating room to have it reinserted under direct visualization.

Complications from Inadequate Local Gastrostomy Tube Care

The most common long-term complication with gastrostomy placement is leakage around the gastrostomy tube site, which may require surgical revision in up to 3.6% of chronically ill children.[64] Avoiding leakage complications is important to maintain a good quality of life for device-dependent children. Leakage may occur from the serial insertion of larger tubes, creating a large tract, improper placement too close to the rib

Table 3
Complications of gastrostomy

Complications	Preventive Measures	Treatments
Injury to adjacent organs	For PEG: confirm indirect visualization of abdominal wall from stomach, aspiration of air with simultaneous visualization with endoscopy, optimize gastric insufflation; consider laparoscopic-assisted PEG, laparoscopic or open gastrostomy if any difficulties	Primary repair vs resection depending on injury
Esophageal or gastric outlet obstruction	Marking location preoperatively to avoid errors in distortion from capnoperitoneum, 1–2 finger breadths below costal margin to allow for growth, greater curvature, and at midclavicular line	Decreasing the amount of water in the balloon; relocate the gastrostomy
Peristomal infections/ cellulitis, dermatitis	Prevent soilage of contents into skin (may need to vent tube), protect skin with barrier/topical agents, treat any fungal infection, avoid leakage, prevent rocking	Antibiotics, temporary gastrostomy removal, operative debridement, or revision if severe
Gastromucosal prolapse	Make sure tube is not too loose, avoid tugging onto tube, disconnect extension	Temporary gastrostomy removal, surgical revision/resiting
Buried bumper syndrome	Avoid having the PEG gastric bumper too tight to the abdominal wall	Surgical revision
Granulation tissue	Minimize trauma using a split gauze or dressing, reduce moisture via stoma powder, stabilize the tube, make sure extension kit is disconnected when not in use, rotate the tube every 4–6 h to prevent pressure necrosis and irritation	Triamcinolone, silver nitrite sticks to amputate excess tissue, surgical debridement
Leakage	Remove tension from the stoma, including disconnecting extension sets, minimize tubes taped in the same position, improper taping, tense taping	Adjust feeds if overfeeding stomach and/or feed over longer time, stoma powder, rule out distal obstruction, treat any motility issues, temporary gastrostomy removal, surgical revision if severe

cage, or a child outgrowing their gastrostomy tube, leading to an improperly placed tube with complications (see **Table 3**). Gastrostomy tube leakage may also lead to cellulitis, abscess, or granulation tissue.[65] To avoid this, skin care is key, including making sure the gastrostomy tube is not too tightly abutting the skin, which may require reducing the amount of liquid in the balloon and/or applying skin barrier protection for compromised irritated skin, such as Calmoseptine ointment. Routine gastrostomy care includes rotating the gastrostomy tube every couple of hours to avoid pressure from tubing attachments, disconnecting the tubing from the feeding supply circuit when not in use, and preventing a child from unnecessarily manipulating the gastrostomy tube, sometimes facilitated by switching to a low-profile gastrostomy tube, such as a Mic-Key button.

PEDIATRIC HERNIAS
Inguinal Hernias

Patient evaluation overview
Inguinal hernias are common in children, with most involving a patent processus vaginalis that fails to obliterate during gestation.[66] Most hernias are repaired without mesh with high ligation of the hernia sac at the level of the internal ring in either open or laparoscopic fashion. For neonates and preterm infants presenting with a reducible inguinal hernia, surgery is typically delayed for several months to minimize need for inpatient monitoring after general anesthesia.[66]

Complications of inguinal hernias repairs
Complications of inguinal hernia repair in children include postoperative hydrocele, wound infection, gonadal atrophy, cryptorchidism, and hernia recurrence (**Table 4**). Recurrence of a previously repaired inguinal hernia occurs in 1.4% of children, with higher rates of 2% to 10% in preterm infants with respiratory comorbidities.[66] In cases of multiple recurrent inguinal hernias, it is important to consider possible genetic predispositions from Ehlers-Danlos syndrome, Marfan syndrome, and other connective tissue disorders.[67] In children and adolescents, there is no agreed-upon indication for the use of prosthetic or biological mesh for inguinal hernia repairs. Rarely, prosthetic mesh repairs may be considered in children with recurrent hernias or connective tissue disorders, but minimal evidence exists, and clinical judgment should largely dictate management.[68]

Table 4 Complications of inguinal hernia repair		
Complications	**Preventive Measures**	**Treatments**
Recurrence	High ligation with delayed-absorption suture (eg, PDS), double ligation, delay repair until no longer requiring supplemental oxygen	Attempt via another approach (if laparoscopic do open or vice versa), consider mesh if history of connective tissue disorder
Postoperative hydrocele or seroma	Obtain absolute hemostasis	If large, consider drainage, otherwise observe
Gonadal atrophy	Define high-risk group and assess flow before surgery (patients with undescended testes or abnormally placed ovaries)	May need orchiectomy or oophorectomy if painful or infected

Testicular or ovarian atrophy after inguinal hernia repairs is a rare complication. Risk factors for testicular atrophy include history of cryptorchidism before or after a repair, strangulation, or an irreducible incarcerated hernia.[69] Girls may also risk compromising their ovary, as they may present with a sliding indirect inguinal hernia containing a prolapsed ovary in up to 12.8% of inguinal hernia repairs.[70,71] Risk of ovarian atrophy is 1.4% in girls presenting with an irreducible hernia and subsequent open repair.[70]

Umbilical Hernias

Patient evaluation overview

Umbilical hernias are common in newborns, but 90% of cases resolve without surgery.[72] General indications for repair include incarceration, strangulation, or pain.[73] In asymptomatic children, many umbilical hernias are followed until after 4 to 5 years, with surgical repair recommended at this time. Primary repair is typically performed without mesh.[74]

Complications of umbilical hernia repair

Complications after umbilical hernia repair are rare but include recurrence, wound infections, seroma, hematoma, and dehiscence.[75] In children, surgery for those under 2 years old is associated with respiratory complications after surgery, and overall complications are higher in children under 4 years old.[72,75] Recurrence of an umbilical hernia after a primary tissue repair is seen in between 0.3% and 2% of children after surgery and is higher in children under 4 years old. Subsequent repair again should be performed without mesh.

CLINICS CARE POINTS

- The general surgical principles of source control with broad-spectrum antibiotics, drainage, and bowel rest can be successfully used to manage most complications after appendectomy in children.

- Nonoperative management of uncomplicated appendicitis is increasing but is associated with an approximately 30% failure rate at 1 year.

- For central venous access, surgeons should prioritize repairing as opposed to replacing existing lines to avoid loss of central venous access points.

- Hypertrophic pyloric stenosis requires appropriate preoperative fluid resuscitation aiming for a chloride greater than 100 mEq/dL, bicarbonate less than 28 mEq/dL to avoid the inability to extubate after surgery.

- Laparoscopic pyloromyotomy has fewer wound-related complications than open surgery.

- Major complications in percutaneous endoscopic gastrostomies can be reduced using a laparoscopic-assisted approach.

- Limiting traction and leakage of gastrostomy tubes will minimize chronic infections and granulation tissue.

- Infants with a history of prematurity or respiratory comorbidities have higher risk of recurrence after inguinal herniorrhaphy.

- Cryptorchidism, incarceration, and strangulation are associated with an increased risk of gonadal atrophy after inguinal hernia repair.

FUNDING

Dr L.I. Kelley-Quon is supported by grant KL2TR001854 from the National Center for Advancing Translational Science (NCATS) of the U.S. National Institutes of Health. The content is solely the responsibility of the authors and does not necessarily represent the official views of the National Institutes of Health.

DISCLOSURE

The authors have nothing to disclose.

REFERENCES

1. Rabbitts JA, Groenewald CB. Epidemiology of pediatric surgery in the United States. Paediatr Anaesth 2020;30(10):1083–90.
2. Somme S, Bronsert M, Morrato E, et al. Frequency and variety of inpatient pediatric surgical procedures in the United States. Pediatrics 2013;132(6):e1466–72.
3. Pennell C, Meckmongkol T, Arthur LG, et al. A standardized protocol for the management of appendicitis in children reduces resource utilization. Pediatr Qual Saf 2020;5(6):e357.
4. Anderson JE, Bickler SW, Chang DC, et al. Examining a common disease with unknown etiology: trends in epidemiology and surgical management of appendicitis in California, 1995-2009. World J Surg 2012;36(12):2787–94.
5. St Peter SD, Snyder CL. Operative management of appendicitis. Semin Pediatr Surg 2016;25(4):208–11.
6. Rolle U, Fahlenbach C, Heidecke CD, et al. Rates of complications after appendectomy in children and adolescents: pediatric surgical compared to general surgical hospitals. J Surg Res 2021;260:467–74.
7. Sauerland S, Jaschinski T, Neugebauer EA. Laparoscopic versus open surgery for suspected appendicitis. Cochrane Database Syst Rev 2010;10:CD001546.
8. Kaselas C, Molinaro F, Lacreuse I, et al. Postoperative bowel obstruction after laparoscopic and open appendectomy in children: a 15-year experience. J Pediatr Surg 2009;44(8):1581–5.
9. Schurman JV, Cushing CC, Garey CL, et al. Quality of life assessment between laparoscopic appendectomy at presentation and interval appendectomy for perforated appendicitis with abscess: analysis of a prospective randomized trial. J Pediatr Surg 2011;46(6):1121–5.
10. St Peter SD, Aguayo P, Fraser JD, et al. Initial laparoscopic appendectomy versus initial nonoperative management and interval appendectomy for perforated appendicitis with abscess: a prospective, randomized trial. J Pediatr Surg 2010;45(1):236–40.
11. Vargas HI, Averbook A, Stamos MJ. Appendiceal mass: conservative therapy followed by interval laparoscopic appendectomy. Am Surg 1994;60(10):753–8.
12. Lee SL, Islam S, Cassidy LD, et al. Antibiotics and appendicitis in the pediatric population: an American Pediatric Surgical Association Outcomes and Clinical Trials Committee Systematic Review. J Pediatr Surg 2010;45(11):2181–5.
13. Shawyer AC, Hatchell AC, Pemberton J, et al. Compliance with published recommendations for postoperative antibiotic management of children with appendicitis: a chart audit. J Pediatr Surg 2015;50(5):783–5.
14. Puapong D, Lee SL, Haigh PI, et al. Routine interval appendectomy in children is not indicated. J Pediatr Surg 2007;42(9):1500–3.
15. Howell EC, Dubina ED, Lee SL. Perforation risk in pediatric appendicitis: assessment and management. Pediatr Heal Med Ther 2018;9:135–45.
16. Zhang Z, Wang Y, Liu R, et al. Systematic review and meta-analysis of single-incision versus conventional laparoscopic appendectomy in children. J Pediatr Surg 2015;50(9):1600–9.

17. Aziz O, Athanasiou T, Tekkis PP, et al. Laparoscopic versus open appendectomy in children: a meta-analysis. Ann Surg 2006;243(1):17–27.
18. Blakely ML, Williams R, Dassinger MS, et al. Early vs interval appendectomy for children with perforated appendicitis. Arch Surg 2011;146(6):660–5.
19. Miftaroski A, Kessler U, Monnard E, et al. Two-step procedure for complicated appendicitis with perityphlitic abscess formation. Swiss Med Wkly 2017;147(1314):w14422.
20. Zhang Y, Stringel G, Bezahler I, et al. Nonoperative management of periappendiceal abscess in children: a comparison of antibiotics alone versus antibiotics plus percutaneous drainage. J Pediatr Surg 2020;55(3):414–7.
21. Versleijen MW, Huisman-de Waal GJ, Kock MC, et al. Arteriovenous fistulae as an alternative to central venous catheters for delivery of long-term home parenteral nutrition. Gastroenterology 2009;136(5):1577–84.
22. Gee SC, Hagemann TM. Palatability of liquid anti-infectives: clinician and student perceptions and practice outcomes. J Pediatr Pharmacol Ther 2007;12(4):216–23.
23. Jones BA, Slater BJ. Non-operative management of acute appendicitis in a pediatric patient with concomitant COVID-19 infection. J Pediatr Surg Case Rep 2020;59:101512.
24. Minneci PC, Mahida JB, Lodwick DL, et al. Effectiveness of patient choice in nonoperative vs surgical management of pediatric uncomplicated acute appendicitis. JAMA Surg 2016;151(5):408–15.
25. Minneci PC, Hade EM, Lawrence AE, et al. Association of nonoperative management using antibiotic therapy vs laparoscopic appendectomy with treatment success and disability days in children with uncomplicated appendicitis. JAMA 2020;324(6):581–93.
26. Ullman AJ, Marsh N, Mihala G, et al. Complications of central venous access devices: a systematic review. Pediatrics 2015;136(5):e1331–44.
27. Pittiruti M, Hamilton H, Biffi R, et al. ESPEN Guidelines on Parenteral Nutrition: central venous catheters (access, care, diagnosis and therapy of complications). Clin Nutr 2009;28(4):365–77.
28. Paterson RS, Chopra V, Brown E, et al. Selection and insertion of vascular access devices in pediatrics: a systematic review. Pediatrics 2020;145(Supplement 3):S243–68.
29. Templeton A, Schlegel M, Fleisch F, et al. Multilumen central venous catheters increase risk for catheter-related bloodstream infection: prospective surveillance study. Infection 2008;36(4):322–7.
30. Askegard-Giesmann JR, Caniano DA, Kenney BD. Rare but serious complications of central line insertion. Semin Pediatr Surg 2009;18(2):73–83.
31. Rey C, Alvarez F, De La Rua V, et al. Mechanical complications during central venous cannulations in pediatric patients. Intensive Care Med 2009;35(8):1438–43.
32. Casado-Flores J, Barja J, Martino R, et al. Complications of central venous catheterization in critically ill children. Pediatr Crit Care Med 2001;2(1):57–62.
33. Sansivero GE. Features and selection of vascular access devices. Semin Oncol Nurs 2010;26(2):88–101.
34. Tsai M-H, Lien R, Wang J-W, et al. Complication rates with central venous catheters inserted at femoral and non-femoral sites in very low birth weight infants. Pediatr Infect Dis J 2009;28(11):966–70.
35. Debourdeau P, Kassab Chahmi D, Le Gal G, et al. 2008 SOR guidelines for the prevention and treatment of thrombosis associated with central venous catheters

in patients with cancer: report from the working group. Ann Oncol 2009;20(9): 1459–71.

36. Chan AP, Baldivia PS, Reyen LE, et al. Central venous catheter repair is highly successful in children with intestinal failure. J Pediatr Surg 2019;54(3):517–20.

37. Baskin KM, Mermel LA, Saad TF, et al. Evidence-based strategies and recommendations for preservation of central venous access in children. JPEN J Parenter Enter Nutr 2019;43(5):591–614.

38. Biffi R, Orsi F, Grasso F, et al. Catheter rupture and distal embolisation: a rare complication of central venous ports. J Vasc Access 2000;1(1):19–22.

39. Bawazir O, Banoon E. Efficacy and clinical outcome of the port-a-cath in children: a tertiary care-center experience. World J Surg Oncol 2020;18(1):134.

40. Chow LM, Friedman JN, Macarthur C, et al. Peripherally inserted central catheter (PICC) fracture and embolization in the pediatric population. J Pediatr 2003; 142(2):141–4.

41. Gill AE, Shivaram GM. Managing systemic venous occlusions in children. CVIR Endovasc 2020;3(1):59.

42. Rodrigues AF, van Mourik ID, Sharif K, et al. Management of end-stage central venous access in children referred for possible small bowel transplantation. J Pediatr Gastroenterol Nutr 2006;42(4):427–33.

43. Modi BP, Jaksic T. Pediatric intestinal failure and vascular access. Surg Clin North Am 2012;92(3):729–43, x.

44. Kelley-Quon LI, Tseng C-H, Jen HC, et al. Hospital type predicts surgical complications for infants with hypertrophic pyloric stenosis. Am Surg 2012;78(10): 1079–82.

45. Jobson M, Hall NJ. Contemporary management of pyloric stenosis. Semin Pediatr Surg 2016;25(4):219–24.

46. Aspelund G, Langer JC. Current management of hypertrophic pyloric stenosis. Semin Pediatr Surg 2007;16(1):27–33.

47. van den Bunder F, van Woensel JBM, Stevens MF, et al. Respiratory problems owing to severe metabolic alkalosis in infants presenting with hypertrophic pyloric stenosis. J Pediatr Surg 2020;55(12):2772–6.

48. Kelay A, Hall NJ. Perioperative complications of surgery for hypertrophic pyloric stenosis. Eur J Pediatr Surg 2018;28(2):171–5.

49. Katz MS, Schwartz MZ, Moront ML, et al. Prophylactic antibiotics do not decrease the incidence of wound infections after laparoscopic pyloromyotomy. J Pediatr Surg 2011;46(6):1086–8.

50. Sola JE, Neville HL. Laparoscopic vs open pyloromyotomy: a systematic review and meta-analysis. J Pediatr Surg 2009;44(8):1631–7.

51. Mullassery D, Pedersen A, Robb A, et al. Incisional hernia in pediatric surgery - experience at a single UK tertiary centre. J Pediatr Surg 2016;51(11):1791–4.

52. Sathya C, Wayne C, Gotsch A, et al. Laparoscopic versus open pyloromyotomy in infants: a systematic review and meta-analysis. Pediatr Surg Int 2017;33(3): 325–33.

53. Hall NJ, Eaton S, Seims A, et al. Risk of incomplete pyloromyotomy and mucosal perforation in open and laparoscopic pyloromyotomy. J Pediatr Surg 2014;49(7): 1083–6.

54. Royal RE, Linz DN, Gruppo DL, et al. Repair of mucosal perforation during pyloromyotomy: surgeon's choice. J Pediatr Surg 1995;30(10):1430–2.

55. Anwar MO, Al Omran Y, Al-Hindi S. Erratum: laparoscopic pyloromyotomy: a modified simple technique. J Neonatal Surg 2016;5(2):26.

56. Warren MG, Do B, Das A, et al. Gastrostomy tube feeding in extremely low birth-weight infants: frequency, associated comorbidities, and long-term outcomes. J Pediatr 2019;214:41–6.e5.

57. Merli L, De Marco EA, Fedele C, et al. Gastrostomy placement in children: percu-taneous endoscopic gastrostomy or laparoscopic gastrostomy? Surg Laparosc Endosc Percutan Tech 2016;26(5):381–4.

58. Sheir HM, Wafa TA, Elshafey A, et al. A simplified laparoscopic-assisted gastro-stomy technique: a single center experience. Ann Pediatr Surg 2020;16:1–5.

59. Liu R, Jiwane A, Varjavandi A, et al. Comparison of percutaneous endoscopic, laparoscopic and open gastrostomy insertion in children. Pediatr Surg Int 2013;29(6):613–21.

60. Wragg RC, Salminen H, Pachl M, et al. Gastrostomy insertion in the 21st century: PEG or laparoscopic? Report from a large single-centre series. Pediatr Surg Int 2012;28(5):443–8.

61. Lee TH, Lin JT. Clinical manifestations and management of buried bumper syn-drome in patients with percutaneous endoscopic gastrostomy. Gastrointest En-dosc 2008;68(3):580–4.

62. Chaplen C. Parents' views of caring for children with gastrostomies. Br J Nurs 1997;6(1):34–8.

63. Pennington C. To PEG or not to PEG. Clin Med 2002;2(3):250–5.

64. Di Leo G, Pascolo P, Hamadeh K, et al. Gastrostomy placement and manage-ment in children: a single-center experience. Nutrients 2019;11(7):1555.

65. Vervloessem D, van Leersum F, Boer D, et al. Percutaneous endoscopic gastro-stomy (PEG) in children is not a minor procedure: risk factors for major complica-tions. Semin Pediatr Surg 2009;18(2):93–7.

66. Ramachandran V, Edwards CF, Bichianu DC. Inguinal hernia in premature infants. Neoreviews 2020;21(6):e392–403.

67. Harrison B, Sanniec K, Janis JE. Collagenopathies-implications for abdominal wall reconstruction: a systematic review. Plast Reconstr Surg Glob Open 2016; 4(10):e1036.

68. Girotto JA, Malaisrie SC, Bulkely G, et al. Recurrent ventral herniation in Ehlers-Danlos syndrome. Plast Reconstr Surg 2000;106(7):1520–6.

69. Abes M, Bakal U, Petik B. Ascending testis following inguinal hernia repair in chil-dren. Eur Rev Med Pharmacol Sci 2015;19(16):2949–51.

70. Merriman TE, Auldist AW. Ovarian torsion in inguinal hernias. Pediatr Surg Int 2000;16(5–6):383–5.

71. Esposito C, Gargiulo F, Farina A, et al. Laparoscopic treatment of inguinal ovarian hernia in female infants and children: standardizing the technique. J Laparoendosc Adv Surg Tech A 2019;29(4):568–72.

72. Halleran DR, Minneci PC, Cooper JN. Association between age and umbilical hernia repair outcomes in children: a multistate population-based cohort study. J Pediatr 2020;217:125–30.e4.

73. Papagrigoriadis S, Browse DJ, Howard ER. Incarceration of umbilical hernias in children: a rare but important complication. Pediatr Surg Int 1998;14(3):231–2.

74. Zendejas B, Kuchena A, Onkendi EO, et al. Fifty-three-year experience with pe-diatric umbilical hernia repairs. J Pediatr Surg 2011;46(11):2151–6.

75. Zens TJ, Rogers A, Cartmill R, et al. Age-dependent outcomes in asymptomatic umbilical hernia repair. Pediatr Surg Int 2019;35(4):463–8.

Prevention and Management of Complications of Tissue Flaps

Travis J. Miller, MD[a], Christopher V. Lavin, BS[b],
Arash Momeni, MD[a,b], Derrick C. Wan, MD[a,b,c],*

KEYWORDS

- Free flap • Complications • Radial forearm flap • Fibula flap • Anterolateral thigh flap
- Transverse rectus abdominis flap • Reconstruction • Plastic surgery

KEY POINTS

- Accurate design of the ALT flap allows for utility in reconstructing defects throughout the body.
- The radial forearm flap is versatile, but a prior Allen's test should be performed to avoid catastrophic hand ischemia.
- Leave sufficient proximal and distal bone with fibula harvest to avoid nerve injury and to maintain ankle stability.
- Proper selection of perforators with DIEP flap harvest can reduce risk of partial flap necrosis.

INTRODUCTION

Free tissue transfer, first described clinically in the 1970s, revolutionized reconstructive options throughout the body.[1,2] Numerous flaps have been described for reconstruction after tissue loss, allowing reconstructive surgeons to transfer substitutes for defects of skin, muscle, nerve, fascia, and bone. The employment of free flaps has allowed surgeons to be more aggressive for resections of cancers and to provide better care for trauma patients by allowing reconstructions that were not previously conceivable. The reliability of free flaps has also increased gradually over time as techniques and methods of flap monitoring have improved. The success rate of free flaps

[a] Division of Plastic and Reconstructive Surgery, Department of Surgery, Stanford University School of Medicine, 770 Welch Road, Suite 400, Stanford, CA 94305, USA; [b] Hagey Laboratory for Pediatric Regenerative Medicine, Stanford University School of Medicine, 257 Campus Drive West, Stanford, CA 94305, USA; [c] Department of Surgery, Stanford University School of Medicine, 257 Campus Drive West, GK103, Stanford, CA 94305, USA
* Corresponding author. Department of Surgery, Stanford University School of Medicine, 257 Campus Drive West, GK103, Stanford, CA 94305.
E-mail address: dwan@stanford.edu

Surg Clin N Am 101 (2021) 813–829
https://doi.org/10.1016/j.suc.2021.06.009
0039-6109/21/© 2021 Elsevier Inc. All rights reserved.
surgical.theclinics.com

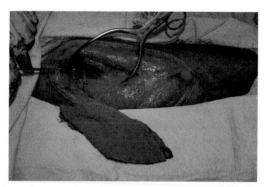

Fig. 1. Demonstration of an ALT flap elevated on its source vessel.

in high volume centers is often cited to exceed 90% for lower extremity reconstructions, and over 98% and 99% for head and neck and trunk/breast reconstruction, respectively.[3,4]

Principles of reconstruction dictate that a donor site should not lead to significant morbidity in contrast to the defect being reconstructed. Thus, with proper design and execution, the most commonly used free flaps have a low expected morbidity profile. In this article, we will discuss the most commonly used free flaps in reconstructive surgery, their indications, complications for the donor and recipient sites, and complication avoidance. Some complications are common to all types of flap surgery (anastomotic issues, flap failure, infection, hematoma), but in this article, we will focus on unique complications for each flap type.

ANTEROLATERAL THIGH FLAP

The anterolateral thigh flap (ALT) has become a mainstay for the reconstruction of soft tissue defects.[5] The ALT has a robust, predictable blood supply that allows for a long pedicle length via the lateral femoral circumflex artery (LFCA) as a large caliber source vessel (**Fig. 1**). The ALT provides abundant skin, fascia, and fat; in addition, the flap is highly customizable, allowing for multiple skin paddles, inclusion of muscle, the possibility for a sensate flap, and the option to fold or tubularize the flap (**Fig. 2**). The flap thus has numerous indications for the reconstruction of external defects, including phalloplasty, and can also be used for oral/visceral reconstructions such as the tongue and esophagus.

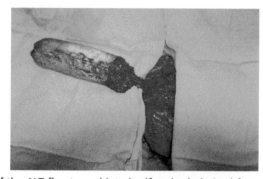

Fig. 2. Example of the ALT flap turned into itself and tubularized for a phalloplasty.

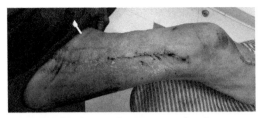

Fig. 3. Primary closure result after an ALT harvest 6 weeks after surgery.

Donor Site Complications

Closure
Primary closure of the donor site can be achieved with widths up to 8 cm, and often skin grafts are not necessary (**Fig. 3**). However, complications can occur if closures are unduly tight, including wound dehiscence and/or compartment syndrome.[6] If significant tension is placed on the wound with attempted closure, it is advisable to place a split-thickness skin graft instead. Flaps of large size may necessitate skin grafting of the donor site (**Fig. 4**).

Lateral thigh paresthesia
Thigh paresthesia is the most commonly reported complication and previously has been described as an expected outcome; however, technique refinement over time with preservation of lateral femoral cutaneous nerve (LFCN) branches to remnant skin has decreased the incidence to under 25%.[7]

Musculocutaneous dysfunction
LFCA perforator anatomy is highly variable. If the perforators are musculocutaneous, a portion of the vastus lateralis will inevitably be damaged during skeletonization of the vessel (**Fig. 5**). In addition, branches of the femoral nerve to the quadriceps may also be damaged during dissection. Knee extension can thus be impaired when significant muscle is taken or denervated. Although there is typically a measurable extension lag postoperatively, activities of daily living are typically not impaired, even with total vastus harvest.[8]

Recipient Site Complications

Head and neck
Resections in this area can lead to significant anatomic challenges and complications for reconstruction. Carotid blowout is estimated to occur in 2% to 5% of patients who undergo interventions for head and neck cancer; this dreaded complication carries a

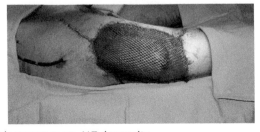

Fig. 4. Skin graft placement to an ALT donor site.

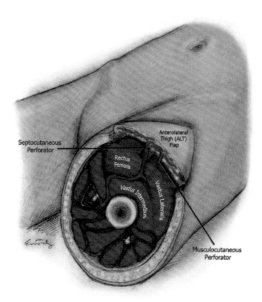

Fig. 5. Schematic representation of septocutaneous and musculocutaneous perforators for the ALT flap.

40% mortality rate.[9] Careful dissection around critical vessels must be used. The skin of the ALT is a great option for lining reconstruction, and with vastus lateralis inclusion in the flap, bulk can be provided around vessels to prevent exposure and saliva contamination (**Fig. 6**). Meticulous microsurgical technique and postoperative monitoring are critical in the head and neck because flap failure has serious implications in this region. When a free flap is unsuccessful or partial necrosis threatens exposure of a critical structure, the surgeon should act expediently on a secondary plan to provide wound coverage. A pedicled pectoralis flap can be used as salvage in the event of flap failure.

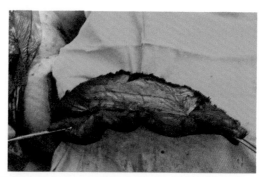

Fig. 6. Harvest of the vastus lateralis in the addition to the overlying fasciocutaneous ALT paddle. In this photo, the vastus is sutured to the fasciocutaneous paddle to prevent shearing between the flap components.

Again, the ALT is pliable and can be used to create 3D structures. One downside to using the ALT in esophageal reconstruction, however, is a longer skin-to-mucosa healing time as compared with mucosa-to-mucosa healing seen in intestinal autotransplant.[10] This can potentiate salivary leaks and may contribute to a comparably higher stricture rate.

Flap thinning

In some instances where a tubularized flap is necessary, such as head and neck defects, the ALT may be too bulky. In these cases, the flap may be thinned to make it useable. However, there is no consensus method for optimal flap thinning, and flap necrosis and total flap failure are possibilities.[11] Subfascial dissection and the preservation of as much deep fascia around the perforators, especially when thinned, helps to lower the risk of negative outcomes. Secondary thinning can also be considered to limit the risk of flap necrosis.

Key points

- The ALT flap is highly customizable and provides generous skin, fat, and fascia for reconstruction. The flap can also be innervated.
- Consider skin grafting for tight closures of the thigh.
- Harvest of the ALT may affect quadriceps function, though this morbidity is typically well-tolerated.
- ALT use in the head and neck is often to cover sensitive structures; accurate design of the ALT and meticulous technique are crucial in optimizing outcome.

RADIAL FOREARM FLAP

The radial forearm flap (RFF) is an extraordinarily versatile flap.[12] Similar to the ALT, the RFF provides skin, subcutaneous tissue, and fascia, and the flap can be shaped into complex structures. The RFF provides less surface area and bulk than the ALT, but the RFF is more easily shaped given its thinness. The option to include tendon (palmaris longus) and vascularized bone (distal radius segment) makes the RFF useful for sling construction for facial reanimation/symmetry procedures and maxillary/mandibular reconstruction. RFFs may be innervated through the inclusion of antebrachial cutaneous nerve branches. The source vessel, the radial artery, allows for a long, wide-caliber pedicle, and the flap can also be used as a flow-through design if needed (**Fig. 7**).

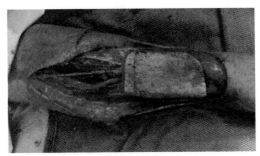

Fig. 7. Example of radial forearm flap after elevation. The hand is present on the right side of the photo. The radial artery and cephalic vein can be seen entering the flap on the left. Dorsal radial sensory branches can be seen entering the dorsal hand distal to the flap.

Donor Site Complications

Hand devascularization

The radial and ulnar arteries provide a dual blood supply to the hand, and in most cases, the radial artery can be harvested without detriment. However, in some cases, the superficial palmar arch may not be complete, and in these patients, radial artery sacrifice may lead to hand ischemia. An Allen's test demonstrating adequate blood flow through the ulnar system should be performed before proceeding with RFF harvest. Alternatively, a "surgical Allen's test" can be performed intraoperatively through direct radial artery clamping to determine if hand perfusion is sufficient through the ulnar system. Computed tomography angiograms (CTAs) and even formal angiograms may not demonstrate dynamic flow of these arterial systems and should not be relied on for this determination.[13] If hand ischemia is a concern intraoperatively, it is prudent to reconstruct the radial artery with a reversed vein graft.

Fracture

A concern after the harvest of an osteocutaneous RFF is the structural integrity of the distal radius. Pathologic fractures have historically been a cause for dismissal of this flap, though interest has increased recently for craniofacial defects.[14,15] The maximum size of the bone wedge is 12 cm long by 1.5 cm wide taken from between the insertions of the brachioradialis and pronator teres (**Fig. 8**). The segment must be unicortical. Prophylactic internal plate fixation of the radius at the time of harvest has proven to be an effective countermeasure, though placement must be precise to prevent complications of malposition such as tendon wear.

Nerve injury

At the volar wrist, the palmar cutaneous nerve may be at risk during flap harvest. This sensory nerve commonly travels at the ulnar side of the flexor carpi radialis subsheath and emerges through the antebrachial fascia 5 cm proximal to the wrist crease and may be injured during dissection.[16] In addition, the superficial branch of the radial nerve is routinely encountered as it emerges from under the brachioradialis 8 cm proximal to the radial styloid.[17] Care must be taken to preserve these nerves during harvest to avoid paresthesia and potential neuroma formation.

Closure

Skin grafting is required in almost all instances. Care must be taken to preserve paratenon around tendons during harvest, and desiccation must be avoided

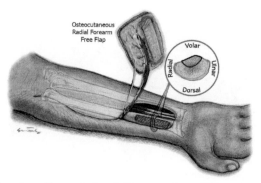

Fig. 8. Schematic drawing of harvest of radial forearm flap with a unicortical bone segment. The perforators to the bone must be preserved during harvest.

intraoperatively. Limited suturing of muscle bellies over exposed tendons may assist in skin graft take. Raising the flap suprafascially can also provide a uniform vascularized wound surface. Use of negative pressure therapy for bolstering will also optimize graft take.[18]

Functional impairment

Data suggest that objective decreases in hand sensation and function are measurable after harvest but do not lead to clinically relevant sequelae.[19] However, at least one study reported impaired wrist motion as a chief factor for dissatisfaction after surgery.[20] To avoid this complication, flap dissection should be kept 2 cm proximal from the wrist crease, and patients should be encouraged to resume light hand activity after skin grafts have healed.

Aesthetics

The forearm is a conspicuous donor site (**Fig. 9**). Using split-thickness sheet grafts is standard in preventing a meshed appearance after healing. Patients should be prepared for a permanent contour deformity in the forearm due to lack of adipose tissue; using full-thickness grafts or synthetic dermal matrices to thicken forearm coverage has not led to promising esthetic results.[21]

Recipient Site Complications

As the indications and recipient sites for the RFF are similar to the ALT, some complications are shared. Below are special considerations for the RFF flap.

Bone complications

Use of an osteocutaneous flap in maxillomandibular reconstruction after resection or osteoradionecrosis opens the possibility for hardware issues and nonunion of the flap to the recipient bone. Tobacco use is a major risk factor.[22] It must be kept in mind that the bone provided by an RFF is unicortical and small volume, and thus the bony portion is usually not suitable for significant weight-bearing or dental implants.

Midfacial reconstruction

Special considerations must be taken in this area; for orbital reconstruction, adequate height must be provided by the osseous-plate construct to match the contralateral orbit or diplopia may result. It is also crucial to suspend the soft tissue of the flap to deeper structures, such as periosteum, when midface skin is being replaced to prevent lower lid malposition.

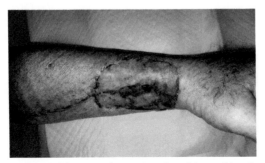

Fig. 9. Demonstration of radial forearm donor site after skin grafting 2 weeks after surgery.

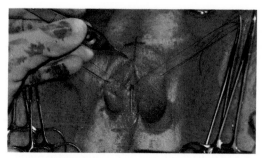

Fig. 10. Demonstration of fistula with an associated stricture after radial forearm phalloplasty.

Tubularized flaps

The RFF faces similar rates of stricture and fistula as the ALT for pharyngoesophageal reconstruction.[23] One special consideration for RFF use is for phalloplasty where the RFF is used as a double-tube, creating skin and urethral lining. Urethral fistulae and strictures are common after phalloplasty, but the RFF has a much lower complication profile than ALT flaps for this indication due to increased pliability and superior vascular supply.[24] Most of these issues can be managed conservatively with wound care and urinary diversion, though in some instances, urethral resurfacing with buccal grafts is required (**Fig. 10**).

Key points

- The RFF has similar indications to the ALT flap, though the RFF soft tissue is thinner and more pliable. Bone can also be taken with the RFF flap.
- Hand ischemia is an unacceptable complication after RFF harvest. An Allen's test is considered mandatory before harvest.
- Wrist flexibility limitations are possible after harvest. The harvest site is conspicuous from an esthetic standpoint.

FREE FIBULA FLAP

Since its description in 1975, this flap has become the workhorse for the reconstruction of long bone gaps.[25] The fibula flap is extremely versatile, and harvest with a skin paddle is optional. Originally thought to be unreliable, further understanding of perforator anatomy has demonstrated that a skin paddle can be reliably harvested with proper design.[26] The fibula can also be cut into many different configurations (such as double barreling), allowing for great customization in the reconstruction of head and neck and extremity defects.[27] (**Fig. 11**) The abundant cortical bone stock also affords dental implants when used for mandibular and maxillary reconstruction (**Fig. 12**).

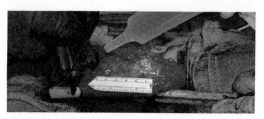

Fig. 11. Fibula flap shaping and customization.

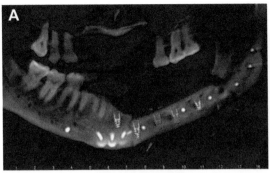
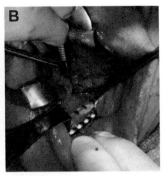

Fig. 12. Dental implant placement. (*A*) Presurgical planning allows for projected placement of the dental implant. (*B*) Intraoperative view of dental fixtures in a single-barrel fibula reconstruction.

Donor Site Complications

Nerve injury

The most common neural complications reported are decreased flexion power of the big toe and paresthesia/dysesthesia to the foot dorsum due to common peroneal nerve neuropraxia. Tourniquet use may also contribute to neuropraxic phenomena.[28] Such symptoms will resolve over time. More rarely, injury to the common peroneal nerve may occur, leading to persistent numbness and permanent weakness of foot dorsiflexion. Some surgeons recommend subperiosteal dissection of the fibula superiorly at the start of harvest to ensure the nerve is protected during exposure, though this is not common practice.[29] Leaving 6 cm of the proximal fibula is likely sufficient to ensure the deep peroneal nerve is protected during the proximal osteotomy.

Ankle instability

A sufficient length (6 cm) of fibula must be left distally to avoid ankle instability. This complication is more common in children; it is advisable to leave longer residual fibula lengths up to 9 cm if possible in this population.[30] Tibiofibular synostosis may be required if instability develops and should be considered prophylactically if insufficient length is preserved.

Foot devascularization

This potential consequence is devastating in the case of a peroneal arteria magna, which is estimated to be present in around 5% of patients.[31] This complication can be easily avoided by obtaining preoperative imaging.

Skin flap survival

Proper design will ensure skin flap viability. Designing the skin paddle center on the posterior axis of the fibula will increase the chance of septocutaneous perforators being captured during harvest (**Fig. 13**). In addition, a cuff of soleus or flexor hallucis longus on the flap may be included if there are concerns about maintaining perforators to the skin paddle.

Closure

Skin grafting should be performed in almost all cases when a skin paddle is harvested; imbrication of the peroneal tendons under muscle will prevent poor skin graft take and tendon exposure. In general, skin grafts should be performed if donor skin paddle width is 6 cm or more, but surgeons should be liberal in grafting this area. There is

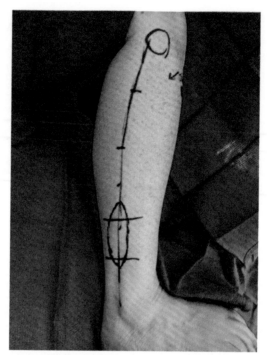

Fig. 13. Example of fibula flap design. Note that the skin paddle is centered on the posterior aspect of the fibula.

limited skin laxity in this area, and compartment syndrome after tight primary closure is possible.[32] **(Fig. 14)**

Recipient Site Complications

Postoperative monitoring
For all recipient sites, harvest of a skin paddle has the advantage of providing an ability to monitor the bone. The bone flap may be able to tolerate venous thrombosis for up to

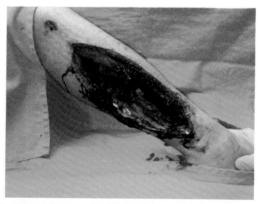

Fig. 14. Attempted primary closure of a fibula donor site with resultant compartment syndrome. The prior suture line has been released, and necrotic muscle required debridement.

24 hours due to bleeding from the medullary canal, though the skin paddle will not tolerate prolonged disruption of vascular inflow and outflow. In many cases where circulation cannot be re-established, the bone may be left as a graft and sufficient osseointegration occurs. Hyperbaric oxygen therapy can be considered to aid in bone graft survival, especially in radiated fields.[33]

Head and neck

When used for oral reconstruction, dehiscence or necrosis of the mandibular skin paddle may occur intraorally. Most small wounds can be managed conservatively (ie, chlorhexidine/bicarbonate rinses). If critical structures such as the pedicle are exposed, however, washout and re-closure, potentially with an additional soft tissue flap, may be required.

Complications concerning bone integrity may also occur when the fibula is used for oral reconstruction. Plate and/or neomandibular/neomaxillary fracture may occur when patients resume masticatory activities. Prior studies show no difference between the use of miniplates or heavier recon plates in predicting postoperative fractures, though some authors advocate the use of heavier plates when reconstructing the angle because of the stress distribution in this area.[33] The use of dental implants also carries risks; it is estimated that around 80% of attempted implant placements into a reconstructed mandible survive, but occasionally implants are lost because of peri-implantitis.[34] A single-barreled fibula may also not allow enough bone stock for a favorable crown-to-implant height for implant use, and implant placement will have less reliable long-term results in these patients. Double-barreling the fibula may circumvent these problems.[35]

Extremity

The fibula is often used for the reconstruction of long bone defects. In many cases, the diameter of the bone to be reconstructed is much larger than that of the fibula (eg, humerus, femur, or tibia). It would seem intuitive that a limb reconstructed with the smaller diameter fibula would be more prone to fracture, though there is a paucity of long-term studies for such cases. Several case series provide excellent outcomes with fibula flaps for long bone reconstruction with and without massive bone allografts (Capanna technique).[36,37] Painful heterotopic ossification is also a potential complication that may occur at the donor or recipient site, and this may cause pain and discomfort. Trimming excessive fibular periosteum at donor and recipient sites may help avoid this outcome.[38]

Key points

- The fibula is a versatile flap that provides bone and soft tissue and is commonly used in the head and neck and extremities.
- Most donor site issues can be avoided by ensuring sufficient remnant bone length and liberal skin grafting.
- In the event of flap failure, the fibula can be used as a bone graft.

DEEP INFERIOR EPIGASTRIC PERFORATOR/FREE TRAVERSE RECTUS ABDOMINIS MYOCUTANEOUS

The free TRAM (traverse rectus abdominis myocutaneous) flap, based on the inferior epigastric artery, and its muscle-sparing equivalent, the DIEP (deep inferior epigastric perforator) flap, have been cemented as the standard free flaps for breast reconstruction. In 1979, Holmstrom demonstrated that discarded abdominoplasty tissue could be used as a free tissue transplant for breast reconstruction, and the use of the free

TRAM steadily gained popularity over its pedicled equivalent because of decreased rates of ischemic complications.[39]

Koshima subsequently developed the muscle-sparing method of harvest, leading to the popularization of DIEP flaps, which are touted to have decreased abdominal bulging compared with the free TRAM flap.[40] Both are commonly used for breast reconstruction, and the free TRAM/DIEP is an option for any type of defect that requires a large volume of soft tissue including fat, skin, or fascia. Large facial, chest wall, extremity, and even buttock defects are all indications for use.

Donor Site Complications

Hernia or bulging

All or a portion of the rectus abdominis muscle must be taken with the free TRAM flap, leaving a segment of the abdominal wall without innervated muscle that may cause hernias or bulging. This may be circumvented by performing a DIEP flap; however, intramuscular dissection may still lead to areas of denervation, and incisions of the anterior rectus sheath are still required for both techniques. Blondeel described that DIEP flaps had a decreased rate of bulging and patients had objectively higher abdominal flexion strengths compared with free TRAM.[41] However, subsequent authors have refuted that the DIEP flap has clinically significant advantages.[42] Taking only a portion of the muscle around the necessary perforator(s) (a muscle-sparing TRAM) is now standard for the TRAM flap and reduces abdominal morbidity (**Fig. 15**). The use of mesh for the abdominal closure also decreases the rate of hernia/bulges.[43]

Closure

Wound healing issues of the donor site occur in an estimated 12% to 39% of cases.[44] A large portion of skin is harvested with the flap (often around the level of the umbilicus to near the pubis), and an overly aggressive harvest can lead to undue tension and wound breakdown (**Fig. 16**). It is critical that the surgeon design the flap such that the wound can be closed without significant tension. Drain use is also routine to help prevent seromas and hematomas. Umbilical necrosis occurs in an estimated 3.2% of cases. These wound complications are more likely in patients with higher body mass index (BMI) and smokers.[45]

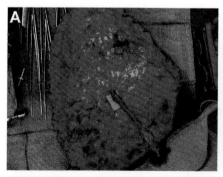 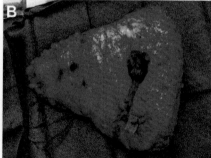

Fig. 15. DIEP versus muscle-sparing TRAM flaps. (*A*) Example of a DIEP with minimal rectus muscle excised. (*B*) Example of a muscle-sparing TRAM flap with a small cuff of muscle around the main perforator to the flap.

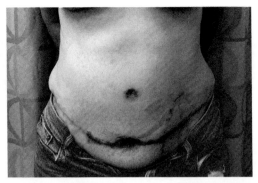

Fig. 16. Delayed wound healing after muscle-sparing TRAM harvest present 4 weeks after surgery.

Nerve injury

The LFCN is potentially within the field of dissection when harvesting a free TRAM/DIEP as it approaches the medial aspect of the anterior superior iliac spine and pierces the iliac fascia. Injury to the nerve may lead to meralgia paresthetica, a condition of dysesthesia or anesthesia to the thigh. The course of these patients is unpredictable, with symptoms resolving spontaneously or lasting for several years.[46] Leaving a layer of sub-Scarpa's fat when dissecting around the iliac crest will prevent injury to this nerve (**Fig. 17**).

Recipient Site Complications

Partial flap necrosis

Give the large volume of tissue provided by the free TRAM/DIEP, occasionally the blood supply from selected perforators is insufficient. This commonly manifests as fat necrosis (hardened nodules within the flap), which is visible on mammograms. Selecting an adequate number of perforators for harvest should circumvent this complication. Higher BMI patients with larger flaps are more susceptible to these complications, and perforator selection should account for this fact.[47] Preoperative abdominal CTA/MRA will aid with perforator selection, and these imaging modalities have been associated with decreased operative time.[48]

Vascular insufficiency

Although the deep inferior epigastric system is usually dominant for abdominal flaps, in some cases, flaps may be reliant on the superficial system, particularly for venous

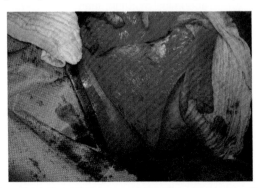

Fig. 17. Preservation of sub-Scarpa's fat around the iliac crest during TRAM/DIEP harvest.

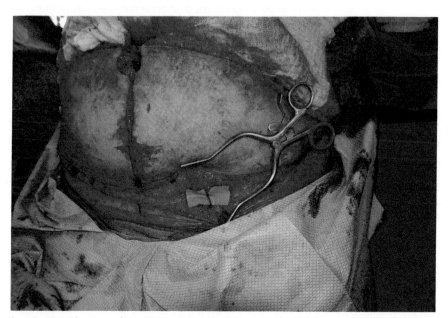

Fig. 18. Identification of the SIEV in DIEP/TRAM harvest. The SIEV can be found one-third of the distance from the pubic tubercle to the anterior superior iliac crest in the supra-Scarpa's fat.

drainage. The estimated incidence is around 1% of free TRAM flaps and 3.3% of DIEP flaps.[49] It is crucial to save the superficial inferior epigastric vein during dissection in all cases as a lifeboat if flap congestion occurs (**Fig. 18**).

Chest wall injury

The most commonly selected recipient vessels for chest/breast reconstruction are the internal mammary vessels, and inadvertent pleural injury is a possible risk of vessel preparation. If recognized intraoperatively, most pleural injuries can be successfully managed with placement of a suction catheter within the defect followed by withdrawal and closure of the injury using a purse-string absorbable suture. Postoperative chest radiographs should be obtained and the patient provided oxygen; in rare instances, a pneumothorax may not resolve, and a chest tube may be necessary.

Key points

- The DIEP flap has less abdominal morbidity than a free TRAM. If a free TRAM is to be performed, abdominal complications can be minimized by muscle and fascial sparing techniques and mesh closure.
- Tension of the donor site must allow for primary closure. Dissection over the iliac crests should spare a layer of fat to avoid LFCN injury.
- Flaps must have sufficient blood supply to match their size to avoid partial flap necrosis.
- The superficial epigastric system should be preserved during dissection in case flap congestion occurs intraoperatively.

SUMMARY

Most commonly used flaps in reconstructive surgery are reliable in the hands of skilled microsurgeons. Flap failure is always a concern with free tissue transfer, but with meticulous surgical planning and execution, such occurrences are rare. Similarly, specific donor and recipient site complications can be reduced by anticipation of potential outcomes and preparation of adequate backup plans.

ACKNOWLEDGMENTS

The authors would like to thank Dr Bauback Safa, Dr Andrew Watt, Dr Mang Chen, and Dr David Perrault for use of photographs in this article. The authors would additionally like to thank Dr Evan Fahy for illustrations provided in this article.

CONFLICT OF INTEREST STATEMENT

The authors have no conflicts of interest to declare for topics discussed in this article.

REFERENCES

1. Antia NH, Buch VI. Transfer of an abdominal dermo-fat graft by direct anastomosis of blood vessels. Br J Plast Surg 1971;24(1):15–9.
2. McLean DH, Buncke HJ. Autotransplant of omentum to a large scalp defect, with microsurgical revascularization. Plast Reconstr Surg 1972;49(3):268–74.
3. Pu LLQ. A Comprehensive Approach to Lower Extremity Free-tissue Transfer. Plast Reconstr Surg Glob Open 2017;5(2). https://doi.org/10.1097/GOX. 0000000000001228.
4. Stranix JT, Lee Z-H, Jacoby A, et al. Forty Years of Lower Extremity Take-Backs: Flap Type Influences Salvage Outcomes. Plast Reconstr Surg 2018;141(5): 1282–7.
5. Song YG, Chen GZ, Song YL. The free thigh flap: a new free flap concept based on the septocutaneous artery. Br J Plast Surg 1984;11:149–59.
6. Addison PD, Lannon D, Neligan PC. Compartment syndrome after closure of the anterolateral thigh flap donor site: a report of two cases. Ann Plast Surg 2008; 60(6):635–8.
7. Collins J, Ayeni O, Thoma A. A systematic review of anterolateral thigh flap donor site morbidity. Can J Plast Surg 2012;20(1):17–23.
8. Weise H, Naros A, Blumenstock G, et al. Donor site morbidity of the anterolateral thigh flap. J Craniomaxillofac Surg 2017;45(12):2105–8.
9. Liang NL, Guedes BD, Duvvuri U, et al. Outcomes of interventions for carotid blowout syndrome in patients with head and neck cancer. J Vasc Surg 2016; 63(6):1525–30.
10. Chen HC, Tang YB. Microsurgical reconstruction of the esophagus. Semin Surg Oncol 2000;19(3):235–45.
11. Agostini T, Lazzeri D, Spinelli G. Anterolateral thigh flap thinning: techniques and complications. Ann Plast Surg 2014;72(2):246–52.
12. Megerle K, Sauerbier M, Germann G. The evolution of the pedicled radial forearm flap. Hand (N Y) 2010;5(1):37–42.
13. Miller TJ, Safa B, Watt AJ, et al. An abnormal clinical Allen's Test is not a contraindication for free radial forearm flap. Clin Case Rep 2020. https://doi.org/10. 1002/ccr3.3093.
14. Connolly TM, Sweeny L, Greene B, et al. Reconstruction of midface defects with the osteocutaneous radial forearm flap: Evaluation of long term outcomes including patient reported quality of life. Microsurgery 2017;37(7):752–62.

15. Arganbright JM, Tsue TT, Girod DA, et al. Outcomes of the Osteocutaneous Radial Forearm Free Flap for Mandibular Reconstruction. JAMA Otolaryngol Neck Surg 2013;139(2):168–72.
16. Jeong YH, Choi JH, Choi HS, et al. Risk Assessment of Injury to Palmar Cutaneous Branch of the Median Nerve Using High-Resolution Ultrasound. Ann Rehabil Med 2019;43(4):458–64.
17. Folberg CR, Ulson H, Scheidt RB. THE SUPERFICIAL BRANCH OF THE RADIAL NERVE: A MORPHOLOGIC STUDY. Rev Bras Ortop 2015;44(1):69–74.
18. Clark JM, Rychlik S, Harris J, et al. Donor site morbidity following radial forearm free flap reconstruction with split thickness skin grafts using negative pressure wound therapy. J Otolaryngol Head Neck Surg 2019;48(1):21.
19. Orlik JR, Horwich P, Bartlett C, et al. Long-term functional donor site morbidity of the free radial forearm flap in head and neck cancer survivors. J Otolaryngol Head Neck Surg 2014;43(1):1.
20. Deleyiannis FW-B, Sacks JM, McLean KM, et al. Patient Self-Report of Disability of the Upper Extremity following Osteocutaneous Radial Forearm Free Flap Harvest. Plast Reconstr Surg 2008;122(5):1479–84.
21. Ho T, Couch M, Carson K, et al. Radial Forearm Free Flap Donor Site Outcomes Comparison by Closure Methods. Otolaryngol Neck Surg 2006;134(2):309–15.
22. Day KE, Desmond R, Magnuson JS, et al. Hardware Removal after Osseous Free Flap Reconstruction. Otolaryngol Head Neck Surg 2014;150(1):40–6.
23. Cho BC, Kim M, Lee JH, et al. Pharyngoesophageal reconstruction with a tubed free radial forearm flap. J Reconstr Microsurg 1998;14(8):535–40.
24. Ascha M, Massie JP, Morrison SD, et al. Outcomes of Single Stage Phalloplasty by Pedicled Anterolateral Thigh Flap versus Radial Forearm Free Flap in Gender Confirming Surgery. J Urol 2018;199(1):206–14.
25. Taylor GI, Miller GD, Ham FJ. The free vascularized bone graft. A clinical extension of microvascular techniques. Plast Reconstr Surg 1975;55(5):533–44.
26. Yu P, Chang EI, Hanasono MM. Design of a reliable skin paddle for the fibula osteocutaneous flap: perforator anatomy revisited. Plast Reconstr Surg 2011;128(2):440–6.
27. Shroff SS, Nair SC, Shah A, et al. Versatility of Fibula Free Flap in Reconstruction of Facial Defects: A Center Study. J Maxillofac Oral Surg 2017;16(1):101–7.
28. Thiele OC, Scuto I, Allamprese F, et al. Intermediate short-term tourniquet use during the preparation of a free vascularised fibula flap for mandibular reconstruction. A case report. Minerva Stomatol 2008;57(1–2):53–5, 56–7.
29. Salgado CJ, Chim H, Moran SL, et al. Fibula Flap. In: Flaps and Reconstructive Surgery. 2nd ed. ; 2017:596-612.e2. Available at: https://www-clinicalkey-com.laneproxy.stanford.edu/#!/content/book/3-s2.0-B9780323243223000523. Accessed August 16, 2020.
30. Nathan SS, Hung-yi L, Cordeiro PG, et al. Instability After Vascularized Fibular Harvest for Tumor Reconstruction. Ann Surg Oncol 2004;12(1):57–64.
31. Rosson GD, Singh NK. Devascularizing Complications of Free Fibula Harvest: Peronea Arteria Magna. J Reconstr Microsurg 2005;21(08):533–8.
32. Kerrary S, Schouman T, Cox A, et al. Acute compartment syndrome following fibula flap harvest for mandibular reconstruction. J Craniomaxillofac Surg 2011;39(3):206–8.
33. van Gemert JTM, Abbink JH, van Es RJJ, et al. Early and late complications in the reconstructed mandible with free fibula flaps. J Surg Oncol 2018;117(4):773–80.

34. Attia S, Wiltfang J, Pons-Kühnemann J, et al. Survival of dental implants placed in vascularised fibula free flaps after jaw reconstruction. J Craniomaxillofac Surg 2018;46(8):1205–10.
35. Ishii N, Shimizu Y, Ihara J, et al. Analysis of Fibular Single Graft and Fibular Double-barrel Graft for Mandibular Reconstruction. Plast Reconstr Surg Glob Open 2016;4(8):e1018.
36. Houdek MT, Wagner ER, Stans AA, et al. What Is the Outcome of Allograft and Intramedullary Free Fibula (Capanna Technique) in Pediatric and Adolescent Patients With Bone Tumors? Clin Orthop 2016;474(3):660–8.
37. Wee C, Ruter D, Schulz S, et al. Reconstruction of extremity long bone defects with vascularized fibula bone grafts. Plast Aesthet Res 2019;2019. https://doi.org/10.20517/2347-9264.2019.02.
38. Kim BB, Kaleem A, Alzahrani S, et al. Modified fibula free flap harvesting technique for prevention of heterotopic pedicle ossification. Head Neck 2019;41(7): E104–12.
39. Holmström H. The free abdominoplasty flap and its use in breast reconstruction. An experimental study and clinical case report. Scand J Plast Reconstr Surg 1979;13(3):423–7.
40. Koshima I, Soeda S. Inferior epigastric artery skin flaps without rectus abdominis muscle. Br J Plast Surg 1989;42(6):645–8.
41. Blondeel N, Vanderstraeten GG, Monstrey SJ, et al. The donor site morbidity of free DIEP flaps and free TRAM flaps for breast reconstruction. Br J Plast Surg 1997;50(5):322–30.
42. Jeong W, Lee S, Kim J. Meta-analysis of flap perfusion and donor site complications for breast reconstruction using pedicled versus free TRAM and DIEP flaps. Breast 2018;38:45–51.
43. Wan DC, Tseng CY, Anderson-Dam J, et al. Inclusion of mesh in donor-site repair of free TRAM and muscle-sparing free TRAM flaps yields rates of abdominal complications comparable to those of DIEP flap reconstruction. Plast Reconstr Surg 2010;126(2):367–74.
44. Lindenblatt N, Gruenherz L, Farhadi J. A systematic review of donor site aesthetic and complications after deep inferior epigastric perforator flap breast reconstruction. Gland Surg 2019;8(4):389–98.
45. Ricci JA, Kamali P, Becherer BE, et al. Umbilical necrosis rates after abdominal-based microsurgical breast reconstruction. J Surg Res 2017;215:257–63.
46. Ivins GK. Meralgia Paresthetica, The Elusive Diagnosis. Ann Surg 2000;232(2): 281–6.
47. Mulvey CL, Cooney CM, Daily FF, et al. Increased Flap Weight and Decreased Perforator Number Predict Fat Necrosis in DIEP Breast Reconstruction. Plast Reconstr Surg Glob Open 2013;1(2):1–7.
48. Mohan AT, Saint-Cyr M. Advances in imaging technologies for planning breast reconstruction. Gland Surg 2016;5(2):242–54.
49. Kim D-Y, Lee TJ, Kim EK, et al. Intraoperative venous congestion in free transverse rectus abdominis musculocutaneous and deep inferior epigastric artery perforator flaps during breast reconstruction: A systematic review. Plast Surg 2015;23(4):255–9.

Ear, Nose, and Throat Surgery

Postoperative Complications After Selected Head and Neck Operations

Joshua D. Smith, MD[a], Jason A. Correll, MS[b],
Chaz L. Stucken, MD[a], Emily Z. Stucken, MD[a],*

KEYWORDS

- Otolaryngology • ENT • Postoperative • Complications • Head and neck

KEY POINTS

- Ear, nose, and throat (ENT) surgery, or otolaryngology, is a diverse specialty that manages a variety of surgical problems of the head and neck.
- ENT surgery is characterized by anatomic complexity, proximity of critical neurovascular structures, and unique esthetic importance of the face and neck.
- Postoperative complications after ENT surgeries have unique cosmetic and functional consequences.
- Possible complications after ENT surgeries range from minor bleeding and wound healing issues to cranial nerve injury, damage to sensory organs, and disfiguring esthetic alterations.
- Management of ENT surgical complications demands prompt recognition and may necessitate return to the operating room for definitive management.

INTRODUCTION

Ear, nose, and throat (ENT) surgery, also known as "otolaryngology," "otorhinolaryngology," or "otolaryngology—head and neck surgery," is recognized as the oldest specialty in the history of American surgery, with origins dating to the 1840s.[1] The modern otolaryngologist dutifully manages a wide variety of surgical problems of the head and neck, including those of a neoplastic, congenital, infectious, sensory, esthetic, iatrogenic, and idiopathic nature. The otolaryngologist's anatomic domain is complex and encompasses myriad structures critical to human form and function (**Box 1**).

---

[a] Department of Otolaryngology–Head and Neck Surgery, University of Michigan, 1500 East Medical Center Drive, Ann Arbor, MI 48109, USA; [b] University of Michigan Medical School, 1301 Catherine Street, Ann Arbor, MI 48109, USA
* Corresponding author. Department of Otolaryngology–Head and Neck Surgery, University of Michigan, 1500 East Medical Center Drive, SPC 5312, Ann Arbor, MI 48109-5312.
E-mail address: estucken@med.umich.edu

Surg Clin N Am 101 (2021) 831–844
https://doi.org/10.1016/j.suc.2021.06.010
0039-6109/21/© 2021 Elsevier Inc. All rights reserved.

surgical.theclinics.com

Box 1
Important anatomic structures frequently encountered in ENT surgery

Lymphovascular
  Common carotid artery
  Internal carotid artery & branches
  External carotid artery & branches
  Vertebral artery
  Internal jugular vein
  Dural venous sinuses (eg, sigmoid sinus)
  Thoracic duct

Nervous
  Cranial nerves
  Phrenic nerve
  Cervical sympathetic chain
  Brachial plexus
  Anterior & middle cranial fossa dura

Sense & Communication Organs
  Olfactory system
  Globe
  Cochlea
  Balance organs (ie, semicircular canals, utricle, saccule)
  Vocal cords

Viscera
  Hypopharynx & cervical esophagus
  Larynx & trachea

Endocrine Organs
  Thyroid gland
  Parathyroid glands

Since its advent nearly two hundred years ago, ENT surgery overall has become much safer to perform because of improvements in preoperative patient selection and advances in surgical techniques, technologies, and perioperative care standards. Nevertheless, surgical complications still do occur and carry with them important functional, esthetic, and psychological consequences unique to otolaryngologic surgery.[2] For the purposes of the ensuing discussion, a useful definition of "complication" is "any deviation from the normal postoperative course."[3] A complication is then distinct from a surgical sequela (ie, anticipated "after-effect" of surgery) or a "failure to cure," as defined by Clavien and Dindo.[3] Surgical complications can be variably classified according to nature (eg, infectious or wound), time-course (eg, temporary or permanent), frequency, and severity (**Table 1**).[3]

Herein, we provide a brief but cogent review of postoperative complications after otolaryngologic surgery. Owing to the breadth and depth of the field, the discussion is organized by subspecialty, focusing on selected operations whose potential complications highlight the complexity and diversity of ENT surgery (**Fig. 1**).

HEAD AND NECK ONCOLOGIC SURGERY

The surgical extirpation of malignancies of the oral cavity, oropharynx, hypopharynx, larynx, nasal cavity and paranasal sinuses, nasopharynx, and salivary glands carries unique risks for Clavien-Dindo Grade III to V complications, for several reasons. First, patients with mucosal malignancies of the upper aerodigestive tract frequently have

Table 1
Clavien-Dindo classification of surgical complications[3]

Complication Grade	Description
Grade 1	Complication without need for pharmacologic, surgical, endoscopic, or radiological interventions
Grade II	Complication requiring pharmacologic treatment (eg, blood transfusion)
Grade III	Complication requiring surgical, endoscopic, or radiological intervention
Grade IIIa	Intervention not under general anesthesia
Grade IIIb	Intervention under general anesthesia
Grade IV	Life-threatening complication requiring ICU management
Grade IVa	Single organ dysfunction
Grade IVb	Multiorgan dysfunction
Grade V	Patient death

comorbid chronic obstructive pulmonary disease, coronary artery disease, hypertension, diabetes mellitus, and tobacco and alcohol use.[4] Second, curative resections are often extensive, near critical neurovascular structures of the head and neck, and invariably impact human swallowing, breathing, and phonation. Third, extirpative defects often require free tissue transfer with microvascular anastomosis, making donor site wound, bleeding, and functional complications possible.[5]

Fig. 2 depicts a breakdown of possible postoperative complications after head and neck oncologic surgery by anatomic site. Pictorial examples of select complications are shown in **Fig. 3**. For additional reading relevant to complications after head and neck oncologic surgery, we refer the interested reader to chapters 4 (complications after endocrine surgery of the neck) and 7 (complications of tissue flaps) of this issue.

Parotidectomy: Indications and Practices

Excision of a parotid gland may be recommended for salivary gland stones (sialolithiasis), infection (sialadenitis), or neoplasms, including primary salivary gland neoplasms or metastatic cutaneous malignancies. Anatomically, each parotid gland resides in the preauricular cheek adjacent to the angle of the mandible and is bisected into superficial and deep lobes by the facial nerve (CN VII).

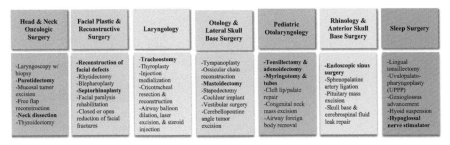

Fig. 1. Major subspecialties of ENT surgery with examples of their representative surgical procedures. Operations discussed in this article are highlighted in bold.

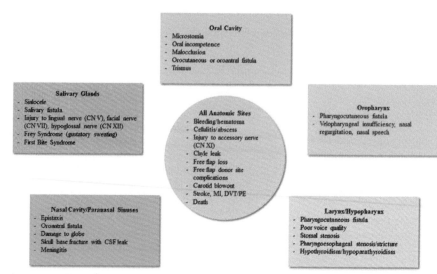

Fig. 2. Possible postoperative complications after head and neck oncologic surgery by anatomic site of malignancy.

Parotidectomy: complications and management

The most feared complication after parotidectomy is facial nerve injury, which may lead to hemifacial weakness, asymmetry, oral incompetence, dry eye, and exposure keratitis. Temporary, mild weakness of facial nerve branches may be seen in more than 20% of patients after parotidectomy.[6] Fortunately, permanent weakness is much less common, occurring after roughly 1% of operations.[6] Electrophysiologic facial nerve monitoring during parotidectomy may help with the identification of facial

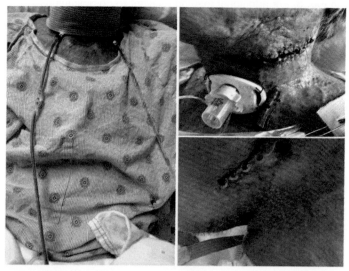

Fig. 3. Examples of postoperative complications after head and neck oncologic surgery. Salivary fistula with abnormal connection between the pharynx and neck soft tissues. Blue dye was swallowed by the patient and appeared in the right neck drain (*left panel*). Dehiscence of surgical wound after neck dissection (*top right panel*). Breakdown of skin with exposure of titanium plate reconstructing the jaw (*bottom right panel*).

nerve branches in the operative field, particularly in revision operations.[7] However, it has not been shown to reduce rates of permanent facial nerve weakness after parotidectomy underscoring the importance of proper anatomic knowledge of the facial nerve course.[8]

Whether temporary or permanent, facial nerve injury may cause reduced lacrimation and eyelid paralysis, which contribute to corneal exposure, desiccation, and trauma. Rigorous lubrication of the eye with artificial tears or ointments and protection with an eye shield is paramount. For permanent facial paralysis after parotidectomy, there are several beneficial surgical procedures aimed at static or dynamic facial reanimation.[9]

Frey syndrome, or "gustatory sweating," is a peculiar complication caused by aberrant regeneration of postganglionic, parasympathetic nerve fibers after parotidectomy. Patients with Frey syndrome experience preauricular flushing and focal perspiration in response to gustatory stimuli. Symptoms can be quite detrimental to the quality of life. Options for management, including topical application of antiperspirant or anticholinergic medications (eg, scopolamine) or injection of botulinum toxin, are variably effective.[10]

Neck dissection: indications and practices

Neck dissection, or cervical lymphadenectomy, removes lymph nodes and fibrofatty tissue from one or more anatomic levels of the neck. The principle indication for neck dissection is the excision of regional metastases from malignancies of the head and neck.

Neck dissection: complications and management

Neck dissection may be complicated by hematoma, seroma, wound infection or dehiscence, injury to marginal mandibular (CN VII), vagus (CN X), accessory (CN XI), hypoglossal (XII), or cervical sympathetic nerves, or chylous fistula.[11] In selective and nerve-sparing, modified radical neck dissections, injury to the accessory nerve (CN XI) as it traverses the level II and IV neck may be particularly debilitating. CN XI dysfunction destabilizes the ipsilateral trapezius and scapula, leading to weakened shoulder abduction, chronic shoulder pain, and deformity.[12] Though existing studies are conflicting, factors such as history of chemoradiation[13] and extent of level II dissection may predispose patients to iatrogenic CN XI injury. For all patients in whom CN XI injury is suspected postoperatively, immediate physical therapy to rehabilitate shoulder mobility is recommended.[14]

Chylous fistula, a particularly dreaded complication of neck dissection, occurs with inadvertent injury to the thoracic duct that returns lymph and chyle to venous circulation in the left level IV neck. Despite meticulous surgical technique, chylous fistula complicates 1% to 2% of neck dissections.[15] Chyle extravasation into the neck can lead to impaired wound healing, dehydration, electrolyte disturbance, and malnutrition. Management of chylous fistula is typically multimodal and may consist of closed drainage, pressure dressings, no-fat diet or total parenteral nutrition, somatostatin analogs (eg, octreotide), or surgical exploration.[15]

FACIAL PLASTIC AND RECONSTRUCTIVE SURGERY

Facial plastic and reconstructive surgery (FPRS) is a dynamic subspecialty concerned primarily with correcting structural and esthetic defects of the face. As facial appearance is central to human identity, self-esteem, and social interaction, complications after cosmetic or reconstructive operations are quite visible and can cause significant psychological distress to patients.[16] The distinction between "complication" and "failure to cure" is particularly crucial for this discussion, as optimal esthetic and functional outcomes often require multiple staged procedures. Fortunately, most postoperative complications after FPRS can be classified as Clavien-Dindo Grade I to III (**Box 2**).

Reconstruction of Facial Defects: Indications and Practices

Skin cancers are the most common malignancy in the United States, and their incidence continues to climb due in part to an aging population with increased cumulative UV light exposure.[17] Extirpative facial defects are typically created by Mohs micrographic surgery or wide local excision for nonmelanoma skin cancers or melanomas (in situ or invasive), respectively. In order of increasing complexity, reconstructive techniques include healing by secondary intention, primary closure, skin grafting, and local, regional, and free flaps.[17]

Reconstruction of facial defects: complications and management

Skin and soft tissue complications (see **Box 2**) are the most prevalent after primary closure, skin grafting, or local or regional flap reconstruction of facial defects. Accurate prevalence rates of individual complications are elusive, though certainly fall well below 5% to 10% of operations.[18] Various factors may increase the risk of postoperative skin and soft tissue complications, including diabetes mellitus, tobacco use, antiplatelet and anticoagulant medications, and defect size and extent.[19]

Dependent on severity and risk of flap necrosis, postoperative hematoma and surgical site infection may be managed expectantly or with a combination of incision and drainage and oral antibiotics. Surgical sites with dehiscence or flap/graft necrosis may

---

Box 2
Potential complications of facial plastic and reconstructive surgery

Skin & Soft Tissue
  Bleeding/hematoma
  Infection
  Wound dehiscence
  Local flap deformities (eg, pincushioning, trapdoor, standing cone)
  Flap/graft necrosis
  Skin irregularities/discoloration
  Asymmetry (eg, hairline, brow)
  Scarring (eg, hypertrophic scar, keloid)

Nervous
  Cutaneous anesthesia
  Paresis/paralysis of CN V branches
  Paresis/paralysis of CN VII branches

Ocular
  Ptosis
  Diplopia
  Ocular injury, retrobulbar hemorrhage, vision loss

Nasal
  Epistaxis
  Nasal septal hematoma, abscess, perforation
  Nasal airway dysfunction
  Nasal deformities (eg, saddle nose, polly beak)
  Cerebrospinal fluid leak

Oral
  Malocclusion
  Oral incompetence
  Vermillion border misalignment

be left to granulate or alternative skin grafts or local flaps may be used in a secondary operation. Finally, ancillary tools such as intralesional steroid injections, pulse dye laser, or dermabrasion may be used to remedy unsightly skin irregularities, discoloration, and hypertrophic scarring.[20]

Septorhinoplasty: Indications and Practices

Septorhinoplasty is a generic term encompassing several intricate surgical techniques to manipulate the bony and cartilaginous framework of the nose and nasal septum. Septorhinoplasty may be functional (eg, to improve nasal airflow), esthetic (eg, to correct nasal asymmetry or prominence), or both. We refer the interested reader to a much more detailed textbook chapter on septorhinoplasty techniques.[21]

Septorhinoplasty: complications and management

Uniquely, complications after septorhinoplasty may manifest in the immediate postoperative period or may only become apparent years later. Early postoperative complications include epistaxis, septal hematoma, abscess, or perforation, and iatrogenic skull base fracture with cerebrospinal fluid (CSF) leak.[22] Late postoperative complications include autologous cartilage graft malposition, visibility, and absorption and named deformities such as "saddle nose," "polly beak," and "inverted-v" requiring revision rhinoplasty.[22] In a recent large series, the overall complication rate after rhinoplasty was 0.7%, with minor bleeding and surgical site infection the most common.[23] The only factors predictive of complications included patient age $\geq$40 years and multiple procedures (eg, septorhinoplasty and facelift).[23]

Technical expertise in septorhinoplasty is paramount to minimize risk of complications and to skillfully remedy them when they do occur. Septal hematoma and abscess require immediate incision and drainage to prevent septal cartilage necrosis and perforation. Iatrogenic CSF leak, while exceedingly rare in septorhinoplasty, demands bed rest, stool softeners, head elevation, and prophylactic antibiotics and may require lumbar drain placement or operative repair.[23] Finally, late complications including graft malposition, visibility, and absorption often require revision rhinoplasty with autologous ear or rib cartilage grafting.[22]

LARYNGOLOGY

Laryngology is a rapidly growing, multidisciplinary field concerned with the medical and surgical management of disorders of the airway, voice, and swallowing. The scope of diseases treated by laryngologists includes disorders of vocal cord motion (eg, paralysis) and vibration (eg, nodules, cysts), degenerative neurologic disorders (eg, Parkinson's), airway stenoses (eg, subglottic stenosis), laryngopharyngitis, and structural pharyngeal disorders (eg, Zenker's diverticulum). Management of these conditions is multifaceted, including pharmacologic, surgical, and ancillary (ie, speech-language therapy) modalities.

The breadth of postoperative complications after laryngologic procedures is beyond the scope of this introductory text. However, we wish to highlight that certain procedures carry unique and tangible risks for postoperative airway compromise that demands immediate reintubation or tracheostomy to prevent devastating hypoxic sequelae.

Tracheostomy: Indications and Practices

Tracheostomy, the surgical creation of a stable airway in the anterior neck, is one of the oldest and most storied operations in head and neck surgery.[24] Tracheostomy is most often performed to facilitate prolonged mechanical ventilation, but may also be done to bypass upper airway obstruction due to head and neck malignancy, bilateral vocal cord paralysis, or laryngotracheal stenosis. In the United States, more than 100,000 tracheostomies are performed yearly, a number that is sure to rise with the ongoing COVID-19 pandemic.[25]

Tracheostomy may be performed via an open surgical procedure or a percutaneous dilational technique by otolaryngologists, general surgeons, or interventional pulmonologists or intensivists. Tracheostomy is the "gold-standard" procedure for the management of airway pathology.

Tracheostomy: complications and management

Complications after tracheostomy may best be separated into early and late complications, though neither classification is well-defined.[26] In the first 5 to 7 days after tracheostomy, "false passage" of the tube may lead to dissection of air into the anterior soft tissues of the neck with resultant subcutaneous emphysema, pneumomediastinum, pneumothorax, and loss of airway patency or support. A deep trachea and excessive neck adiposity may increase the risk of accidental tracheostomy dislodgement and false passage. Management of this complication demands prompt replacement of the tracheostomy tube within the tracheal lumen and confirmation of correct positioning with bedside flexible tracheoscopy. Subsequent pneumothorax may necessitate emergent needle decompression and chest tube placement.

The most feared late complication of tracheostomy, tracheoinnominate fistula, is caused by tracheostomy tube erosion of the anterior tracheal wall with the formation of a fistulous connection to the brachiocephalic artery (**Fig. 4**). In this rare condition, a "sentinel" bleed typically precedes massive hemoptysis and, in over 50% of individuals, rapid asphyxiation and death.[26] For any patient presenting with tracheostomy site bleeding, a high index of suspicion for a sentinel bleed from tracheoinnominate fistula is paramount for timely endovascular intervention. Once massive hemoptysis occurs, interventions such as blood and fluid resuscitation and endovascular or surgical control of hemorrhage are often unsuccessful.

Tracheal stenosis or malacia may occur as late complications of tracheostomy in approximately 1% to 2% of patients (see **Fig. 4**).[27] Factors such as traumatic emergency tracheostomy, cuff pressure necrosis, and mucosal trauma from aggressive suctioning may predispose to these complications. Depending on the severity of stenosis or malacia and patient symptoms, management may include placement of a longer tracheostomy tube to bypass the diseased segment or segmental tracheal resection and reconstruction.[27] Subglottic stenosis may occur after cricothyroidotomy

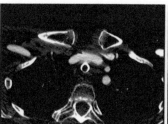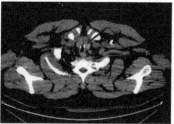

Fig. 4. Examples of postoperative complications after tracheostomy. Contrast-enhanced computed tomography (CT) angiogram showing luminal irregularity and evidence of fistulous tract between innominate artery and trachea (tracheoinnominate fistula, *left panel arrow*). Contrast-enhanced CT showing a tracheal "A-frame" stenosis (*right panel arrow*) that developed months after a tracheostomy.

if a tracheostomy tube is left in place across the cricothyroid membrane rather than the preferred location between the second and third tracheal rings (tracheostomy). For this reason, it is recommended that a cricothyroidotomy (which may be performed in an emergency setting) be converted to a formal tracheostomy.

OTOLOGY AND LATERAL SKULL BASE SURGERY

Benign and malignant processes of the outer, middle, and inner ear and lateral skull base uniquely impair human communication and social interaction through their impact on hearing, balance, and facial function. The principle domain of the otologic surgeon is the temporal bone, a pyramidal-shaped component of the lateral skull base that houses several precious neurovascular structures and sensory organs. Inadvertent surgical injury to any of these structures, including the sigmoid sinus, jugular bulb, internal carotid artery, facial nerve (CN VII), cochlea and semicircular canals, and temporal lobe dura, can cause tremendous morbidity and even death (**Box 3**).[28] Herein, we review complications of mastoidectomy, a common and representative otologic operation used in the surgical management of numerous temporal bone pathologies.

Mastoidectomy: Indications and Practices

Mastoidectomy may be indicated for the treatment of acute mastoiditis, chronic otitis media, and cholesteatoma, or may be performed for access to the deeper portions of the ear as required for cochlear implantation or treatment of diseases of the cerebellopontine angle and petrous apex of the temporal bone.[28] Performed for either scenario, a mastoidectomy entails the careful drill-out of bone and air cells of the mastoid cavity, respecting the integrity of the adjacent sigmoid sinus, skull base, temporal lobe, facial nerve, chorda tympani nerve, and ossicles.[28]

Box 3
Potential complications of otology and lateral skull base surgery

Sensory Organs
  Hearing loss due to cochlear injury (eg, drill acoustic trauma, labyrinthine fistula)
  Vertigo, disequilibrium, imbalance due to semicircular canal injury (eg, labyrinthine fistula)

Nervous
  Facial anesthesia, hypoesthesia, pain (CN V)
  Facial paralysis (CN VII)
  Taste disturbance (chorda tympani)
  Lower cranial nerve injury (CN IX, X)

Intracranial
  Dural tear
  CSF leak
  Brain abscess
  Subdural empyema
  Meningitis

Vascular
  Lateral sinus thrombosis
  Injury to sigmoid sinus, jugular bulb, internal carotid artery causing hemorrhage

Structural
  Ossicular chain disruption
  Tympanic membrane perforation
  External auditory canal stenosis

Mastoidectomy: complications and management

Owing to the heterogeneity of mastoidectomy approaches and indications, precise rates of individual postoperative complications are elusive. In many series, mastoidectomy is associated with the highest rate of iatrogenic facial nerve injury among any otologic surgery.[29] Revision surgeries, improper surgical technique, and anatomic variation in the course of the nerve through the mastoid may all predispose to iatrogenic nerve injury.[29] When an injury does occur, it often leads to disfiguring hemifacial paralysis. Prompt recognition is essential to allow for decompression of the nerve if transection has not occurred, or microsurgical repair or grafting of the nerve in cases of partial or complete transection. As stated previously, rigorous eye care is the foremost concern after iatrogenic facial nerve injury.

Other feared consequences of the middle ear or mastoid surgery include hearing loss and/or vestibular dysfunction. The prevalence of profound hearing loss or vestibular dysfunction after mastoidectomy for ear cholesteatoma is roughly 1% to 3%.[30] When these complications occur, early hearing rehabilitation with amplification or cochlear implant is warranted. Concomitant vertigo, imbalance, and disequilibrium warrant aggressive vestibular therapy.

PEDIATRIC OTOLARYNGOLOGY

In children of all ages, disorders of the ears, nose, and throat are among the most common reasons for primary care and emergency department visits and ambulatory surgeries.[31] General and pediatric otolaryngologists thus play a critical role in childhood health and development by treating a wide range of prevalent conditions, including hearing loss and otitis media, adenoid hypertrophy, upper respiratory infections, obstructive sleep apnea (OSA), and congenital craniofacial and airway abnormalities. Obtaining the trust of both the child and parent(s) is paramount in pediatric otolaryngology, as emotion, anxiety, and fear are high in the perioperative period. As such, unanticipated complications of ENT surgeries in children not only provokes physical pain and disability but also significant psychological distress to the entire family.

Tonsillectomy and Adenoidectomy: Indications and Practices

In the United States, combined excision of the palatine and adenoid tonsils remains one of the most common surgical procedures in children and adolescents.[32] The two principle indications for tonsillectomy and adenoidectomy are obstruction (OSA or sleep-disordered breathing) and infection (recurrent streptococcal pharyngitis or recurrent otitis media).

Tonsillectomy and adenoidectomy: complications and management

Expected sequelae of tonsillectomy and adenoidectomy include pain, reduced oral intake and activity level, and emotional irritability. True complications of tonsillectomy and adenoidectomy may include dehydration, hemorrhage, and respiratory compromise. Often the most important feared complication discussed, post-tonsillectomy hemorrhage occurs in 0.1% to 3% of children.[33] Postoperative bleeding may be more common in adolescents and is most likely to occur within 24 hours of surgery or on postoperative days 7 to 10.[34]

Children with mild post-tonsillectomy bleeding should at minimum be admitted for observation, as some bleeding will cease spontaneously. Those with significant bleeding should be taken to the operating room urgently for intubation and hemorrhage control with electrocautery due to risk of asphyxiation. For severe hemorrhage, aggressive fluid resuscitation, blood transfusion, and inhaled or topical tranexamic acid may be warranted.

Myringotomy and Tubes: Indications and Practices

Myringotomy and tympanostomy tube placement is indicated when long-term ventilation of the middle ear space is needed to treat recurrent acute or chronic otitis media and/or Eustachian tube dysfunction. Myringotomy and tympanostomy tube placement is a relatively benign procedure with potential tremendous benefit to the patient. The procedure effectively cures chronic ear disease in many patients, reduces pain of recurrent ear infections, and improves hearing during a crucial time for speech, language, and cognitive development.

Myringotomy and tubes: complications and management

Most complications of myringotomy and tube placement are mild, including transient tube otorrhea, premature tube extrusion, and persistent tympanic membrane perforation. Tube otorrhea, caused by a recurrent middle ear infection, occurs in roughly one-third of children.[35] Most cases are readily resolved with topical fluoroquinolone antibiotic drops.

Persistent tympanic membrane perforation after tympanostomy tube extrusion or removal occurs in 2% to 15% of patients.[35] Initially, observation may be appropriate, as most perforations will close spontaneously within 1 year. For persistent perforations and those causing hearing loss or recurrent middle ear infection, surgical repair with autologous fascia and/or cartilage may be warranted.

RHINOLOGY AND ANTERIOR SKULL BASE SURGERY

In the past several decades, tremendous advancements in endoscopic imaging and instrumentation have expanded the utility and safety of minimally invasive surgical approaches to the nasal cavity, paranasal sinuses, nasopharynx, and anterior skull base. Today, a diverse range of sinonasal pathologies including chronic rhinosinusitis, epistaxis, CSF leak, pituitary adenoma, and other benign and malignant tumors are treated with endoscopic surgical techniques by subspecialty-trained ENT surgeons. In rhinology and anterior skull base surgery, the most concerning postoperative complications relate to anatomic proximity of the orbit and optic nerve, anterior skull base and frontal lobe dura, and internal and external carotid artery vascular systems.

Endoscopic Sinus Surgery: Indications and Practices

With over 250,000 cases performed annually, endoscopic sinus surgery has rapidly become one of the commonest operations performed by otolaryngologists in the United States.[36] Endoscopic sinus surgery aims to restore normal mucosal health, drainage, and aeration of the nasal cavity and paranasal sinuses in carefully selected patients with chronic rhinosinusitis. Most commonly an ambulatory procedure, endoscopic sinus surgery usually permits a rapid postoperative recovery with minimal discomfort.

Endoscopic sinus surgery: complications and management

Most complications after endoscopic sinus surgery (eg, epistaxis, intranasal scarring, reduced smell) are minor and transient. Major complications are rare (ie, ≤1%) and can be separated into 3 groups based on anatomic structures involved: hemorrhage, orbit and optic nerve injury, and skull base and CSF leak.[37] Hemorrhage from the anterior ethmoidal or sphenopalatine artery may rarely occur postoperatively, leading to profuse epistaxis or periorbital hemorrhage with rapid compromise of vision. Anterior ethmoidal or sphenopalatine artery hemorrhage necessitates immediate return to the operating room for control of bleeding. Orbital complications of endoscopic sinus surgery include retrobulbar hematoma and direct injury to the extraocular muscles, nasolacrimal duct, globe, or optic nerve. Inadvertent fracture of the anterior skull base may lead to iatrogenic CSF leak and meningitis.[37] Prevention of all major complications of endoscopic sinus surgery relies on extensive knowledge of anatomic variation in bony and vascular anatomy and meticulous surgical technique. Complex sinus surgery is often performed with the aid of an image-guidance surgical navigation system to improve safety. When major complications do occur, prompt recognition is paramount. Typically, major complications require operative intervention (ie, Clavien-Dindo Grade III), often in consultation with ophthalmologic and neurosurgical specialists.

SLEEP SURGERY

OSA is defined by repeated episodes of upper airway collapse during sleep with associated sleep fragmentation and oxygen desaturations. The impact of OSA on quality of life and physical health is profound. Continuous positive airway pressure is extremely effective as first-line treatment for OSA, though compliance with routine use is challenging in many patients. A variety of sleep surgeries may be performed to treat OSA, depending on the level of obstruction identified. These include pharyngeal or lingual tonsillectomy, radiofrequency ablation of the tongue base, uvulopalatopharyngoplasty, septoplasty, genioglossus advancement with hyoid suspension, tracheostomy, and implantation of a hypoglossal nerve stimulator. Common complications of sleep surgeries include bleeding, which may be minor and self-limited, or may be dramatic requiring emergent return to the operating room to secure the airway and control hemorrhage. Sleep surgeries share important postoperative risks of cardiac and respiratory complications owing to altered physiology in patients affected by OSA, as well as common medical comorbidities.

Hypoglossal Nerve Stimulator: Indications and Practices

Hypoglossal nerve stimulator (CN XII) is one of the newest and most innovative surgical procedures in ENT surgery. In appropriately selected patients with OSA, hypoglossal nerve stimulator counteracts posterior collapse of the tongue base that contributes to upper airway obstruction during sleep.[38]

Hypoglossal nerve stimulator: complications and management

The vast majority of complications of hypoglossal nerve stimulator are minor and transient. In a recent randomized, controlled trial, tongue weakness (18%), tongue discomfort with stimulation (40%), and tongue soreness (21%) were the most common complications.[39] Most of these symptoms resolved after several months with adjustment of device settings.[39] Device malfunction and electrode dislodgement requiring repositioning or explant is rare.

SUMMARY

ENT surgery is an incredibly diverse surgical specialty with a storied history. Over the past two centuries, tremendous advancements in surgical training, expertise, and instrumentation and evidence-based approaches to appropriate patient selection have made ENT surgeries very safe and impactful for afflicted patients. However, when postoperative complications do occur, they may lead to visible disfigurement, cranial nerve deficits, hemorrhage, and impaired breathing, swallowing, voicing, hearing, and balance, among other profound effects.

DISCLOSURE

The authors have no conflicts of interest to disclose relevant to this article.

REFERENCES

1. Fenton RA. A brief history of otolaryngology in the United States from 1847 to 1947. Arch Otolaryngol 1947;46(2):153–62.
2. Bernal-Sprekelsen M, Carrau RL, Dazert S, et al. Complications in otolaryngology – head and neck surgery. New York: Thieme; 2013. p. 1–352.
3. Dindo D, Demartines N, Clavien P. Classification of surgical complications: a new proposal with evaluation in a cohort of 3663 patients and results of a survey. Ann Surg 2004;240(2):205–13.
4. Johnson DE, Burtness B, Leemans CR, et al. Head and neck squamous cell carcinoma. Nat Rev Dis Prim 2020;6:92.
5. Kovatch KJ, Hanks JE, Stevens JR, et al. Current practices in microvascular reconstruction in otolaryngology – head and neck surgery. Laryngoscope 2019; 129(1):138–45.
6. Ruohoalho J, Makitie AA, Aro K, et al. Complications after surgery for benign parotid gland neoplasms: a prospective cohort study. Head Neck 2017;39(1):170–6.
7. Haring CT, Ellsperman SE, Edwards BM, et al. Assessment of intraoperative nerve monitoring parameters associated with facial nerve outcome in parotidectomy for benign disease. JAMA Otolaryngol Head Neck Surg 2019;145(12):1137–43.
8. Sood AJ, Houlton JJ, Nguyen SA, et al. Facial nerve monitoring during parotidectomy: a systematic review and meta-analysis. Otolaryngol Head Neck Surg 2015; 152(4):631–7.
9. Joseph AW, Kim JC. Management of flaccid facial paralysis of less than two years' duration. Otolaryngol Clin North Am 2018;51(6):1093–105.
10. Li C, Wu F, Zhang Q, et al. Interventions for the treatment of Frey's syndrome. Cochrane Database Syst Rev 2015;3:CD009959.
11. Robbins KT, Medina JE, Wolfe GT, et al. Standardizing neck dissection terminology: official report of the Academy's Committee for Head and Neck Surgery and Oncology. Arch Otolaryngol Head Neck Surg 1991;117(6):601–5.
12. Remmler D, Byers R, Scheetz J, et al. A prospective study of shoulder disability resulting from radical and modified neck dissections. Head Neck Surg 1986;8: 280–6.
13. Proctor E, Robbins KT, Vieira F, et al. Postoperative complications after chemoradiation for advanced head and neck cancer. Head Neck 2004;26(3):272–7.
14. Harris AS. Do patients benefit from physiotherapy for shoulder dysfunction following neck dissection? A systematic review. J Laryngol Otol 2020;134(2): 104–8.
15. Crumley RL, Smith JD. Postoperative chylous fistula prevention and management. Laryngoscope 1976;86:804–13.
16. Chuang J, Barnes C, Wong BJF. Overview of facial plastic surgery and current developments. Surg J 2016;2:e17–28.
17. Joseph AW, Joseph SS. Mohs reconstruction and scar revision. Otolaryngol Clin N Am 2019;52:461–71.
18. Namin A, Shokri T, Vincent A, et al. Complications in facial esthetic surgery. Semin Plast Surg 2020;34:272–6.
19. Miller MQ, David AP, McLean JE, et al. Association of Mohs reconstructive surgery timing with postoperative complications. JAMA Facial Plast Surg 2018; 20(2):122–7.

20. Neuner RA, Sclafani AP, Minkis K, et al. Patient, defect, and surgical factors influencing use of ancillary procedures after facial Mohs repairs. Facial Plast Surg 2021. https://doi.org/10.1055/s-0040-1721100.
21. Sclafani AP, Thomas JR, Tardy ME. Rhinoplasty. In: Cumming's otolaryngology head and neck surgery. Philadelphia: Elsevier; 2021. p. 470–509.
22. Surowitz JB, Most SP. Complications of rhinoplasty. Facial Plast Surg Clin N Am 2013;21:639–51.
23. Layliev J, Gupta V, Kaoutzanis C, et al. Incidence and preoperative risk factors for major complications in aesthetic rhinoplasty: analysis of 4978 patients. Aesth Surg J 2017;37(7):757–67.
24. Jackson C. Tracheotomy. Laryngoscope 1909;19(4):285–90.
25. Cheung NH, Napolitano LM. Tracheostomy: epidemiology, indications, timing, technique, and outcomes. Respir Care 2014;59(6):895–919.
26. Spataro E, Durakovic N, Kallogjeri D, et al. Complications and 30-day hospital readmission rates of patients undergoing tracheostomy: a prospective analysis. Laryngoscope 2017;127(12):2746–53.
27. Streitz JM Jr, Shapshay SM. Airway injury after tracheotomy and endotracheal intubation. Surg Clin North Am 1991;71:1211–30.
28. Mancini F, Taibah AK, Falcioni M. Complications and their management in tympanomastoid surgery. Otolaryngol Clin North Am 1999;32:567–83.
29. Hohman MH, Bhama PK, Hadlock TA. Epidemiology of iatrogenic facial nerve injury: a decade of experience. Laryngoscope 2013;124(1):260–5.
30. Prinsley P. An audit of "dead ear" after ear surgery. J Laryngol Otol 2013;127(12): 1177–83.
31. Montalbano A, Rodean J, Kangas J, et al. Urgent care and emergency department visits in the pediatric Medicaid population. Pediatrics 2016;137(4): e20153100.
32. Hall MJ, Schwartzman A, Zhang J, et al. Ambulatory surgery data from hospitals and ambulatory surgery centers: United States, 2010. Natl Health Stat Rep 2017; 102:1–15.
33. De Luca Canto G, Pacheco-Pereira C, Aydinoz S, et al. Adenotonsillectomy complications: A meta-analysis. Pediatrics 2015;136(4):702–18.
34. Chang JE, Shapiro NL, Bhattacharyya N. Do demographic disparities exist in the diagnosis and surgical management of otitis media? Laryngoscope 2018; 128(12):2898–901.
35. Kay DJ, Nelson M, Rosenfeld RM. Meta-analysis of tympanostomy tube sequelae. Otolaryngol Head Neck Surg 2001;124(4):374–80.
36. Pynnonen MA, Davis MM. Extent of sinus surgery, 2000 – 2009: a population-based study. Laryngoscope 2014;820–5.
37. Stankiewicz JA, Lal D, Connor M, et al. Complications in endoscopic sinus surgery for chronic rhinosinusitis: a 25-year experience. Laryngoscope 2011;121: 2684–701.
38. Yu JL, Thaler ER. Hypoglossal nerve (cranial nerve XII) stimulation. Otolaryngol Clin North Am 2020;53(1):157–69.
39. Strollo PJ Jr, Soose RJ, Maurer JT, et al. Upper-airway stimulation for obstructive sleep apnea. N Engl J Med 2014;370:139–49.

Breast Surgery
Management of Postoperative Complications Following Operations for Breast Cancer

Zahraa Al-Hilli, MD, FRCSI*, Avia Wilkerson, MD

KEYWORDS

- Breast cancer surgery • Axillary surgery • Postoperative complications • Morbidity

KEY POINTS

- Breast cancer surgery without reconstruction postoperative complications will be reviewed in this chapter.
- Complications from breast cancer surgery may occur within the breast, at the lumpectomy or mastectomy site, or within the axilla after axillary surgery.
- Severity and prevalence of postoperative complications related to breast cancer surgery is variable and significantly procedure-related.
- Management of postoperative complications may be conservative or operative depending on severity of symptoms and their impact on patients' quality of life.

INTRODUCTION

Breast cancer is the most common cancer diagnosed among women in the Unites States and globally.[1] The American Cancer Society has estimated that 333,490 new cases of breast cancer (invasive and in situ) will be diagnosed in women and men and an estimated 44,130 breast cancer deaths will be recorded in 2021.[2]

The therapeutic options and management strategies for breast cancer are complex and ever evolving.[3] Despite advances in adjuvant therapeutic options, surgery remains the mainstay treatment for patients with early-stage and locally advanced breast cancer. The surgical options for the management of breast cancer include lumpectomy or mastectomy, in addition to axillary staging (sentinel) lymph node biopsy (SLNB) or axillary lymph node dissection (ALND). The equivalence of survival outcomes for mastectomy compared with breast-conserving therapy (lumpectomy with whole-breast irradiation) has been established in multiple prospective randomized trials with long-term follow-up.[4–7] Patient preference is a critical component of the decision-making process for surgery, and a multidisciplinary approach is paramount in achieving optimal oncologic and surgical outcomes. Both lumpectomy and

Department of General Surgery, Digestive Diseases and Surgery Institute, Cleveland Clinic, 9500 Euclid Avenue /A80, Cleveland, OH 44195, USA
* Corresponding author.
E-mail address: alhillz@ccf.org

Surg Clin N Am 101 (2021) 845–863
https://doi.org/10.1016/j.suc.2021.06.014
0039-6109/21/© 2021 Elsevier Inc. All rights reserved.

surgical.theclinics.com

mastectomy may be coupled with reconstructive options to enhance cosmetic outcomes and improve quality of life for patients.

Breast cancer surgery is associated with low rates of surgical morbidity. However, it is important to acknowledge that accurate acute and chronic complication rates may be challenging to identify because of variations in reporting and duration of follow-up. The management of postoperative complications related to breast and axillary surgery for breast cancer are reviewed here. Breast cancer surgery with reconstruction has expanded in recent years; however, the management of specific reconstruction-related complications is not discussed in this article.

POSTOPERATIVE COMPLICATIONS ASSOCIATED WITH BREAST SURGERY

The reported complication rates after breast cancer surgery are low, with rates ranging from 2% to 50%, and are reportedly more common when performed in conjunction with axillary surgery and immediate breast reconstruction.[8–11] A breakdown by procedure type has shown morbidity rates between 5% and 50% after mastectomy and from 3% to 35% after lumpectomy with or without reconstruction.[12–14]

Seroma

Seroma after breast surgery is defined as a collection of fluid that develops in the dead space beneath the mastectomy skin flaps, within the lumpectomy cavity, or within nodal sampling site of the axilla. The cause of seroma formation is hypothesized to be multifactorial.[15–22] Acute inflammation from surgical trauma may result in fibrinolytic activity in the serum and lymph, inciting the formation of exudate. In addition, factors such as use of electrocautery, extent of dissection, body mass index, lymph node status and number of nodes removed, duration and amount of drainage, and prolonged shoulder immobilization have also been revealed as contributors.[15–23]

Seroma is a common finding after breast surgery, with rates ranging from 3% to 85%.[24–29] In addition to patient discomfort and anxiety, seroma formation poses a risk for wound breakdown, skin flap necrosis, infection, decreased shoulder mobility, and delay in adjuvant treatment. Therefore, the prevention or management of a significant seroma remains a goal for all breast surgeries. Several techniques have been used to eliminate dead space after breast and axillary surgery in order to reduce seroma formation. These techniques include the use of external compression, suction drainage, quilting/flap fixation, fibrin sealants, and shoulder immobilization.

From an operative perspective, the use of cautery and thermal devices has been identified as contributing to the development of seroma to varying degrees.[16] This link has been shown in several randomized trials and retrospective reviews comparing electrocautery with scalpel.[17] Some studies have also investigated the use of laser scalpels, argon diathermy, and ultrasonic scalpel, which reduced or caused no seroma formation.[30,31]

The data regarding the application of mechanical pressure have been conflicting.[32] Despite this, many surgeons recommend postoperative mechanical pressure using wraps or compression in addition to limitation of arm abduction greater than 90° and delay in extensive physical activity.[33,34]

Suction drains are frequently used to prevent seroma formation after mastectomy and ALND and uncommonly in the setting of lumpectomy and SLNB. This practice is supported by trials showing that the omission of drains was associated with higher seroma formation and recurrence rates as well as greater seroma volumes. In contrast, other studies have suggested no difference seroma formation in drain-free mastectomy compared with suction drain usage.[35,36] There has been no benefit shown with the use of 1 versus multiple drains or low-suction versus high-suction drainage.[37–39] The optimal timing for drain removal remains controversial, although it is generally dictated by the volume of drainage before removal. Most surgeons prefer volumes lower than 20 to 50 mL within 24 to 48 hours.

Quilting or flap fixation is another commonly used technique for the prevention of seroma after mastectomy. Several techniques have been described, and each essentially involves fixing the skin flaps to the underlying pectoralis muscle with sutures with the goal of minimizing dead space. These methods have been shown to successfully reduce seroma rates compared with controls, from 29% to 81% in control cases to 10% to 36%.[40–44] The combination of suction drainage and quilting has shown reduction in seroma formation as well as potential for omitting the use of suction drains.

Fibrin sealants are biologic hemostasis agents that influence the coagulation cascade. They have been found in some cases to aid in obliterating dead space; however, data supporting their use have been inconclusive. As such, they are not widely used.

There is limited data guiding a standard management strategy for established seromas.[45] Typically, smaller asymptomatic seromas may be observed. The presence of symptoms such as discomfort or increasing swelling can prompt the need for aspiration. This procedure can be performed by clinical palpation guidance or, more commonly and precisely, with ultrasonography guidance. Repeat aspiration may be indicated for recurrent seromas. It must be acknowledged that the risk associated with seroma aspiration or repeated aspiration is the introduction of pathogens, resulting in potential infection at the aspiration site. Several studies have suggested a causal relationship between the duration of drainage and need for multiple aspirations with the development of a surgical site infection.[24,46] An infected seroma requires definitive drainage and antibiotics. In some instances, seromas become chronic despite repeat aspirations, and their management can be challenging. In this setting, reinsertion of a drain, use of agents to promote adhesion of the cavity, or surgical intervention may be warranted. Sclerosing agents have been injected into seroma cavities to promote adhesion to the chest wall with varying or limited benefit. Examples of such agents include talc, tetracycline, saline, and iodine.[47–50] Failure of seroma resolution and persistence of symptoms warrants surgical intervention, including scoring or diathermy of the capsule or excision and repeat closure.[51]

Infection

Surgical site infections (SSIs) account for 2% to 19% of breast surgery–related complications.[11,52] The rates may vary according to type of surgery, reporting accuracy, and patient-related factors (obesity, diabetes, smoking, renal failure, prior radiation, skin disorders). The occurrence of this complication can result in prolonged hospitalization, poor patient satisfaction, delay in treatment time for adjuvant therapy, and increase in cost of treatment.

Although surgeries involving the breast are generally considered clean procedures, SSI rates are found to range from 1.4% to 19% after breast cancer surgery.[53–58] A study by de Blacam and colleagues,[54] using data from the National Surgical Quality Improvement Program (NSQIP) and evaluating 26,988 patient outcomes after lumpectomy and mastectomy, showed that the overall 30-day morbidity rate after all procedures was 5.6%, with the most common complication being superficial and deep SSIs. Independent risk factors for development of any wound infection in patients undergoing mastectomy were high body mass index (BMI), smoking, and diabetes (odds ratios [ORs] = 1.8, 1.6 and 1.8 respectively). Similarly, high BMI and smoking were also associated with increased risk of infection in patients undergoing lumpectomy (ORs = 1.7 and 1.9).

Previous data have shown that prophylactic antibiotics can decrease risk for SSIs. Within breast surgery, data from randomized trials and other studies addressing the use of prophylactic antibiotics have been conflicting.[59,60] Recommendations for antibiotics prophylaxis include the administration within 1 hour of surgical incision, use of an antibiotic consistent with published guideless, and discontinuation within 24 hours postoperatively.[61] Recommendations by the American Society of Breast Surgeons (ASBrS) regarding the use of perioperative prophylactic antibiotics in breast surgery are summarized in **Box 1**.[62]

SSI after breast surgery may present with minor cellulitis at the incision site that is amenable to treatment with a course of oral antibiotics. In the setting of more severe infection that presents with more extensive cellulitis or systemic symptoms, intravenous antibiotics are necessary. If there is clinical concern, it is imperative to rule out the presence a deep collection or abscess, which may be apparent on clinical examination with detection of fluctuance, tenderness, and swelling at the site. Breast ultrasonography is helpful; however, clinicians must be cognizant that the appearance of a collection or abscess can mimic that of a hematoma or organizing seroma. In this setting, a diagnostic aspiration may confirm the diagnosis. The management of an abscess requires incision, drainage, and allowing the wound to then heal by secondary intention. Microbiology assessment and culture of the fluid can guide further antibiotic treatment.

Box 1

American Society of Breast Surgeons consensus recommendations on preoperative antibiotics and surgical site infection in breast surgery[63]

ASBrS consensus recommendations on preoperative prophylactic antibiotics (PPAs) and SSI in breast surgery.

1. PPAs are indicated in patients undergoing mastectomy, with or without any type of axillary dissection or reconstruction, to lower the risk of SSI.

2. PPAs may be indicated in patients undergoing partial mastectomy for cancer, with or without sentinel lymph node biopsy or axillary dissection.

3. Oral antibiotics or PPAs may be considered in patients undergoing brachytherapy catheter device placement for accelerated partial breast irradiation.

4. PPAs may be used in patients undergoing simple surgical excisional biopsy, especially if specific patient or clinical risk factors for SSI are present.

5. A first-generation cephalosporin is the PPA of choice, unless the patient is allergic or has a history of prior infection with methicillin-resistant *Staphylococcus aureus*.

6. Continuation of antibiotics after the initial PPA is discouraged unless there is a specific clinical indication.

7. If SSI occurs, aerobic and anaerobic cultures should be obtained and sensitivity of any available SSI fluid should be determined. Culture and sensitivity reports should prompt appropriate changes in antibiotic management.

8. If SSI rates are used as a quality measure (QM), then standardized ascertainment measures and definitions should be used, as well as appropriate risk adjustment.

9. The ASBrS supports enrollment of patients into well-designed clinical trials regarding methods to improve the rate of breast-related SSI because reported breast SSI rates are usually higher than other "clean" cases.

Hematoma

A hematoma may accumulate within a surgical bed once wound edges have been reapproximated and sutured close. Although currently less common than before the standard use of electrocautery devices, postoperative bleeding remains the most common cause of reoperation after surgery for breast cancer, reported in up to 11% of patients.[64] An NSQIP data study found that 1.3% of patients who underwent breast cancer surgery required re-operation for bleeding (0.4% for lumpectomy without reconstruction, 1.9% for mastectomy without reconstruction, 1.9% for mastectomy with immediate reconstruction, and 1.2% for lumpectomy with reconstruction).[65] The mean number of days from the index operation to reoperation was slightly less than 4 days for hematoma compared with 17 days for seroma, infection, and other wound complications.

Risk for postoperative bleeding must be balanced with need for thromboembolic prophylaxis in the setting of malignancy and need for nonnarcotic analgesia. For example, use of low-molecular-weight heparin was found to be significantly associated with postoperative hematoma.[66] In addition to venous thromboembolism (VTE) prophylaxis, other medications, such as aspirin and nonsteroidal antiinflammatory drugs, have been shown to increase postoperative bleeding when used in the perioperative setting.[33,67] Although some studies have suggested increased risk for postoperative bleeding with increasingly used intravenous ketorolac (Toradol), other studies failed to find an increased bleeding risk of statistical significance compared with patient cohorts that did not receive this analgesic postoperatively.[68]

Management of postoperative breast hematomas is contingent on the extent of bleeding.[69] Although small hematomas typically do not require surgical intervention and reabsorb over time, larger hematomas resulting from active bleeding or significant oozing within the surgical site may quickly expand and necessitate return to the operating room for breast exploration, hematoma evacuation, and attainment of hemostasis.[70] Actively bleeding vessels are ligated, but are often not found during reoperation. After hemostasis is achieved, the surgical wound is irrigated copiously and then closed. Close monitoring of postoperative breast hematomas is essential, because they carry a higher risk for wound infection.

Mastectomy Flap Necrosis

Mastectomy flap necrosis (MSFN) is a common complication that presents either as partial-thickness or full-thickness flap necrosis. Its reported incidence within the literature ranges from 5% to 30%, in part because of its variable onset and presentation.[71] MSFN results when the supply of blood flow from perforators of the axillary, internal thoracic artery, and second through fourth intercostal arteries, which coalesce to form a subdermal arterial plexus, does not meet the metabolic demand of the skin flaps.[72] Significant postoperative morbidity may result from MSFN, such as infection or extrusion of reconstructive implants, as well as significant challenges to patient management, such as delay in the initiation of adjuvant therapy.

Given the heterogeneity of MSFN with regard to depth and severity of necrosis, the SKIN (Skin Ischemia and Necrosis) scoring system was developed by Lemaine and colleagues[73] for patients following mastectomy with reconstruction. SKIN scores for depth are divided into 4 categories ranging from A (no skin flap injury) to D (full-thickness necrosis). A score of B indicates cyanosis or erythema of the skin flap indicating ischemia without necrosis. A score of C indicates partial-thickness necrosis with at least epidermal sloughing. For surface area, SKIN scores are divided into 4 categories with regard to the breast skin or nipple areolar complex: 1 (none), 2 (1%–10%), 3

(11%–30%), and 4 (>30%). In the study that established this scoring system, SKIN scores offered significant discrimination in predicting need for reoperation for MSFN. No participants with composite scores of A1 to B4 required operation compared with 44.1% and 57.1% of those with composite scores of D3 and D4.

Several risk factors for MSFN have been identified, including smoking, because nicotine propagates vasoconstriction and inhibits endothelial cell–dependent vasodilation, putting skin flaps with already fragile blood supply at significant risk.[71] Accordingly, smoking cessation should be emphasized. Patients who underwent ipsilateral lumpectomy before mastectomy have also shown to have increased risk; this is thought to be caused by dermal changes from previous radiation. In addition to smoking and preoperative radiation, other studies found that BMI greater than 30, history of breast augmentation, diabetes, and nipple-sparing mastectomy were risk factors for MSFN.[9,74] Surgical technique may also increase MSFN risk. For example, Wise pattern incisions, decreased flap thickness, immediate reconstruction for large breast volumes, and use of nipple-sparing mastectomy techniques have all shown higher risk for MSFN.[71] As such, patient selection and optimization as well as meticulous surgical planning based on patient factors and history should be considered.

Nonoperative management remains the preferred treatment of MSFN following simple mastectomy.[71] A conservative management strategy involves permitting areas of necrosis to slough and heal via secondary intention. Dressing changes and topical agents such as silver nitrate to minimize bacterial burden may be used to promote improvement in wound appearance.[75] Eschar covering smaller surface areas may be debrided in an outpatient setting. Wound management systems and hyperbaric oxygen have shown success in previous studies. Skin grafts are reserved for cases in which there is massive skin necrosis. Operative management involves debridement of necrotic tissue with reparative wound closure, including primary closure via suturing versus skin grafting depending on the extent of skin loss.

Wound Dehiscence

The partial or complete separation of approximated surgical wound edges, wound dehiscence, is one of the most prevalent noninfectious wound complications after mastectomy; it is the most common after hematoma.[76] Wound dehiscence is more prevalent after mastectomy with flap creation plus reconstructive implant, followed by mastectomy plus reconstructive implant alone. Similarly, it is expectedly more common with simple mastectomy than partial mastectomy/lumpectomy. Of note, wound dehiscence can be precipitated by aforementioned complications such as seroma superinfection, which may cause flap necrosis that results in the separation of wound edges. As such, avoidance of seroma formation and preservation of adequate blood supply of the remaining breast skin are important practices in reducing risk for wound dehiscence. Both patient-related and treatment-related factors that affect tissue remodeling and wound healing may predispose patients to wound dehiscence.[77] For example, patient-related factors affecting tissue integrity, such as advanced age, malnutrition, obesity, smoking, immunocompromised state, and use of steroidal or immunosuppressive drugs, may increase risk for poor wound healing, as may technical factors such as inadequate preservation of skin perfusion and excessive tension at approximated wound edges.[78] Other postoperative complications, such as SSI, can also predispose patients to wound separation.

Wound dehiscence most often occurs 5 to 8 days postoperatively. Secondary closure has shown to foster faster healing time and requires shorter postoperative follow-up than healing by secondary intention.[79] Although negative pressure wound systems may improve outcomes for healing by secondary intension, there is insufficient data to conclude the efficacy of this strategy compared with secondary closure.[80]

Persistent Breast Pain

Persistent postsurgical pain (PPSP) after breast cancer surgery refers to clinical patient discomfort that lasts more than 2 months postsurgery in the absence of primary causes such as chronic infection or localized pain that preceded the surgery. The quality and intensity of PPSP are largely different than postoperative pain, often characterized by burning or lancing sensations. Of breast cancer operations, PPSP has classically been associated with mastectomy, inspiring establishment of the term postmastectomy pain syndrome.[81,82] However, it is notably also common after lumpectomy. A recent meta-analysis of PPSP after breast cancer surgery found that 46% of patients experienced PPSP at any involved location, with about 27% of those women developing PPSP with severity classified as moderate to severe.[83] PPSP is more common after ALND, likely because of injury or sacrificing of the intercostobrachial nerve.[82] Preservation of the intercostobrachial nerve was found to diminish the likelihood of developing postmastectomy pain syndrome, reduce the pain intensity in those who did go on to develop PPSP, and reduce the incidence of sensory deficits after ALND.

Previously identified risk factors for PPSP have included younger age at diagnosis and treatment, high BMI, large tumor size, adjuvant radiation and/or chemotherapy, poor coping skills, and depression.[84] Several management strategies may be used to prevent or treat PPSP after breast cancer surgery.[85] For example, paravertebral blocks in addition to general anesthesia may be used preoperatively and perioperatively.[86] Exercise therapy, psychological or behavioral interventions, serotonin reuptake inhibitors, and other antidepressants such as amitriptyline have all been used with some, but inconsistent, success in treating patients with PPSP.[87,88]

Mondor Disease

Mondor disease is a syndrome characterized by sclerosing superficial thrombophlebitis of the anterior thoracic wall venous structures, most commonly involving the superior epigastric vein, which produces a palpable cord in the lower outer breast quadrant.[89,90] The cause is diverse and has ranged from idiopathic to local trauma or surgery involving the breast and/or chest wall to conditions resulting in damage or stagnation of involved veins, such as excessively compressive brassiers.[89] Mondor disease may involve not only breast but the axilla as well (known as axillary web syndrome) and has been documented following ALND as well as SLNB of the axilla.[91]

The natural history of Mondor disease is self-limiting.[92] Diagnosis may be achieved clinically via patient history and physical examination but may also be aided with ultrasonography of the palpable and/or tender area in cases that are less clear. Positive cases show ultrasonographic evidence of a hypoechoic structure representing the affected superficial vein. Doppler should show an absence of flow within the affected vein with or without the presence of an intraluminal thrombus.[93] Of note, Mondor disease may be variable in presentation but never involves the upper inner portion of the breast. Treatment is supportive and includes warm compresses, use of nonsteroidal inflammatory medications for pain control, and avoidance of compressive clothing and exacerbating activities. Treatment with antiplatelet therapy such as aspirin or anticoagulation with heparin is typically not warranted.

Fat Necrosis

Fat necrosis represents scar tissue that forms secondary to a localized ischemia of breast tissue and resulting nonviable adipose cells.[94] Although most commonly resulting from trauma, it may also result from breast biopsies or surgeries, both oncologic and elective. It often presents as a benign palpable nodule. Notably, fat necrosis may also occur independent of any breast trauma or instrumentation, such as secondary to malignancy-related inflammation.[95] The clinical significance of fat necrosis ranges from suboptimal cosmetic outcomes to its potential to complicate the interpretation of breast imaging and the development of palpable masses, which may be particularly distressing for this patient cohort. The prevalence and significance of fat necrosis may differ according to the oncologic procedure performed. For example, mastectomy and reconstruction with autologous flaps is associated with higher rates of fat necrosis after radiation than simple mastectomy or lumpectomy.[96]

The natural history of fat necrosis is variable, because some lesions resolve spontaneously or regress whereas others remain stable or enlarge. Surgical intervention is typically not required unless the lesion causes significant pain or distortion of the breast contour. Fat necrosis can be followed with imaging. If imaging is concerning and suspicion for malignancy is high, a core needle biopsy should be performed, with subsequent excisional biopsy if pathology is indeterminate or discordant with imaging findings. Aspiration may alleviate discomfort if fat necrosis is associated with oily material known as an oil cyst, which represents degenerate adipose tissue.

Venous Thromboembolism

VTE following breast surgery is very uncommon, with reported postoperative deep venous thrombosis rates between 0.16% and 0.4%.[97,98] Similar to other surgery types, the longer duration of operation associated with mastectomy and autologous reconstruction or mastectomy with immediate reconstruction confers a higher risk of VTE than lumpectomy.[99,100] Other risk factors include older age (>65 years), obesity, history of chemotherapy, increased duration of hospital stay, and recent surgery within 30 days.[101,102] There is a lack of evidence on the effectiveness and benefit of VTE prophylaxis for breast cancer surgery. It is recommended that decisions regarding VTE prophylaxis are individualized and take into consideration type of procedure, duration, anesthesia type, prior history of VTE, hypercoagulability, and risk of bleeding.[62] Patients in the ambulatory setting who undergo procedures with local or regional anesthesia do not require VTE prophylaxis. Early ambulation and sequential compression devices should be routine. Prophylactic anticoagulation should be considered for procedures lasting longer than 3 hours, in patients with increased Caprini scores (>5) who are not high risk for bleeding complications, and for patients undergoing mastectomy with immediate reconstruction. VTE prophylaxis is recommended for all patients undergoing mastectomy with autologous reconstruction unless there is a specific medical contraindication.[62] The relationship between VTE prophylaxis and risk of hematoma formation, reoperation, and need for transfusion is unclear. The risk of unplanned return to the operating room for a hematoma (~2%) should be weighed against the benefit of VTE prophylaxis.[65]

POSTOPERATIVE COMPLICATIONS ASSOCIATED WITH AXILLARY SURGERY

Axillary surgery staging and management options include SLNB and ALND. The postoperative complications related to these procedures include seroma, infection, lymphedema, nerve injury, and shoulder/arm morbidity. The overall rate of complications related to axillary surgery may be confounded by the type of breast surgery performed.

Seroma

ALND carries greater association with seroma development than SLNB. Furthermore, extent of breast surgery (mastectomy vs breast conservation) can also contribute to differences in rates of seroma formation. In a study by Boostrom and colleagues,[24] the overall seroma rate among 561 patients undergoing breast or axillary surgery was 8.4%. By procedure, rate of seroma formation was 2.1% for SLNB alone and 5.7% for ALND alone. The rate for mastectomy with SLNB was 16.2% compared with 7.7% with mastectomy and ALND. Patients in the mastectomy and SLNB group were considered to have seromas at the mastectomy site rather than within the axilla.

Management strategies for seromas in the axilla are similar to those described for breast seromas. Suction drainage at the axilla is usually initiated at the time of surgery for patients undergoing ALND, but is not typically used for SLNB. In a systematic review of randomized controlled trials evaluating the efficacy of drain use after ALND, He and colleagues[103] showed that axillary drain usage after breast surgery resulted in a reduction of seroma formation (OR, 0.36; 95% confidence interval [CI], 0.16–0.81, $P = .001$), volume of aspiration when required ($P = .008$), and frequency of aspiration ($P<.00001$). In patients undergoing mastectomy, 1 drain is typically placed in the axillary bed and a second drain in the mastectomy cavity. If an axillary seroma is identified postoperatively, repeat aspiration is the most commonly used approach, with drain placement, sclerotherapy, or capsulotomy reserved for recurrent/persistent seromas.

Lymphedema

Breast cancer–related lymphedema (BCRL) represents a significant source of postoperative morbidity, affecting quality of life and increasing health care–related costs. Lymphedema results from the obstruction or destruction of the lymphatic system during cancer-related treatment, resulting in the accumulation of interstitial fluid and the development of soft tissue edema and distortion.[104] The reported incidence of BCRL varies, with rates up to 40% in patients undergoing combination therapy with surgery, radiation, and systemic therapy.[105–112] Rates in patients undergoing tumor resection and SLNB alone have been reported up to 8%.[108–112]

Lymphedema awareness and education is increasingly accepted as an important component of survivorship for patients with breast cancer. Several societies have advocated for patient evaluation by lymphedema professionals where indicated and for the incorporation of exercise for those at risk or who experience lymphedema.[113] Stages of lymphedema as described by the International Society of Lymphology are shown in **Table 1**.[114]

Several techniques can be used for diagnosis, including bioimpedance spectroscopy, circumferential tape measurement, perometry, tissue dielectric constant,

Table 1 International Society of Lymphology lymphedema staging[114]	
Stage	Evidence
0	Subclinical; absence of edema in risk development patient
1	Presence of edema reduced by treatment or arm elevation (pitting edema)
2	Edema partially reduced by treatment (pitting and nonpitting edema), intractable and progressive
3	Elephantiasis with skin lesions and relapsing infections

ultrasonography, and water displacement methods. Baseline measurements preoperatively with follow-up measurements of both the ipsilateral and contralateral arms postoperatively are recommended.[105]

Lymphedema prevention strategies at the time of surgery are increasingly used. Axillary reverse mapping (ARM) is one of the more commonly used techniques and involves mapping the upper arm lymphatics with blue dye at the time of SLNB or ALND in order to differentiate between the breast nodes (nodes draining technetium-99) and preserve the arm nodes (blue dye).[115] This technique has been found to reduce the rate of lymphedema development compared with other standard approaches.[116,117] A caution and limitation of this technique is that crossover nodes carry a risk of harboring lymph node metastases.[117] In addition to preservation of arm lymphatics, this technique allows for the possibility of reapproximation of the afferent and efferent lymphatics after removal of lymph nodes.

Primary prevention surgery techniques are showing great promise and are increasingly adopted for patients undergoing planned ALND. Lymphaticovenous bypass is a microsurgical technique that reroutes lymphatic fluid into the venous system via anastomosis of divided lymphatics with proximal recipient veins and has also been used for the treatment of established lymphedema. Immediate lymphatic reconstruction has evolved, with a current goal of reestablishing upper extremity lymphatic drainage at the time of initial axillary surgery. This technique involves the identification of target veins and assessing for size match, proximity to lymphatic structure, excursion, and valvular competency.[118] Transected blue dye containing lymphatics are carefully mobilized under high-power loupe or microscopic visualization. In the instance of precise size match and availability of a single transected lymphatic, an end-to-end microanastomotic technique is used. When significant size discrepancy exists between the lymphatic and recipient vein (1:3), or if there are multiple transected lymphatics in proximity to a recipient vein, an intussusception technique is used for the anastomosis. A systematic review and meta-analysis of studies treating patients with prophylactic lymphovenous anastomoses showed a reduction in lymphedema incidence (relative risk [RR], 0.33; 95% CI, 0.19–0.56) compared with patients receiving no prophylactic treatment ($P<.0001$).[119]

The lymphatic microsurgical preventive healing approach (LYMPHA) is another described approach. This techniques involved dunking the transected main blue lymphatics trunks identified using ARM into a lateral branch of the axillary vein distal to a competent valve.[120] Reports of this technique have shown lower lymphedema rates compared with controls.[120,121] Although necessitating increased operative time, the techniques described here are not associated with significant complications.

The development of lymphedema after breast cancer surgery can be managed with combined decongestive therapy, which consists of manual lymphatic drainage, gradient compression bandaging, therapeutic exercises, and skin care (see **Table 1**).[113,122] Lymphaticovenous bypass surgery and lymph node transfer procedures have been described in conjunction with these techniques in comprehensive management strategies for lymphedema.[122–124]

Nerve Injury

The risk of nerve injury after ALND is low. Potential nerve injuries include injury to the long thoracic nerve resulting in winged scapula, injury to the thoracodorsal nerve resulting in weakness of shoulder adduction and internal rotation, injury to the medial pectoral nerve resulting in atrophy of the lateral aspect pectoralis muscle, and transection of the intercostobrachial nerves, which can result in numbness and paresthesia of the upper inner arm. Meticulous surgical technique with careful identification and avoidance of these structures can prevent these injuries.

Arm Morbidity

Arm/shoulder-related morbidity is a common and underreported complication following axillary surgery. Shoulder stiffness is a common complaint that can result from limited range of movement after surgery. This stiffness can affect quality of life and ability to complete activities of daily living. A study by Kwan and colleagues[125] aimed to determine the prevalence of contributing factors for chronic arm morbidity after breast cancer treatment and to measure the impact of impaired arm morbidity on quality of life. In 744 patients with at least 2 years of follow-up, approximately half of all screened patients were symptomatic for arm or shoulder problems, with ALND and radiation therapy found to be significantly related to the occurrence of arm symptoms (detected in up to 70%). Similar findings have been reported by other groups, with the most common symptoms including numbness, pain, weakness, and decreased function.[126–129] Physical therapy and exercise programs after breast cancer surgery are helpful in the prevention and management of decreased arm and shoulder function.

Axilla web is another finding that can be seen after axillary surgery. These webs are bands of scar tissue that develop after ALND and present in a cordlike fashion throughout the axilla and surgical bed, and can extend toward the forearm or thumb. Physical therapy and massage therapy can be helpful in managing this problem.

Blue dye complications

Sentinel lymph node biopsy is the standard of care for axillary staging in clinically node-negative breast cancer. Tracers used for sentinel lymph node mapping include technetium-99–labeled colloid, diluted methylene blue dye, isosulfan blue, or newer agents such as indocyanine green. Side effects associated with methylene blue dye include temporary tattooing of the skin and skin necrosis after subdermal injection.[130–133] Risk for this complication may be minimized by dilution of methylene blue with normal saline.[134] Other reported blue dye–related complications have included implant-altered oxygen saturation, capsular contracture, mycoplasma breast infection, pulmonary edema, and serotonin syndrome in patients who take serotonergic medications.[135–138]

Lymphazurin, or isosulfan blue, has also long been used for sentinel lymph node mapping. However, its cost, availability, and potential for severe allergic reaction (0.1%–1.1%) have decreased its use.[109,139,140] Routine prophylaxis is not recommended, although steroid use before or after induction of anesthesia has been shown to decrease the severity of such adverse reactions.[140]

SUMMARY

Overall, morbidity associated with breast cancer surgery is low. The most common complications related to breast cancer surgery without reconstruction include infection, seroma formation, and bleeding. Complications may present in the breast or axilla, with risks varying significantly by the cancer surgery performed. Preoperative planning, mitigation of patient-related risk factors, use of prophylactic treatment, and meticulous surgical technique are critical in order to reduce complication rates.

CLINICS CARE POINTS

- Overall, morbidity associated with breast cancer surgery is low.
- The most common complications related to breast cancer surgery without reconstruction include infection, seroma formation, and bleeding.

- Complications may present in the breast or axilla, with risks varying significantly by the cancer surgery performed.
- Preoperative planning, mitigation of patient-related risk factors, use of prophylactic treatment, and meticulous surgical technique are critical in order to reduce complication rates.

DISCLOSURE

None.

REFERENCES

1. U.S Breast cancer statistics. Available at: https://www.breastcancer.org/symptoms/understand_bc/statistics. Accessed April 10, 2021.
2. Cancer facts & figures 2021. Available at: https://www.cancer.org/content/dam/cancer-org/research/cancer-facts-and-statistics/annual-cancer-facts-and-figures/2021/cancer-facts-and-figures-2021.pdf. Accessed April 10, 2021.
3. NCCN clinical practice guidelines in oncology (NCCN guidelines) breast cancer. Version 3.2021. Available at: https://www.nccn.org/guidelines/guidelines-detail?category=1&id=1419. Accessed on 4.19.2021
4. Rodrigo Arriagada B, Le MG, Rochard F. Conservative treatment versus mastectomy in early breast cancer: patterns of failure with 15 years of follow-up data patients and methods trial design. J Clin Oncol 1979;14(5):1558–64.
5. Clarke M, Collins R, Darby S, et al. Effects of radiotherapy and of differences in the extent of surgery for early breast cancer on local recurrence and 15-year survival: an overview of the randomised trials. Lancet 2005;366(9503):2087–106.
6. Veronesi U, Cascinelli N, Mariani L, et al. Twenty-year follow-up of a randomized study comparing breast-conserving surgery with radical mastectomy for early breast cancer. N Engl J Med 2002;347(16):1227–32.
7. Fisher B, Anderson S, Bryant J, et al. Twenty-year follow-up of a randomized trial comparing total mastectomy, lumpectomy, and lumpectomy plus irradiation for the treatment of invasive breast cancer. N Engl J Med 2002;347(16):1233–41.
8. Degnim AC, Throckmorton AD, Boostrom SY, et al. Surgical site infection after breast surgery: impact of 2010 CDC reporting guidelines. Ann Surg Oncol 2012;19(13):4099–103.
9. Garwood ER, Moore D, Ewing C, et al. Total skin-sparing mastectomy. Ann Surg 2009;249(1):26–32.
10. Mansel RE, Fallowfield L, Kissin M, et al. Randomized multicenter trial of sentinel node biopsy versus standard axillary treatment in operable breast cancer: the ALMANAC trial. JNCI J Natl Cancer Inst 2006;98(9):599–609.
11. El-Tamer MB, Ward BM, Schifftner T, et al. Morbidity and mortality following breast cancer surgery in women. Ann Surg 2007;245(5).
12. Olsen MA, Lefta M, Dietz JR, et al. Risk factors for surgical site infection after major breast operation. J Am Coll Surg 2008;207(3):665–71.
13. Vinton AL, Traverse LW, Jolly PC. Wound complications after modified radical mastectomy compared with tylectomy with axillary lymph node dissection. Am J Surg 1991;161(5):584–8.
14. Schilling PL, Dimick JB, Birkmeyer JD. Prioritizing quality improvement in general surgery. J Am Coll Surg 2008;207(5):698–704.

15. Kuroi K, Shimozuma K, Taguchi T, et al. Evidence-based risk factors for seroma formation in breast surgery. Jpn J Clin Oncol 2006;36(4):197–206.
16. Srivastava V, Basu S, Shukla VK. Seroma formation after breast cancer surgery: what we have learned in the last two decades. J Breast Cancer 2012;15(4):373–80.
17. Porter K, O'Connor S, Rimm E, et al. Electrocautery as a factor in seroma formation following mastectomy. Am J Surg 1998;176(1):8–11.
18. Keogh GW, Doughty JC, McArdle CSM, et al. Seroma formation related to electrocautery in breast surgery: a prospective randomized trial. The Breast 1998;7(1):90050–9.
19. Tejler G, Aspegren K. Complications and hospital stay after surgery for breast cancer: a prospective study of 385 patients. Br J Surg 2005;72(7):542–4.
20. Bonnema J, Ligtenstein DA, Wiggers T, et al. The composition of serous fluid after axillary dissection. Eur J Surg 1999;165(1):9–13.
21. Oertli D, Laffer U, Haberthuer F, et al. Perioperative and postoperative tranexamic acid reduces the local wound complication rate after surgery for breast cancer. Br J Surg 2005;81(6):856–9.
22. Watt-Boolsen S, Nielsen VB, Jensen J, et al. Postmastectomy seroma. A study of the nature and origin of seroma after mastectomy. Dan Med Bull 1989;36(5):487–9.
23. Zieliński J, Jaworski R, Irga N, et al. Analysis of selected factors influencing seroma formation in breast cancer patients undergoing mastectomy. Arch Med Sci 2013;1:86–92.
24. Boostrom SY, Throckmorton AD, Boughey JC, et al. Incidence of clinically significant seroma after breast and axillary surgery. J Am Coll Surg 2009;208(1):148–50.
25. Abe M, Iwase T, Takeuchi T, et al. A randomized controlled trial on the prevention of seroma after partial or total mastectomy and axillary lymph node dissection. Breast Cancer 1998;5(1):67–9.
26. Woodworth PA, McBoyle MF, Helmer SD, et al. Seroma formation after breast cancer surgery: incidence and predicting factors. Am Surg 2000;66(5):444–50.
27. Gonzalez EA, Saltzstein EC, Riedner CS, et al. Seroma formation following breast cancer surgery. Breast J 2003;9(5):385–8.
28. Coveney EC, O'Dwyer PJ, Geraghty JG, et al. Effect of closing dead space on seroma formation after mastectomy–a prospective randomized clinical trial. Eur J Surg Oncol 1993;19(2):143–6.
29. Anand R, Skinner R, Dennison G, et al. A prospective randomised trial of two treatments for wound seroma after breast surgery. Eur J Surg Oncol 2002;28(6):620–2.
30. Currie A, Chong K, Davies GL, et al. Ultrasonic dissection versus electrocautery in mastectomy for breast cancer – A meta-analysis. Eur J Surg Oncol 2012;38(10):897–901.
31. Khan S, Khan S, Chawla T, et al. Harmonic scalpel versus electrocautery dissection in modified radical mastectomy: a randomized controlled trial. Ann Surg Oncol 2014;21(3):808–14.
32. Chen CY, Hoe AL, Wong CY. The effect of a pressure garment on post-surgical drainage and seroma formation in breast cancer patients. Singapore Med J 1998;39(9):412–5.
33. Vitug AF, Newman LA. Complications in breast surgery. Surg Clin North Am 2007;87(2):431–51.

34. Schultz I, Barholm M, Gröndal S. Delayed shoulder exercises in reducing seroma frequency after modified radical mastectomy: a prospective randomized study. Ann Surg Oncol 1997;4(4):293–7.

35. Taylor JC, Rai S, Hoar F, et al. Breast cancer surgery without suction drainage: The impact of adopting a 'no drains' policy on symptomatic seroma formation rates. Eur J Surg Oncol 2013;39(4):334–8.

36. Troost MS, Kempees CJ, de Roos MAJ. Breast cancer surgery without drains: No influence on seroma formation. Int J Surg 2015;13:170–4.

37. Chintamani SV, Singh J, Bansal A, et al. Half versus full vacuum suction drainage after modified radical mastectomy for breast cancer- a prospective randomized clinical trial[ISRCTN24484328]. BMC Cancer 2005;5(1):11.

38. Bonnema J, van Geel AN, Ligtenstein DA, et al. A prospective randomized trial of high versus low vacuum drainage after axillary dissection for breast cancer. Am J Surg 1997;173(2):76–9.

39. Petrek JA, Peters MM, Cirricione C, et al. A prospective randomized trial of single versus multiple drains in the axilla after lymphadenectomy. Surg Gynecol Obstet 1992;175(5):405–9.

40. van Bastelaar J, Beckers A, Snoeijs M, et al. Flap fixation reduces seroma in patients undergoing mastectomy: a significant implication for clinical practice. World J Surg Oncol 2016;14(1):66.

41. Ouldamer L, Caille A, Giraudeau B, et al. Quilting suture of mastectomy dead space compared with conventional closure with drain. Ann Surg Oncol 2015; 22(13):4233–40.

42. ten Wolde B, van den Wildenberg FJH, Keemers-Gels ME, et al. Quilting prevents seroma formation following breast cancer surgery: closing the dead space by quilting prevents seroma following axillary lymph node dissection and mastectomy. Ann Surg Oncol 2014;21(3):802–7.

43. van Bastelaar J, van Roozendaal L, Granzier R, et al. A systematic review of flap fixation techniques in reducing seroma formation and its sequelae after mastectomy. Breast Cancer Res Treat 2018;167(2):409–16.

44. Cong Y, Cao J, Qiao G, et al. Fascia suture technique is a simple approach to reduce postmastectomy seroma formation. J Breast Cancer 2020;23(5):533–41.

45. H Turner EJ, Benson JR, Winters ZE. Techniques in the prevention and management of seromas after breast surgery. Futur Oncol 2014;10(6):1049–63.

46. Vilar-Compte D, Jacquemin B, Robles-Vidal C, et al. Surgical site infections in breast surgery: case-control study. World J Surg 2004;28(3):242–6.

47. Rice DC, Morris SM, Sarr MG, et al. Intraoperative topical tetracycline sclerotherapy following mastectomy: a prospective, randomized trial. J Surg Oncol 2000;73(4):224–7.

48. Saeb-Parsy K, Athanassoglou V, Benson JR. Talc Seromadesis: a novel technique for the treatment of chronic seromas following breast surgery. Breast J 2006;12(5):502–4.

49. Gruver DI. Hypertonic saline for treatment of seroma. Plast Reconstr Surg 2003; 112(3):934.

50. Throckmorton AD, Askegard-Giesmann J, Hoskin TL, et al. Sclerotherapy for the treatment of postmastectomy seroma. Am J Surg 2008;196(4):541–4.

51. Stanczyk M, Grala B, Zwierowicz T, et al. Surgical resection for persistent seroma, following modified radical mastectomy. World J Surg Oncol 2007; 5(1):104.

52. Pastoriza J, McNelis J, Parsikia A, et al. Predictive factors for surgical site infections in patients undergoing surgery for breast carcinoma. Am Surg 2021;87(1): 68–76.
53. Eck DL, Koonce SL, Goldberg RF, et al. Breast surgery outcomes as quality measures according to the NSQIP database. Ann Surg Oncol 2012;19(10): 3212–7.
54. de Blacam C, Ogunleye AA, Momoh AO, et al. High body mass index and smoking predict morbidity in breast cancer surgery. Ann Surg 2012;255(3):551–5.
55. Amland PF, Andenaes K, Samdal F, et al. A prospective, double-blind, placebo-controlled trial of a single dose of azithromycin on postoperative wound infections in plastic surgery. Plast Reconstr Surg 1995;96(6):1378–83.
56. Davis GB, Peric M, Chan LS, et al. Identifying risk factors for surgical site infections in mastectomy patients using the National Surgical Quality Improvement Program database. Am J Surg 2013;205(2):194–9.
57. Bold RJ, Mansfield PF, Berger DH, et al. Prospective, randomized, double-blind study of prophylactic antibiotics in axillary lymph node dissection. Am J Surg 1998;176(3):239–43.
58. Gupta R, Sinnett D, Carpenter R, et al. Antibiotic prophylaxis for post-operative wound infection in clean elective breast surgery. Eur J Surg Oncol 2000;26(4): 363–6.
59. Jones DJ, Bunn F, Bell-Syer SV. Prophylactic antibiotics to prevent surgical site infection after breast cancer surgery. Cochrane Database Syst Rev 2014. https://doi.org/10.1002/14651858.CD005360.pub4.
60. Platt R, Zaleznik DF, Hopkins CC, et al. Perioperative Antibiotic Prophylaxis for Herniorrhaphy and Breast Surgery. N Engl J Med 1990;322(3):153–60.
61. Bratzler DW, Hunt DR. Healthcare epidemiology: the surgical infection prevention and surgical care improvement projects: national initiatives to improve outcomes for patients having surgery. Clin Infect Dis 2006;43(3):322–30.
62. The American Society of Breast Surgeons Official Statement. Consensus guideline on venous thromboembolism (VTE) prophylaxis for patients undergoing breast operations.; 2016. https://www.breastsurgeons.org/docs/statements/Consensus-Guideline-on-Venous-Thromboembolism-VTE-Prophylaxis-for-Patients-Undergoing-Breast-Operations.pdf. Accessed on
63. Bakker XR, Roumen RMH. Bleeding after excision of breast lumps. Eur J Surg 2002;168(7):401–3.
64. Al-Hilli Z, Thomsen KM, Habermann EB, et al. Reoperation for complications after lumpectomy and mastectomy for breast cancer from the 2012 National Surgical Quality Improvement Program (ACS-NSQIP). Ann Surg Oncol 2015;22: 459–69.
65. Friis E, Horby J, Sorensen LT, et al. Thromboembolic prophylaxis as a risk factor for postoperative complications after breast cancer surgery. World J Surg 2004; 28(6):540–3.
66. Klifto KM, Major MR, Leto Barone AA, et al. Perioperative systemic nonsteroidal anti-inflammatory drugs (NSAIDs) in women undergoing breast surgery. Cochrane Database Syst Rev 2019. https://doi.org/10.1002/14651858.CD013290.
67. Rojas KE, Fortes TA, Flom P, et al. Intraoperative ketorolac use does not increase the risk of bleeding in breast surgery. Ann Surg Oncol 2019;26(10):3368–73.
68. Kilbride K. Surgical complications and management. In: Keurer's breast surgical oncology. Kuerer H.M.(Ed.), (2010). Kuerer's Breast Surgical Oncology. McGraw Hill. https://accesssurgery-mhmedical-com.ccmain.ohionet.org/content.aspx?bookid=428&sectionid=39936122. Accessed April 19, 2021

69. Mahoney MC, Ingram AD. Breast emergencies: types, imaging features, and management. Am J Roentgenol 2014;202(4):W390–9.

70. Robertson S, Jeevaratnam J, Agrawal A, et al. Mastectomy skin flap necrosis: challenges and solutions. Breast Cancer Targets Ther 2017;9:141–52.

71. Palmer JH, Taylor GI. The vascular territories of the anterior chest wall. Br J Plast Surg 1986;39(3):287–99.

72. Lemaine V, Hoskin TL, Farley DR, et al. Introducing the SKIN score: a validated scoring system to assess severity of mastectomy skin flap necrosis. Ann Surg Oncol 2015;22(9):2925–32.

73. Margulies AG, Hochberg J, Kepple J, et al. Total skin-sparing mastectomy without preservation of the nipple-areola complex. Am J Surg 2005;190(6):907–12.

74. Patel K, Hill L, Gatti M, et al. Management of massive mastectomy skin flap necrosis following autologous breast reconstruction. Ann Plast Surg 2012;69(2):139–44.

75. Uçkay I, Agostinho A, Belaieff W, et al. Noninfectious wound complications in clean surgery: epidemiology, risk factors, and association with antibiotic use. World J Surg 2011;35(5):973–80.

76. Wernick B, Nahirniak P, Stawicki SP. Impaired wound healing 2021. Available at: http://www.ncbi.nlm.nih.gov/pubmed/29489281.

77. Spira JAO, Borges EL, Silva PAB, et al. Factors associated with complex surgical wounds in breast and abdomen: a case-control observational study. Rev Lat Am Enfermagem 2018;26:E3052.

78. Dodson MK, Magaan EF, Meeks GR. A randomized comparison of secondary closure and secondary intention in patients with superficial wound dehiscence. Obs Gynecol 1992;80(3):321–4.

79. Dumville JC, Owens GL, Crosbie EJ, et al. Negative pressure wound therapy for treating surgical wounds healing by secondary intention. Cochrane Database Syst Rev 2015. https://doi.org/10.1002/14651858.CD011278.pub2.

80. Richebé P, Capdevila X, Rivat C. Persistent postsurgical pain. Anesthesiology 2018;129(3):590–607.

81. Vilholm OJ, Cold S, Rasmussen L, et al. The postmastectomy pain syndrome: an epidemiological study on the prevalence of chronic pain after surgery for breast cancer. Br J Cancer 2008;99(4):604–10.

82. Wang L, Cohen JC, Devasenapathy N, et al. Prevalence and intensity of persistent post-surgical pain following breast cancer surgery: a systematic review and meta-analysis of observational studies. Br J Anaesth 2020;125(3):346–57.

83. Tasmuth T, Blomqvist C, Kalso E. Chronic post-treatment symptoms in patients with breast cancer operated in different surgical units. Eur J Surg Oncol 1999;25(1):38–43.

84. Carpenter JS, Andrykowski MA, Sloan P, et al. Postmastectomy/Postlumpectomy pain in breast cancer survivors. J Clin Epidemiol 1998;51(12):1285–92.

85. Lin Z-M, Li M-H, Zhang F, et al. Thoracic paravertebral blockade reduces chronic postsurgical pain in breast cancer patients: a randomized controlled trial. Pain Med 2020;21(12):3539–5347.

86. Gilron I. Antidepressant drugs for postsurgical pain: current status and future directions. Drugs 2016;76(2):159–67.

87. Thapa P, Euasobhon P. Chronic postsurgical pain: current evidence for prevention and management. Korean J Pain 2018;31(3):155–73.

88. Amano M, Shimizu T. Mondor's disease: a review of the literature. Intern Med 2018;57(18):2607–12.

89. Wong S, Lai LK, Chan P, et al. Mondor's disease: sclerosing thrombophlebitis of subcutaneous veins in a patient with occult carcinoma of the breast. Hong Kong Med J 2017. https://doi.org/10.12809/hkmj154699.

90. Koehler L, Haddad T, Hunter D, et al. Axillary web syndrome following breast cancer surgery: symptoms, complications, and management strategies. Breast Cancer Targets Ther 2018;11:13–9.

91. Obradovic K, Adzic N, Pavlovic Stankovic D, et al. Superficial thrombophlebitis of the breast (Mondor's Disease): an uncommon localization of common disease. Clin Med Insights Case Rep 2020;13. 1179547620972414.

92. Kim HS, Cha ES, Kim HH, et al. Spectrum of Sonographic Findings in Superficial Breast Masses. J Ultrasound Med 2005;24(5):663–380.

93. Tan PH, Lai LM, Carrington EV, et al. Fat necrosis of the breast—A review. The Breast 2006;15(3):313–8.

94. Kerridge WD, Kryvenko ON, Thompson A, et al. Fat necrosis of the breast: a pictorial review of the mammographic, ultrasound, CT, and MRI findings with histopathologic correlation. Radiol Res Pract 2015;2015. 613139.

95. Lee J, Park HY, Kim WW, et al. Natural course of fat necrosis after breast reconstruction: a 10-year follow-up study. BMC Cancer 2021;21(1):166.

96. Lovely JK, Nehring SA, Boughey JC, et al. Balancing venous thromboembolism and hematoma after breast surgery. Ann Surg Oncol 2012;19(10):3230–5.

97. Andtbacka RHI, Babiera G, Singletary SE, et al. Incidence and prevention of venous thromboembolism in patients undergoing breast cancer surgery and treated according to clinical pathways. Ann Surg 2006;243(1):96–101.

98. Fischer JP, Wes AM, Tuggle CT, et al. Venous thromboembolism risk in mastectomy and immediate breast reconstruction. Plast Reconstr Surg 2014;133(3):263E–73E.

99. Nwaogu I, Yan Y, Margenthaler JA, et al. Venous thromboembolism after breast reconstruction in patients undergoing breast surgery: an american college of surgeons NSQIP analysis. J Am Coll Surg 2015;220(5):886–93.

100. Masoomi H, Paydar KZ, Wirth GA, et al. Predictive risk factors of venous thromboembolism in autologous breast reconstruction surgery. Ann Plast Surg 2014;72(1):30–3.

101. Tran BH, JoAnna Nguyen T, Hwang BH, et al. Risk factors associated with venous thromboembolism in 49,028 mastectomy patients. The Breast 2013;22(4):444–8.

102. He X-D, Guo Z-H, Tian J-H, et al. Whether drainage should be used after surgery for breast cancer? A systematic review of randomized controlled trials. Med Oncol 2011;28(S1):S22–30.

103. Rockson SG. Update on the biology and treatment of lymphedema. Curr Treat Options Cardiovasc Med 2012;14(2):184–92.

104. McLaughlin SA, Staley AC, Vicini F, et al. Considerations for clinicians in the diagnosis, prevention, and treatment of breast cancer-related lymphedema: recommendations from a multidisciplinary expert ASBrS panel. Ann Surg Oncol 2017;24(10):2818–26.

105. Ozcinar B, Guler SA, Kocaman N, et al. Breast cancer related lymphedema in patients with different loco-regional treatments. The Breast 2012;21(3):361–5.

106. Donker M, van Tienhoven G, Straver ME, et al. Radiotherapy or surgery of the axilla after a positive sentinel node in breast cancer (EORTC 10981-22023 AMAROS): a randomised, multicentre, open-label, phase 3 non-inferiority trial. Lancet Oncol 2014;15(12):1303–10.

107. Olson JA, McCall LM, Beitsch P, et al. Impact of immediate versus delayed axillary node dissection on surgical outcomes in breast cancer patients with

positive sentinel nodes: results from American College of Surgeons Oncology Group Trials Z0010 and Z0011. J Clin Oncol 2008;26(21):3530–5.

108. Wilke LG, McCall LM, Posther KE, et al. Surgical complications associated with sentinel lymph node biopsy: results from a prospective international cooperative group trial. Ann Surg Oncol 2006;13(4):491–500.

109. Lucci A, McCall LM, Beitsch PD, et al. Surgical Complications Associated With Sentinel Lymph Node Dissection (SLND) plus axillary lymph node dissection compared with SLND alone in the American College of Surgeons Oncology Group Trial Z0011. J Clin Oncol 2007;25(24):3657–63.

110. Galimberti V, Cole BF, Zurrida S, et al. Axillary dissection versus no axillary dissection in patients with sentinel-node micrometastases (IBCSG 23–01): a phase 3 randomised controlled trial. Lancet Oncol 2013;14(4):297–305.

111. Ashikaga T, Krag DN, Land SR, et al. Morbidity results from the NSABP B-32 trial comparing sentinel lymph node dissection versus axillary dissection. J Surg Oncol 2010;102(2):111–8.

112. McLaughlin SA, DeSnyder SM, Klimberg S, et al. Considerations for clinicians in the diagnosis, prevention, and treatment of breast cancer-related lymphedema, recommendations from an expert panel: part 2: preventive and therapeutic options. Ann Surg Oncol 2017;24(10):2827–35.

113. The diagnosis and treatment of peripheral lymphedema: 2016 consensus document of the International Society of Lymphology. Lymphology 2016;49:170–84.

114. Thompson M, Korourian S, Henry-Tillman R, et al. Axillary Reverse Mapping (ARM): a new concept to identify and enhance lymphatic preservation. Ann Surg Oncol 2007;14(6):1890–5.

115. Tummel E, Ochoa D, Korourian S, et al. Does axillary reverse mapping prevent lymphedema after lymphadenectomy? Ann Surg 2017;265(5):987–92.

116. Ahmed M, Rubio IT, Kovacs T, et al. Systematic review of axillary reverse mapping in breast cancer. Br J Surg 2016;103(3):170–8. https://doi.org/10.1002/bjs.10041.

117. Schwarz GS, Grobmyer SR, Djohan RS, et al. Axillary reverse mapping and lymphaticovenous bypass: lymphedema prevention through enhanced lymphatic visualization and restoration of flow. J Surg Oncol 2019;120(2):160–7.

118. Jørgensen MG, Toyserkani NM, Sørensen JA. The effect of prophylactic lymphovenous anastomosis and shunts for preventing cancer-related lymphedema: a systematic review and meta-analysis. Microsurgery 2018;38(5):576–85.

119. Feldman S, Bansil H, Ascherman J, et al. Single Institution Experience with Lymphatic Microsurgical Preventive Healing Approach (LYMPHA) for the Primary Prevention of Lymphedema. Ann Surg Oncol 2015;22(10):3296–301.

120. Boccardo F, Casabona F, DeCian F, et al. Lymphatic Microsurgical Preventing Healing Approach (LYMPHA) for primary surgical prevention of breast cancer-related lymphedema: over 4 years follow-up. Microsurgery 2014;34(6):421–4.

121. Rogan S, Taeymans J, Luginbuehl H, et al. Therapy modalities to reduce lymphoedema in female breast cancer patients: a systematic review and meta-analysis. Breast Cancer Res Treat 2016;159(1):1–14.

122. Ozturk CN, Ozturk C, Glasgow M, et al. Free vascularized lymph node transfer for treatment of lymphedema: a systematic evidence based review. J Plast Reconstr Aesthet Surg 2016;69(9):1234–47.

123. Penha T, IJsbrandy C, Hendrix N, et al. Microsurgical techniques for the treatment of breast cancer—related lymphedema: a systematic review. J Reconstr Microsurg 2012;29(02):99–106.

124. Kwan W, Jackson J, Weir LM, et al. Chronic arm morbidity after curative breast cancer treatment: prevalence and impact on quality of life. J Clin Oncol 2002; 20(20):4242–8.
125. Ververs JMM, Roumen RM, Vingerhoets AJJ, et al. severity and predictors of physical and psychological morbidity after axillary lymph node dissection for breast cancer. Eur J Cancer 2001;37(8):991–9.
126. Kuehn T, Klauss W, Darsow M, et al. Long-term morbidity following axillary dissection in breast cancer patients – clinical assessment, significance for life quality and the impact of demographic, oncologic and therapeutic factors. Breast Cancer Res Treat 2000;64(3):275–86.
127. Hack TF, Cohen L, Katz J, et al. Physical and psychological morbidity after axillary lymph node dissection for breast cancer. J Clin Oncol 1999;17(1):143–9.
128. Ivens D, Hoe A, Podd T, et al. Assessment of morbidity from complete axillary dissection. Br J Cancer 1992;66(1):136–8.
129. Thevarajah S, Huston TL, Simmons RM. A comparison of the adverse reactions associated with isosulfan blue versus methylene blue dye in sentinel lymph node biopsy for breast cancer. Am J Surg 2005;189(2):236–9.
130. Bleicher RJ, Kloth DD, Robinson D, et al. Inflammatory cutaneous adverse effects of methylene blue dye injection for lymphatic mapping/sentinel lymphadenectomy. J Surg Oncol 2009;99(6):356–60.
131. Stradling B, Aranha G, Gabram S. Adverse skin lesions after methylene blue injections for sentinel lymph node localization. Am J Surg 2002;184(4):350–2.
132. Govaert GAM, Oostenbroek RJ, Plaisier PW. Prolonged skin staining after intradermal use of patent blue in sentinel lymph node biopsy for breast cancer. Eur J Surg Oncol 2005;31(4):373–5.
133. Zakaria S, Hoskin TL, Degnim AC. Safety and technical success of methylene blue dye for lymphatic mapping in breast cancer. Am J Surg 2008;196(2):228–33.
134. El-Tamer M, Komenaka IK, Curry S, et al. Pulse oximeter changes with sentinel lymph node biopsy in breast cancer. Arch Surg 2003;138(11):1257–60.
135. Singh-Ranger G, Mokbel K. Capsular contraction following immediate reconstructive surgery for breast cancer - An association with methylene blue dye. Int Semin Surg Oncol 2004;1(1):3.
136. Reyes FJ, Noelck MB, Valentino C, et al. Complications of methylene blue dye in breast surgery: case reports and review of the literature. J Caner 2010; 8(2):20–5.
137. Teknos D, Ramcharan A, Oluwole SF. Pulmonary edema associated with methylene blue dye administration during sentinel lymph node biopsy. J Natl Med Assoc 2008;100(12):1483–4.
138. Krag DN, Anderson SJ, Julian TB, et al. Technical outcomes of sentinel-lymph-node resection and conventional axillary-lymph-node dissection in patients with clinically node-negative breast cancer: results from the NSABP B-32 randomised phase III trial. Lancet Oncol 2007;8(10):881–8.
139. Raut CP, Hunt KK, Akins JS, et al. Incidence of anaphylactoid reactions to isosulfan blue dye during breast carcinoma lymphatic mapping in patients treated with preoperative prophylaxis. Cancer 2005;104(4):692–9.
140. The American Society of Breast Surgeons Official Statement. Consensus Guideline on Preoperative Antibiotics and Surgical Infection in Breast Surgery. Available at: https://www.breastsurgeons.org/docs/statements/Consensus-Guideline-on-Preoperative-Antibiotics-and-Surgical-Site-Infection-in-Breast-Surgery.pdf. Accessed April 10, 2021.

Complications After Pancreaticoduodenectomy

Robert Simon, MD

KEYWORDS

- Pancreaticoduodenectomy • Whipple • Complications • Pancreatic fistula
- Delayed gastric emptying • Informed consent

KEY POINTS

- Mortality rate for pancreaticoduodenectomies has decreased drastically over the years, but morbidity remains high.
- Grading systems are important to ensure uniform complication assessment and guide therapy.
- Pancreatic fistula is one of the most dreaded complications after pancreaticoduodenectomy.
- Understanding the potential complications is imperative to patient education to set expectations and provide better informed consent.

INTRODUCTION

The first pancreaticoduodenectomy was performed in 1909 by Dr Kausch.[1] The procedure was adapted and popularized by Dr Allen Oldfather Whipple in 1935, who performed only 37 in his career.[2] Pancreaticoduodenectomy was initially performed in a 2-stage operation. The first was the anastomosis stage wherein a cholecystogastrostomy was formed as well as a gastrojejunostomy. The common bile duct was then transected during this stage. Approximately 4 weeks later, the patient was brought back to the operating room for the resection stage of the operation. The duodenum, pancreatic head, and common bile duct were resected, and the pancreatic duct was oversewn.[3] This procedure was performed infrequently because of high in-hospital mortality rate, which approached 25%. In the 1980s the procedure increased in popularity as surgical techniques improved. As surgeon experience went up, the morbidity and mortality rates went down, and although the mortality rate is low, approximately 1% in high-volume centers, there continues to be a high morbidity

General Surgery, Department of Hepatopancreaticobiliary Surgery, Digestive Disease and Surgery Institute, Cleveland Clinic Foundation, 9500 Euclid Avenue, Cleveland, OH 44195, USA
E-mail address: Simonr@ccf.org

Surg Clin N Am 101 (2021) 865–874
https://doi.org/10.1016/j.suc.2021.06.011
0039-6109/21/© 2021 Elsevier Inc. All rights reserved.

surgical.theclinics.com

rate that approaches 50%.[4,5] Understanding the potential complications is important so that one can help recognize when complications do arise and better treat the patient. In addition, it is imperative when having discussions with patients and their families preoperatively to help them truly make an informed decision about whether or not they want to move forward with surgery.

The classic Whipple procedure that is performed to today is a single-stage operation wherein the pancreatic head, duodenum, and common bile duct are resected and 3 new anastomoses are performed with a pancreaticojejunostomy, hepaticojejunostomy, and gastrojejunostomy. There are a few variations on the Whipple operation that have been developed over the years. The primary one is a pylorus-preserving Whipple procedure, wherein the duodenum is transected immediately distal to the pylorus and a duodenojejunostomy is performed. This variation was first described in the 1970s by Traverso and Longmire[6] to try and prevent postgastric symptoms and was popularized in the 1980s.[7–9]

SURGICAL SITE INFECTIONS

After pancreaticoduodenectomy, surgical site infections are one of the most common complications, listed as high as 23.5%, but in the United States, they tend to be lower, around 7% to 13%.[10] Although deep surgical site infections are usually amenable to percutaneous drainage by interventional radiology, sometimes surgery is needed to washout the surgical field. Preoperative bile duct cannulation has been shown to increase the risk of infectious complications; this is likely due to seeding of the bile with enteric bacteria that causes bacteremia, potentially leading to infections. In one study, patients who underwent preoperative stenting of their biliary tree had infectious complications 41% of the time, whereas those who did not undergo stenting had infectious complications only 25% of the time.[11] Another study found that those who were stented preoperatively had an odds ratio of 3.4 for an infectious complication.[12] Although preoperative stenting of the bile duct is technically a modifiable risk factor for infections, it is often unavoidable. If a patient is jaundiced and about to undergo neoadjuvant chemotherapy, a stent is a must, not only to prevent cholangitis but also to make the patients themselves more comfortable as well as improve their nutritional status. Even in patients who are going to receive upfront surgery, if wait times are prolonged then preoperative stenting is indicated.

In terms of preventing infectious complications, wound protectors have been shown to decrease the rate of surgical site infections. A recent article using the American College of Surgeons National Surgical Quality Improvement Program database of more than 11,000 pancreaticoduodenectomies showed that wound protectors decreased the rate of superficial and deep surgical site infections from 9.5% to 5.7%. In those who had preoperative stents placed, the rate dropped from 12.2% to 6.6%, and in those without stenting, the rate dropped from 6.5% to 4.6%.[13] Proper antibiotic selection has also been shown to decrease infections. Ideally, a second-/third-generation cephalosporin combined with metronidazole should be used. When cohorts were compared, those that received the second-/third-generation cephalosporin and metronidazole had fewer overall surgical site infections, 14.8% versus 26.4%. The rate of Clostridium difficile also decreased from 8.1% to 1.9% using this novel antibiotic prophylaxis regimen.[14] Changing gloves and suction tips after all anastomoses are completed, combined with irrigating the abdomen with warm saline, has also been shown to decrease wound complications. Last, there is also some evidence that using negative pressure wound therapy on the incision can reduce the infection rate after pancreaticoduodenectomy.[15]

DELAYED GASTRIC EMPTYING

Delayed gastric emptying (DGE) is a known complication after pancreaticoduodenectomy and is the main reason why nasogastric tubes (NGTs) used to routinely be placed intraoperatively and kept postoperatively. The International Study Group of Pancreatic Surgery (ISGPS) in 2007 developed a standard definition of DGE. In broad terminology, DGE is defined as requiring an NGT for longer than 3 days, having to reinsert an NGT after postoperative day 3, or the inability to tolerate an oral diet after postoperative day 7. DGE is further broken up into 3 grades: grade A, where an NGT is required between 4 and 7 days, or the patient is unable to tolerate an oral diet after 7 days but is able to resume it before day 14; grade B, where an NGT is required between 8 and 14 days, or the patient is unable to tolerate an oral diet after 14 days but is able to resume it before day 21; and last, grade C, where an NGT is required after 14 days and an oral diet is not tolerated after 21 days.[16] Multiple studies have looked into DGE, and although the incidence varies widely, it is considered to occur in about 20% to 30%[5,17] of cases, representing one of the most common complications of pancreaticoduodenectomy. The cause of DGE is multifactorial. One reason is that there is a decrease in the amount of motilin secreted as a result of the duodenum being resected. Another reason is that the vagal and sympathetic innervation of the antrum and pylorus are cut by dissecting along the common hepatic artery and the lesser omentum. Decreased blood flow to the pylorus and antrum due to dissection and mobilization are also thought to be a contributing factor toward DGE. Finally, pancreatic fistulae are also thought to be a potential cause of DGE.

Treatment of DGE is usually simple because it is self-limiting. Nasojejunal feeding tubes are often the only treatment necessary and allow enteral nutrition because the remainder of the intestine is typically working well. Patients are able to go home with these tubes in place and are typically well tolerated. If the patient has DGE for a prolonged period, a gastrostomy tube with jejunal extension can be used to facilitate the patient going home and being more comfortable.

Ultimately the best way to treat DGE is to prevent it in the first place, and there have been a few interventions with some promising results. The first is when reconstructing the enteric anastomosis, it should be performed in an antecolic fashion, because this has been found to have lower rates of DGE when compared with retrocolic anastomoses (9% compared with 33%).[18] Another promising technique that has been suggested to improve DGE rates is a Braun enteroenterostomy. The Braun enteroenterostomy was described by Braun himself in the late 1800s with the purpose of preventing bile reflux and helping divert food from the afferent limb of a loop gastrojejunostomy.[19] The technical aspect involves creating a side-to-side enteroenterostomy 25 cm away from the gastrojejunostomy anastomosis; this can be performed with a stapled or a handsewn technique. A study by the University of Florida from 2010 showed that the rate of DGE decreased from 60% in those without a Braun enteroenterostomy to 36% in those who had a Braun enteroenterostomy performed.[20] A more recent meta-analysis from 2018 looked at 11 studies with more than 1600 patients undergoing pancreaticoduodenectomy. Those who had a Braun enteroenterostomy performed developed DGE 11.5% of the time compared with 26.6% in those without a Braun enteroenterostomy.[21] Another technique that has been evaluated and explored is whether or not to preserve the pylorus. In terms of oncologic outcomes, mortality rate, and risk of other complications such as pancreatic fistulae, there is no significant difference between the pylorus-preserving pancreaticoduodenectomy or the standard pancreaticoduodenectomy.[22] In terms of DGE, though, it has been suggested that resecting the pylorus leads to lower rates of DGE. In one study, pylorus resection was associated with a 15% risk of DGE compared with 42.5% in the pylorus-preserving group.[23]

PANCREATIC FISTULA

One of the most feared complications of pancreaticoduodenectomy is a pancreatic fistula. The pancreas does not typically hold suture well because of its friable nature and as a result is prone to leakage. In the most recent ISGPS guidelines, a pancreatic fistula has been classified into 3 categories. Grade A fistula refers to a biochemical leak defined as drain fluid amylase measured on postoperative day 3 or beyond that is greater than 3 times the serum level and is not clinically relevant. A grade B pancreatic fistula requires a change in the expected postoperative management of the patient. This fistula is more specifically defined as persistent drainage greater than 3 weeks in duration, requirement of percutaneous or endoscopic drainage of amylase-rich fluid collection, bleeding that requires angiography, or infection. Once organ failure occurs, this becomes a grade C pancreatic fistula. Organ failure includes those that require reintubation, hemodialysis, or vasopressor support. In addition, a grade C pancreatic fistula also includes those that require a reoperation for the pancreatic leak, or those that lead to death from the leak. To reiterate, biochemical leaks are clinically insignificant seeing because they do not change the clinical course of the patient. Group B and C pancreatic fistulas have been grouped together into clinically relevant pancreatic fistulas (CR-PF), which is important when interpreting the literature. Although multiple techniques have been developed in an attempt to minimize the incidence of pancreatic fistulae, not one is perfect.[24]

Pancreatic fistulas have also sparked the question of whether or not to place a drain near the pancreatic duct anastomosis. As a result, risk calculators have been developed to help guide surgeons in this regard. The most commonly used calculator was developed by Dr Vollmer and colleagues and uses a 10-point grading scale, dividing patients up into negligible risk, low risk, intermediate risk, and high risk for developing a CR-PF. The variables that go into calculating the risk score include texture of the pancreas itself, whether the pathologic condition is pancreatic in origin or extrapancreatic, the diameter of the main pancreatic duct, and intraoperative blood loss.[25] Those scoring 0 points were placed in the negligible-risk strata and had a 0% risk of developing a CR-PF based on a multiinstitutional validation study. Those scoring 1 to 2 points were in the low-risk group and had a 6.6% risk of developing a CR-PF. Those with a score of 3 to 6 were placed in the intermediate-risk group and had a 12.9% risk of developing a CR-PF, and finally patients scoring between 7 and 10 were placed in the high-risk group and had a 28.6% risk of developing a CR-PF. Complications, length of stay, and readmission rates also had a positive correlation with increasing risk score.[26] A more recently developed pancreatic fistula risk score was developed in 2019, which is an adaptation of the previously described risk score wherein only 3 variables are required: pancreatic gland texture, main pancreatic duct diameter, and body mass index. This scoring system was validated, and it was found that the low-risk group had a less than 5% risk of a pancreatic fistula. The intermediate-risk group had a 5% to 20% risk of a pancreatic fistula, and the high-risk group had a greater than 20% risk of a pancreatic fistula.[27] The clinical applicability of these risk scores is their ease in calculating on the fly a patient's risk of pancreatic fistula formation and whether to leave a drain postoperatively.

From a technical standpoint, there is no one technique that has been shown to be clearly superior in reducing pancreatic fistula. Ultimately it comes down to what the particular surgeon feels comfortable with. One thing that has been shown to reduce pancreatic fistula rates is proper antibiotic prophylaxis. When the antibiotic prophylaxis was changed to a second-/third-generation cephalosporin and metronidazole, the rate of clinically relevant pancreatic fistulas was reduced from 23.4% to 6.0%.[14]

BILIARY COMPLICATIONS

One of the rarer complications after a pancreaticoduodenectomy is a biliary complication. These complications are mainly divided into early complications, manifested as a bile leak, and late complications, manifested as bile duct strictures at the hepaticojejunostomy anastomosis. The rate of bile leaks is generally considered low at less than 5%.[28,29] Owing to it being a rare complication, it is difficult to find statistically significant risk factors, although one study found that small-diameter bile ducts (<5 mm) was a risk factor for bile leaks. In this study, about one-half of the bile leaks sealed spontaneously and did not require any intervention. About one-third of these leaks required a percutaneous drain to be placed into the biloma, and only about one-fourth required a reintervention, either by interventional radiology or reoperation.[28] Another study found that bile leaks resolved spontaneously in about 56% of patients.[29]

Biliary strictures are a rare complication as well, occurring in less than 5% of pancreaticoduodenectomies. It is generally thought that bile leaks can result in the future development of biliary strictures. In one study, one-third of patients with biliary strictures were found to have postoperative bile leaks and the remaining patients were found to have recurrence of their cancer.[30] Another study found that biliary strictures were more common in those who had preoperative percutaneous biliary diversion via a transhepatic catheter, thought to be due to inflammation of the bile duct.[31]

In addition to general principles of performing any anastomosis, such as tension free and ensuring a good blood supply, technical aspects that can minimize bile leaks and strictures are to evenly space the sutures and avoid unnecessary throws into the bile duct. The suture path should be planned well so that the bile duct is not stabbed, and if the suture spacing is inadequate, the needle should be removed and placed in a different spot. It is also important to get good healthy bites of the bile duct so that the suture does not pull through and tear the bile duct.

HEMORRHAGE

Bleeding remains one of the more common complications after pancreaticoduodenectomies. The ISGPS has again helped us develop a grading scale and universal definition, and this helps ensure that surgeons and clinicians are on the same page when discussing patients and reviewing the literature. There are 3 parameters that help define postoperative hemorrhage after pancreaticoduodenectomy. The first parameter is onset of the bleeding, early versus late, early being defined by bleeding within the first 24 hours of the operation and late being greater than 24 hours after the operation. Early bleeding tends to be related to inadequate hemostasis during the index operation or an underlying coagulopathy. Late bleeding tends to result from intestinal ulcerations, erosion of blood vessels from a pancreatic fistula, a tie becoming dislodged, or development of a pseudoaneurysm. The location of the bleeding can be grouped as being intraluminal or extraluminal. Potential intraluminal sources of bleeding can be hemobilia from biliary stents placed preoperatively, bleeding from enteric staple lines or anastomoses, or ulcer formation. Potential extraluminal sources of bleeding can be raw surfaces from dissection planes or pseudoaneurysms. Bleeding severity is classified into 2 groups. Mild hemorrhage does not have any clinical impairment. Severe hemorrhage requires 4 or more units of packed red blood cells to be transfused within a 24-hour period, a hemoglobin level drop greater than 4 g/dL, or an operation or interventional angiography for control.[32]

Understanding the onset, location, and severity of the hemorrhage helps the clinician best treat the patient. For example, many patients are jaundiced or malnourished preoperatively, and this can lead to them being coagulopathic. Therefore recognizing this coagulopathy and treating with vitamin K is critical. If a patient has intraluminal bleeding, then an endoscopy could be warranted, but if the bleeding is extraluminal then endoscopy is unnecessary. It has been shown that pancreatic fistulae, especially combined with a bile leak, can predispose to a gastroduodenal artery stump blowout. Therefore, if bile is noted in the drain with a high amylase level, there should be a high suspicion of a GDA stump.

CHYLE LEAK

Chyle leaks are another complication that the ISGPS has defined, and it has developed a classification system. The definition of a chyle leak is milky fluid output after postoperative day 2 with a triglyceride level greater than or equal to 110 mg/dL. A grade A chyle leak is classified as one that is not clinically relevant, meaning that it does not prolong the hospital length of stay and improves with conservative dietary modifications. A grade B chyle leak is one that requires one of 3 interventions, one being nasojejunal nutrition or total parental nutrition, a second being placement of a percutaneous drain or maintenance of the surgically placed drain for longer than planned, and a third being the use of octreotide. A grade C chyle leak is one that requires invasive treatment; this includes operative exploration for the chyle leak, intensive care unit admission, or interventional radiology involvement for lymphatic embolization. If mortality occurs that is directly related to the chyle leak, this would be classified as a grade C chyle leak.[33]

The occurrence of chyle leaks has been reported in various studies, ranging from as low as 1.3% to as high as 10.4%.[34,35] The clinical relevance of chyle leaks depends on if the chyle leak is contained or if it is causing diffuse ascites. Hospital length of stay is longer in those with chyle leaks, and of those with chyle leaks, it is longer if there is diffuse ascites. Most importantly, though, chylous ascites has been shown to have a lower overall survival, whereas those with contained chyle leaks have a similar overall survival compared with patients with no chyle leak. Risk factors for chyle leaks include higher lymph node harvest and vascular reconstruction.[34]

Frequently chyle can be seen intraoperatively during the dissection, and when this happens, the most important thing is to make an attempt at locating the source and oversewing it. It is often easy to control with 1 or 2 interrupted sutures. Other times, though, there is no chyle seen intraoperatively, and when patients start getting enteral nutrition, milky chylous fluid is seen in the drains. Most chylous leaks resolve after placing patients on a low-fat diet, in particular limiting them to medium-chain fatty acids. According to various studies, this treatment is effective in about 75% to 85% of patients.[34,36,37] Resolution of the chyle leak is confirmed by seeing the drain output turn serous. One can then start reintroducing fats into the patient's diet to ensure that the drain fluid remains serous. Once this occurs, the drain can be safely removed.

NUTRITION

Two of the main functions of the pancreas are insulin production and pancreatic enzyme production. Taking part of the pancreas puts patients at risk of developing diabetes mellitus and exocrine pancreatic insufficiency (EPI). Diabetes mellitus after partial pancreatectomy is also called type 3c diabetes, or pancreatogenic diabetes, and has been reported to be as high as 22% or even 37% after pancreaticoduodenectomy in some studies.[38,39] It is known that the risk of developing diabetes increases with time. As one gets further and further away from their operation, their risk of developing type 3c diabetes increases. In one study by the Mayo Clinic on the development of immediate postresection diabetes after pancreaticoduodenectomy, the investigators found that the incidence was only 4%.[40] It is generally known that the incidence of type 3c diabetes after distal pancreatectomy is higher than after pancreaticoduodenectomy. In studies looking at resections for chronic pancreatitis, the incidence of new-onset diabetes after a distal pancreatectomy was 85% and only 40% after a pancreaticoduodenectomy.[41,42] Even in patients who have normal pancreatic tissue, diabetes after distal pancreatectomy has been found to be as high as 60%.[43] The reason for the lower incidence after pancreaticoduodenectomies could be related to the distribution of beta islet cells, the insulin-producing cell of the pancreas. A cadaveric study examining the islet cell concentrations throughout the pancreas found that the head and body had similar concentrations, whereas the tail had more than 2 times the amount of islet cells.[44]

EPI is found in about 36% of patients after pancreatic resections, with higher incidences after pancreaticoduodenectomies compared with distal pancreatectomies. On average, these patients developed EPI 14 months from surgery.[45] This observation stresses the importance of following these patients long term postoperatively and screening them at every visit for steatorrhea and malabsorption to ensure that they do not require pancreatic enzyme supplementation. Fecal elastase levels can be checked as well to not only help diagnose these patients but also help get insurance approval for the pancreatic enzymes. Also of note, pancreatic enzymes are broken down by acid, and therefore proton pump inhibitors are usually required to help improve the efficacy of the enzymes and reduce the amount of pancreatic enzymes taken by patients. In addition, it is imperative to properly educate patients on the purpose of the enzymes and the correct way to take them. Patients should be instructed to take half of their dose with the first bite of their meal and the remainder halfway through their meal. If they forget to take them, they should not take them after the meal, because it is a waste of the medication. I also tell them that the purpose is to help digest grease and fat, therefore if they are eating a particularly greasy, fatty meal, they may need to take an extra pill or two to help them digest it properly.

SUMMARY

When the pancreaticoduodenectomy was first described and developed in the 1960s and the 1970s, the mortality rate was as high as 25%. In subsequent years, the mortality rate has been lowered significantly, and now it is thought to be around 1.5%; this is thought to result only partially from better operative techniques and skill. Considering that the morbidity rate of pancreaticoduodenectomies remains high, nearing 50% in some studies, a more important aspect of the improvement in mortality is likely due to better postoperative care and management of postoperative complications.[46] For example, silastic drains, feeding tubes, antibiotics, and better percutaneous techniques to control fluid collections and hemorrhage are imperative in taking care of these complex patients.

CLINICS CARE POINTS

- Pancreaticoduodenectomies are a complex operation with a high morbidity rate

- Having an understanding of the definitions is imperative to recognizing and treating complications
- DGE and pancreatic fistulas are among the most common complication after pancreaticoduodenectomies and result in the highest amount of resource use of any of the other complications

DISCLOSURE

The author has nothing to disclose.

REFERENCES

1. Kausch W. Das carcinoma der papilla duodeni und seine radikale entfeinung. Beitr Z Clin Chir 1912;78:439–86.
2. Whipple AO, Parsons WB, Mullins CR. Treatment of carcinoma of the ampulla of Vater. Ann Surg 1935;102:763–79.
3. Whipple AO. A reminiscence: pancreaticduodenectomy. Rev Surg 1963;20: 221–5.
4. Cameron JL, Riall TS, Coleman J, et al. One Thousand Consecutive Pancreatico-duodenectomies. Ann Surg 2006;244(1):10–5.
5. Miedema BW, Sarr MG, van Heerden JA, et al. Complications following pancrea-ticoduodenectomy. Current management. Arch Surg 1992;127(8):945–50.
6. Traverso LW, Longmire WP. Preservation of the Pylorus in Pancreaticoduodenec-tomy a Follow-Up Evaluation. Ann Surg 1980;192(3):306–10.
7. Braasch JW, Gongliang J, Rossi RL. Pancreatoduodenectomy with preservation of the pylorus. World J Surg 1984;8(6):900–5.
8. Kozuschek W. Duodeno-cephalopancreatectomy with Preservation of the Pylo-rus. Zentralbl Chir 1989;114(11):745–54.
9. Jin GL, Yu CF, Wang JH. Pancreaticoduodenectomy with Preservation of the Gastric Pylorus. Zhonghua Wai KeZa Zhi 1985;23(12):729–31.
10. Karim SAM, Abdulla KS, Abdulkarim QH, et al. The Outcomes and Complications of Pancreaticoduodenectomy (Whipple Procedure): Cross Sectional Study. Int J Surg 2018;52:383–7.
11. Povoski SP, Karpeh MS, Conlon KC, et al. Association of preoperative biliary drainage with postoperative outcome following pancreaticoduodenectomy. Ann Surg 1999;230:131–42.
12. Pisters PW, Hudec WA, Hess KR, et al. Effect of preoperative biliary decompres-sion on pancreaticoduodenectomy-associated morbidity in 300 consecutive pa-tients. Ann Surg 2001;234:47–55.
13. Tee MC, Chen L, Franko J, et al. Effect of wound protectors on surgical site infec-tion in patients undergoing whipple procedure. HPB (Oxford) 2020. https://doi.org/10.1016/j.hpb.2020.11.1146.
14. Cengiz TB, Jarrar A, Power C, et al. Antimicrobial Stewardship Reduces Surgical Site Infection Rate, as well as Number and Severity of Pancreatic Fistulae after Pancreatoduodenectomy. Surg Infect (Larchmt) 2020;21(3):212–7.
15. Gupta R, Darby GC, Imagawa DK. Efficacy of negative pressure wound treatment in preventing surgical site infections after whipple procedures. Am Surg 2017; 83(10):1166–9.

16. Wente MN, Bassi C, Dervenis C, et al. Delayed gastric emptying (DGE) after pancreatic surgery: a suggested definition by the International Study Group of Pancreatic Surgery (ISGPS). Surgery 2007;142(5):761–8.
17. Lermite E, Pessaux P, Brehant O, et al. Risk Factors of Pancreatic Fistula and Delayed Gastric Emptying After Pancreaticoduodenectomy with Pancreaticogastrostomy. J Am Coll Surg 2007;204(4):588–96.
18. Hanna MM, Tamariz L, Gadde R, et al. Delayed Gastric Emptying After Pylorus Preserving Pancreaticoduodenectomy-Does Gastrointestinal Reconstruction Technique Matter? Am J Surg 2016;211(4):810–9.
19. Braun H. Ueber die Gastro-enteostomie and Gleichzeutig Ausgeführte. Arch Klin Chir 1893;45:361.
20. Hochwald SN, Grobmyer SR, Hemming AW, et al. Braun enteroenterostomy is associated with reduced delayed gastric emptying and early resumption of oral feeding following pancreaticoduodenectomy. Journ Surg Onc 2010;101: 351–5.
21. Zhou Y, Hu B, Wei K, et al. Braun anastomosis lowers the incidence of delayed gastric emptying following pancreaticoduodenectomy: a meta-analysis. BMC Gastroenterol 2018;18(1):176.
22. Diener MK, Knaebel HP, Heukaufer C, et al. A Systematic Review and Meta-Analysis of Pylorus-Preserving Versus Classical Pancreaticoduodenectomy for Surgical Treatment of Periampullary and Pancreatic Carcinoma. Ann Surg 2007;245(2):187–200.
23. Hackert T, Hinz U, Hartwig W, et al. Pylorus resection in partial pancreaticoduodenectomy: impact on delayed gastric emptying. Am J Surg 2013;206(3):296–9.
24. Bassi C, Marchegiani G, Dervenis C, et al. The 2016 Update of the International Study Group (ISGPS) Definition and Grading of Postoperative Pancreatic Fistula: 11 Years After. Surgery 2017;161(3):584–91.
25. Callery MP, Pratt WB, Kent TS, et al. A prospectively validated clinical risk score accurately predicts pancreatic fistula after pancreatoduodenectomy. J Am Coll Surg 2013;216(1):1–14.
26. Miller BC, Christein JD, Behrman SW, et al. A multi-institutional external validation of the fistula risk score for pancreatoduodenectomy. J Gastrointest Surg 2014; 18(1):172–80.
27. Mungroop TH, van Rijssen LB, van Klaveren D, et al. Alternative Fistula Risk Score for Pancreatoduodenectomy (a-FRS): Design and International External Validation. Ann Surg 2019;269(5):937–43.
28. Duconseil P, Turrini O, Ewald J, et al. Biliary Complications After Pancreaticoduodenectomy: Skinny Bile Ducts are Surgeons' Enemies. World J Surg 2014;38(11): 2946–51.
29. Malgras B, Duron S, Gaujoux S, et al. Early Biliary Complications Following Pancreaticoduodenectomy: Prevalence and Risk Factors. HPB (Oxford) 2016;18(4): 367–74.
30. Parra-Membrives P, Martínez-Baena D, Sánchez-Sánchez F. Late Biliary Complications After Pancreaticoduodenectomy. Am Surg 2016;82(5):456–61.
31. House MG, Cameron JL, Schulick RD, et al. Incidence and Outcome of Biliary Strictures After Pancreaticoduodenectomy. Ann Surg 2006;243(5):571–8.
32. Wente MN, Veit JA, Bassi C, et al. Postpancreatectomy hemorrhage (PPH): an International Study Group of Pancreatic Surgery (ISGPS) definition. Surgery 2007; 142(1):20–5.

33. Besselink MG, van Rijssen LB, Bassi C, et al. Definition and Classification of Chyle Leak After Pancreatic Operation: A Consensus Statement by the International Study Group on Pancreatic Surgery. Surgery 2017;161(2):365–72.

34. Assumpcao L, Cameron JL, Wolfgang CL, et al. Incidence and Management of Chyle Leaks Following Pancreatic Resection: A High Volume Single-Center Institutional Experience. J Gastrointest Surg 2008;12(11):1915–23.

35. Strobel O, Brangs S, Hinz U, et al. Incidence, Risk Factors and Clinical Implications of Chyle Leak After Pancreatic Surgery. Br J Surg 2017;104:108–17.

36. Evans JG, Spiess PE, Kamat AM, et al. Chylous ascites after post-chemotherapy retroperitoneal lymph node dissection: review of the M. D. Anderson experience. J Urol 2006;176(4 Pt 1):1463–7.

37. Baniel J, Foster RS, Rowland RG, et al. Management of chylous ascites after retroperitoneal lymph node dissection for testicular cancer. J Urol 1993;150(5 Pt 1):1422–4.

38. Pappas S, Krzywda E, Mcdowell N. Nutrition and Pancreaticoduodenectomy. Nutr Clin Pract 2010;25(3):234–43.

39. Hamilton L, Jeyarajah DR. Hemoglobin A1c can be Helpful in Predicting Progression to Diabetes After Whipple Procedure. HPB (Oxford) 2007;9:26–8.

40. Ferrara MJ, Lohse C, Kudva YC, et al. Immediate Post-Resection Diabetes Mellitus After Pancreaticoduodenectomy: Incidence and Risk Factors. HPB (Oxford) 2013;15(3):170–4.

41. Hutchins RR, Hart RS, Pacifico M, et al. Long-Term Results of Distal Pancreatectomy for Chronic Pancreatitis in 90 Patients. Ann Surg 2002;236(5):612–8.

42. Huang JJ, Yeo CJ, Sohn TA, et al. Quality of Life and Outcomes After Pancreaticoduodenectomy. Ann Surg 2000;231(6):890–8.

43. Kim KJ, Jeong CY, Jeong SH, et al. Pancreatic Diabetes After Distal Pancreatectomy: Incidence Rate and Risk Factors. Korean J Hepatobiliary Pancreat Surg 2011;15(2):123–7.

44. Wang X, Misawa R, Zielinski MC, et al. Regional Differences in Islet Distribution in the Human Pancreas - Preferential Beta-Cell Loss in the Head Region in Patients with Type 2 Diabetes. PLoS One 2013;8(6):e67454.

45. Kusakabe J, Anderson B, Liu J, et al. Long-Term Endocrine and Exocrine Insufficiency After Pancreatectomy. J Gastrointest Surg 2019;23:1604–13.

46. Cameron JL, He J. Two Thousand Consecutive Pancreaticoduodenectomies. J Am Coll Surg 2015;220(4):530–6.

Failure of Abdominal Wall Closure

Prevention and Management

Samuel J. Zolin, MD*, Michael J. Rosen, MD

KEYWORDS

- Fascial dehiscence • Burst abdomen • Abdominal closure • Fascial closure
- Abdominal closure techniques

KEY POINTS

- Fascial dehiscence is a rare but potentially devastating complication, occurring most commonly in frail patients and often associated with an underlying infectious process.
- A small-bites technique with greater than or equal to 4:1 suture length to wound length ratio using continuous, slowly absorbable monofilament suture is currently recommended for primary fascial closure.
- Prophylactic mesh has been shown to reduce incisional hernia rates and may help to prevent fascial dehiscence in selected patients, although further long-term data are needed.
- In patients with ventral hernias undergoing nonhernia operations, consideration can be given to combined definitive hernia repair.
- When fascia cannot be closed or after fascial dehiscence, multiple management strategies exist; in general, closure with absorbable synthetic mesh is safe and allows for subsequent hernia repair in more optimal conditions.

INTRODUCTION/BACKGROUND

Secure closure of the abdominal wall is imperative after any abdominal operation, with aims of avoiding early fascial dehiscence and long-term incisional hernia. Fascial dehiscence (FD), defined as an unintended acute wound failure at the level of the fascia following primary closure of a laparotomy incision,[1] can lead to dramatic early setbacks and long-term consequences for patients. FD is estimated to occur between 0.3% and 5.5% of the time after laparotomy, most commonly between 4 and 14 days after surgery.[2,3] FD has obvious negative short-term consequences, including need for reoperation, prolonged hospital stay, and increased cost, as well as mortalities of up to 35%.[4] Long-term follow-up indicates that up to 83% of these patients develop incisional hernias and that patients who experience FD have significantly

Cleveland Clinic Foundation, 9500 Euclid Avenue, A100, Cleveland, OH 44195, USA
* Corresponding author.
E-mail address: zolins@ccf.org

Surg Clin N Am 101 (2021) 875–888
https://doi.org/10.1016/j.suc.2021.07.001
0039-6109/21/© 2021 Elsevier Inc. All rights reserved.

lower quality of life with regard to general health, mental health, and social functioning compared with patients who do not experience FD.[5]

NATURE OF THE PROBLEM

In the early postoperative period, the integrity of the abdominal wall depends entirely on the suture and suture-holding capacity of the tissue, because the incised fascia has yet to heal. Wound healing consists of 4 phases, which are coagulation, inflammation, proliferation, and remodeling, and is mediated by interactions between inflammatory cells and the extracellular matrix. Wound strength increases as collagen is deposited and matures during the proliferation and remodeling phases. The proliferation phase can last for about 3 weeks, and by the end of this phase the strength of the abdominal wall is still only approximately 15% to 20% that of unviolated abdominal wall. As time passes, the type 1 to type 3 collagen ratio increases, indicating a more organized extracellular matrix and increased wound strength. The remodeling phase can take months and even a year or more, and healed tissue regains only about 80% of the strength of native tissue.[4,6,7]

In general, a combination of technical and patient-related factors lead to the occurrence of FD, ultimately permitting tension on the abdominal wall to overcome the strength of tissue, suture, or knots. Technical factors may include insecure knots, inadequate suture bites of fascia, excessive distance between fascial sutures, and excessive tension on the closure. Other nontechnical risk factors associated with FD include increasing age, male sex, chronic obstructive pulmonary disease, ascites, jaundice, anemia, emergency surgery, prolonged operative time, and postoperative coughing. Postoperative wound infection is one of the strongest risk factors associated with FD, likely mediated by a prolonged inflammatory phase and release of tissue degradative enzymes by both bacteria and neutrophils.[8,9] Although many of these risk factors are nonmodifiable, the presence of several of these factors in a single patient may indicate substantially higher risk of FD, which some clinicians have used as indications to consider adjuncts to primary fascial closure.[2,10]

FD is difficult to study prospectively because it occurs uncommonly; randomized controlled trials (RCTs) to determine preventive approaches would need to recruit many patients or take place in patients with significantly increased risk of FD to accrue enough instances of FD as an outcome. Therefore, most data to guide prevention of FD come from hernia prevention literature, with the assumption that approaches that prevent long-term hernia development will also prevent short-term FD. Available data have been summarized with expert and societal recommendations in the 2015 European Hernia Society (EHS) Guidelines on the Closure of Abdominal Wall Incisions and the 2018 EHS Clinical Guidelines on the Management of the Abdominal Wall in the Context of the Open or Burst Abdomen, although additional literature on these topics has since been published.

PREOPERATIVE/PREPROCEDURE PLANNING

Avoiding complications related to abdominal wall closure begins before arriving in the operating room (OR). For elective procedures, it is helpful to obtain complete operative records for every patient and to review techniques used for prior abdominal closures, including whether mesh was ever used and its location within the abdominal wall. This point is particularly important if mesh prophylaxis is considered, to avoid or anticipate reoperative planes.

During physical examination and preoperative review of imaging, surgeons should note the presence of any hernias. Small (eg, <2 cm) primary umbilical or epigastric hernias can often be incorporated into incisions used for abdominal access and repaired primarily. Alternatively, if these hernias are asymptomatic and not in a location where they could be incorporated into planned incisions, they may be left alone. A larger incisional hernia should prompt consideration of how the resulting fascial defect will be managed. If the surgeon does not have expertise in hernia repair, the authors recommend preoperative consultation with a hernia specialist to determine whether concomitant definitive hernia repair would be appropriate in the clinical context. Such an approach can allow patients to avoid developing a potentially larger hernia recurrence requiring a second operation. Factors including the degree of intraoperative contamination, length of primary operation and anticipated length of hernia repair, patient body mass index (BMI), hemoglobin A1c level, nutritional status, urgency of the primary operation, and whether subsequent abdominal operations are anticipated (eg, part 1 of a multistage procedure) should be weighed. At our center, we consider definitive hernia repair with permanent synthetic mesh when there is anticipated to be minimal to no contamination, no subsequent operations are planned, and patients otherwise meet criteria for abdominal wall reconstruction (AWR). On the day of surgery, if there are intraoperative complications, if excessive blood loss or contamination occur, or if the operation takes substantially longer than expected and hernia repair would add several hours, we instead close primarily or with an absorbable mesh interposition with plans for later hernia repair.[11] Regardless, preoperative consultation is beneficial so that cosurgeons may review records and imaging and can ensure their availability.

PROCEDURAL APPROACH

A comprehensive review of preoperative surgical site infection (SSI) prevention measures is beyond the scope of this article; however, patients should receive antibiotic prophylaxis with appropriate coverage for the planned procedure. Data indicate that chlorhexidine preparatory solution is associated with decreased SSI rates compared with povidone-iodine in clean and clean-contaminated procedures.[12,13]

From the outset, incisions should be located and sized sufficiently to allow a safe and efficient operation. Disruption of native fascia beyond what is needed for these goals should be avoided. Some data suggest that nonmidline incisions (eg, transverse or paramedian) can reduce the incidence of incisional hernia, and these are recommended by the EHS when possible.[14] However, no significant difference in risk for FD has been shown and these incisions can carry their own morbidity related to transection of the rectus muscle. If a midline incision is used, every effort should be made to stay on midline for the length of the incision when opening, because deviations make fascial closure more difficult. Dissecting directly down to fascia through skin and subcutaneous tissue, instead of obliquely, facilitates fascial exposure at time of closure and may minimize soft tissue trauma. Selection of an abdominal entry site away from prior scar is typically helpful in ensuring safe access.

Intraoperatively, contamination should be minimized. In emergency procedures, contamination may already be present, in which case obtaining rapid source control and avoiding additional spillage are helpful. Multiple RCTs indicate that use of a wound protector, particularly one that is dual ringed, is associated with reduced risk of postoperative SSI.[15,16]

Regardless of technique used to close fascia, abdominal closure should be considered a critical portion of the procedure and receive a proportional amount of attention. Many surgeons tend to devote less time and attention to closure because it occurs at or toward the end of most operations and is perceived as a simple, rote task. Spending a few extra minutes providing patients with a high-quality closure can substantially reduce the risk of short-term and long-term wound failure. Adequate exposure of the full length of the fascial defect ensures that substantial bites of healthy fascia are being taken. "Working in a hole" to avoid a larger skin incision should be avoided if the quality of fascial closure is compromised. Active assistance, including following sutures and retracting to provide better fascial exposure, further expedites closure.

In 2015, the EHS recommended use of a single-layer aponeurotic closure technique with slowly absorbable monofilament suture using a continuous, small-bites technique with suture length/wound length (SL/WL) ratio of greater than or equal to 4:1 for elective surgeries.[14] Continuous suturing of elective midline incisions was recommended based on data suggesting a significantly lower rate of incisional hernia in elective surgery, as well as decreased time to complete closure. A single-layer aponeurotic closure was weakly recommended because no clinical studies directly compared different closure methods. This closure would involve suturing only the abdominal fascia in 1 layer, as opposed to incorporating all layers of the abdominal wall except the skin (mass closure) or closing more than 1 separate layer of fascia (layered closure). Slowly absorbable sutures were recommended rather than nonabsorbable sutures because of decreased risk of suture sinus formation and prolonged wound pain. In addition, rapidly absorbable suture is associated with increased risk of incisional hernia.[17] From a wound healing perspective, this makes sense because the half-life for Vicryl suture is 2 to 3 weeks, overlapping with a period in which the abdominal wall still lacks much of its intrinsic strength.[6] Monofilament sutures were recommended rather than multifilament sutures because multifilament sutures may be more prone to bacterial absorption and infection than monofilament sutures.[4,18] A small-bites technique involves taking bites of fascia 5 to 8 mm from the incision edge and placing stitches every 5 mm along the incision length (**Fig. 1**). Although recommended based on

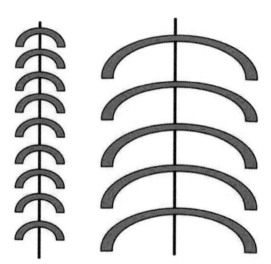

Fig. 1. Small bites versus large bites. Two examples of 4:1 suture length to wound length closure. On the left, a small-bites approach is taken, whereas, on the right, larger bites are taken. To maintain a greater than 4:1 SL/WL ratio, more bites must be taken with the small-bites technique. Data suggest that a small-bites technique is associated with decreased risk of incisional hernia and SSI, likely because less adjacent soft tissue is captured in each bite and placed at risk for necrosis.

data from Millbourn and colleagues,[19] this technique was subsequently strongly supported by the STITCH trial, which showed a 21% rate of incisional hernia at 1-year follow-up with a conventional 1 cm × 1 cm mass closure compared with 13% with a 5 mm × 5 mm closure.[19,20] An SL/WL ratio of greater than or equal to 4:1 has been associated with reduced risk of incisional hernia.[21]

A 2017 Cochrane Review[22] presented more tempered results, concluding that monofilament sutures may reduce risk of incisional hernia compared with multifilament sutures and that absorbable sutures may reduce risk of sinus or fistula tract formation. Otherwise, no major differences were found between mass versus layered closure, or continuous versus interrupted closure for outcomes of wound infection, FD, or incisional hernia at 1 year or more after follow-up. Both the 2015 EHS guidelines and the 2017 Cochrane Review noted issues with design or reporting in several of the reviewed trials: comparator arms differed by multiple aspects of treatment, patient populations were heterogeneous, and different types of incisions were included in single trials. In addition, SL/WL was not recorded in all studies. Further RCTs with long-term follow-up, standardized technique, and capturing all relevant data are needed; however, these recommendations represent the best available evidence.

Despite recommendations for continuous suturing with an SL/WL ratio of greater than or equal to 4:1 with slowly absorbable monofilament suture and small bites, a recent survey study suggests that many surgeons do not apply this method because of lack of technical knowledge of how it is performed, concerns that this technique requires excessive time, or thinking that this technique does not apply to their patient populations. Many surgeons who do attempt to use this technique do not measure the length of suture used or the size of bites taken, raising the question of whether such a technique is being performed adequately to bring about its desired effect.[23] In 2017, Tolstrup and colleagues[24] reported outcomes of implementing a standardized closure technique for emergency laparotomies. This technique was a quality improvement effort wherein surgeons were instructed to use a standardized small-bites technique using continuous 2-0 PDS (polydioxanone) sutures with self-locking knots and received multiple instructional sessions on the new closure technique before implementation. Surgeons were instructed to document the SL/WL ratio. Measured compliance in the postintervention period was 95%. The rate of FD was reduced from 6.6% in the historical cohort of 1079 patients to 3.8% in the postintervention cohort of 494 patients, representing a statistically and clinically significant 42% reduction.[24] This group subsequently published incisional hernia outcomes of this effort, finding incisional hernia rates of 27% in the preintervention group and 15% in the standardized closure group, respectively, although follow-up was slightly longer in the preintervention group.[25] Although nonrandomized, these studies support the applicability of a small-bites technique even in emergency settings, as well as the ability to implement a standardized closure technique with monitoring using prospective, surgeon-collected data for the purposes of quality improvement. Surgeons who are attempting this technique should measure the length of the wound and the length of suture remnants as a method of verifying an adequate SL/WL.

Our institutional preference when primary fascial closure is not possible and the patient is not a candidate for concurrent AWR (eg, highly contaminated field, patient cannot tolerate additional operative time or extensive dissection) is to use an inlay of absorbable polyglactin-based mesh (Vicryl). If omentum is present, this is oriented to cover the bowel before closure. If some fascia can be reapproximated using interrupted figure-of-eight sutures, this is done to limit the bridged area. Then, Vicryl mesh is sewn to intact fascia circumferentially with running, slowly absorbable suture, typically 2-0 PDS. The mesh is doubled over at the edge so that each suture bite incorporates fascia and 2 layers of mesh. Bites are taken at 5-mm intervals and tails are left on the sutures so that sutures can be tied to one another. As much skin and soft tissue are reapproximated over the mesh as possible to maintain a moist healing environment and reduce risk of intestinal fistula. Skin is typically closed with interrupted nylon sutures and/or staples. If soft tissue coverage cannot be obtained completely, then wet-to-dry dressings that are changed 2 to 3 times daily are used to keep the mesh moist. Once granulation tissue has covered the mesh, negative-pressure wound therapy can be applied or skin grafting can be performed.[26] As time goes on, any mesh that does not incorporate into underlying tissue can be debrided carefully so that the wound base granulates. As noted earlier, a concern regarding Vicryl mesh bridging is that of enterocutaneous fistula development. The literature on use of Vicryl mesh bridging consists primarily of retrospective series, which reveal an enteric fistula rate ranging from 0% to 16% (**Table 1**).[26–32] Notably, 1 small randomized controlled trial comparing Vicryl mesh closure with vacuum-assisted closure showed a 5% fistula rate in the Vicryl mesh group and a 21% fistula rate in the vacuum-assisted closure group, although the trial was underpowered for this to reach statistical significance.[33] Although the potential for fistula development cannot be ignored, data suggest that almost all patients undergoing Vicryl mesh closure do not develop a fistula. Clearly, there are tradeoffs with this approach, but, when caring for complex patients with large abdominal wall defects, this technique is highly reproducible even without advanced training, does not require additional returns to the OR, and does not burn bridges for future AWR.

Retention sutures are another technique that has been used historically in patients thought to be at high risk of FD. However, data regarding the utility of retention sutures are sparse, such that no recommendation on their use could be made in the 2015 EHS guidelines.[34,35]

A major emerging topic within the hernia prevention literature is prophylactic mesh (PM) placement for abdominal closure. Given the impact on patients and high costs to the health care system that incisional hernias confer, numerous investigations have taken place to determine whether PM placement at time of abdominal closure reduces rates of incisional hernia. In general, these studies have supported the effectiveness of

Table 1
Rates of enterocutaneous fistula following Vicryl mesh closure of the abdomen

Author, Year	Patients Studied (n)	Fistula Rate (%)
Dayton, et al,[30] 1986	8	0
Ivatury, et al,[31] 1989	7	0
Fabian, et al 1994	27	3.7
Jernigan, et al,[29] 2003	166	8.4
Mayberry, et al,[32] 2004	140	7.1
Bee, et al,[33] 2008	20	5.0
Fischer, et al,[28] 2009	380	8.0
Renard, et al,[27] 2020	57	15.8
Lewis, et al,[26] 2020	61	11.5

Rates of enterocutaneous fistula development following Vicryl mesh closure of the abdomen as reported in the literature. Although fistula development is a serious outcome of this approach, data suggest that this outcome is still uncommon.

PM placement rather than suture closure alone, particularly in high-risk groups for incisional hernia, such as patients with obesity or who are undergoing abdominal aortic aneurysm repair (**Table 2**). In their 2015 guidelines, the EHS stated that "[PM] augmentation is effective in prevention of incisional hernias," but avoided making a strong recommendation regarding its routine use because of lack of larger trials. Several subsequent meta-analyses have further supported the efficacy of prophylactic mesh at reducing rates of incisional hernia.[36,37] However, there are several important questions that remain, including the optimal material and location of PM placement within the abdominal wall, which patients should be selected for this intervention, long-term outcomes in terms of mesh-related morbidity, and degree of surgical skill or training necessary to place these materials optimally in challenging patients.

Table 2
Randomized controlled trials evaluating incisional hernia prevention with prophylactic mesh after midline laparotomy

Author, Year	n	Mesh Type	Mesh Position	Incisional Hernia: Mesh Group (%)	Incisional Hernia: Suture Group (%)	P
Pans, et al,[48] 1998	288	Polyglactin	Intraperitoneal	22.9	28.5	.43
Gutierrez de la Pena, et al,[49] 2003	88	Polypropylene	Onlay	0	11.4	.02
Strzelczyk, et al,[50] 2006	74	Polypropylene	Retromuscular	0	21.1	.005
El-Khadrawy, et al,[51] 2009	40	Polypropylene	Preperitoneal	5	15	.01
Bevis, et al,[52] 2010	80	Polypropylene	Preperitoneal	13.5	37.2	.022
Abo-Ryia, et al,[53] 2013	64	Polypropylene	Preperitoneal	3.1	28.1	<.01
Caro-Tarrago, et al,[54] 2014	160	Polypropylene	Onlay	1.5	35.9	<.01
Sarr, et al,[55] 2014	280	Biologic	Intraperitoneal	17.3	19.5	.6
Bali, et al,[56] 2014	40	Biologic	Onlay	0	31.6	.008
Garcia-Urena, et al,[57] 2015	107	Polypropylene	Onlay	11.3	31.5	.011
Muysoms, et al,[14] 2016	120	Partially absorbable polypropylene	Retromuscular	0	28	<.001
Jairam, et al,[37] 2017	480	Polypropylene	Onlay (188) or retromuscular (185)[a]	15.8	30.8	<.001

RCTs evaluating use of PM for prevention of incisional hernia. Mean follow-up in all trials was at least 1 year, with most having follow-up of at least 2 years. Overall, these data suggest the efficacy of PM placement for prevention of incisional hernia. In many trials, technical details regarding closure methods in the nonmesh group were not recorded, and some of these trials occurred before there were data in support of a small-bites suture technique. Future investigation comparing PM placement with optimal suturing technique are needed, as well as attention to long-term mesh-related outcomes.

[a] This was a 3-armed trial comparing suture with both onlay mesh and retromuscular mesh prophylaxis.

Pertinent to FD, Lima and colleagues[10] recently published an RCT comparing the small-bites suture technique versus the small-bites technique augmented with onlay PM in patients at high risk for FD undergoing emergent midline laparotomy, with FD as the primary outcome. Patients with a Rotterdam risk score greater than or equal to 4.0 or greater than or equal to 2.2 with obesity, malnutrition, malignancy, or smoking were included, whereas patients with existing incisional hernia or presence of mesh, prior recent laparotomy, severe hemodynamic instability, need for open abdomen, or relaxing incisions were excluded. For patients receiving mesh reinforcement, polypropylene mesh with pore diameter 0.8 mm and weight 100 g/m^2 was used and was sized so that at least 3 cm of overlap would be present in all directions from the incision. All patients were imaged at 30 days. FD occurred in 13.5% of patients closed with suture alone, whereas no instances of FD occurred in patients closed with PM reinforcement. Although this difference was statistically and clinically significant, there were also significantly greater rates of nonhealing incisional wounds (23.8% vs 5.8%) and SSIs (20.7% vs 7.7%) in the group receiving PM. In addition, operative time was an average of 50.8 minutes longer in the group receiving PM. Of note, despite the intention of all patients receiving an SL/WL ratio of greater than or equal to 4:1 in this study, only 34.7% of patients in the suture group and 23.7% of patients in the PM group received this.[10]

Ultimately, the decision to place PM at the time of abdominal closure depends on multiple factors, including the patient's baseline risk of developing an incisional hernia, the degree of contamination, and the surgeon's familiarity and comfort level with PM use. If a surgeon intends to use PM, the authors recommend preoperative discussion of this with the patient as part of informed consent and shared decision making. Many patients have concerns regarding mesh use based on negative media portrayals[38] and may reasonably be upset if a permanent implant is placed without prior discussion, even if there is expected benefit.

In addition, patients who are not stable for definitive abdominal closure should be considered. Damage control laparotomy (DCL), where the abdomen is temporarily closed, most often with a vacuum dressing or with skin-only closure, has become a popular and potentially lifesaving technique for physiologically unstable patients in trauma and emergency general surgery settings. Use of DCL after initial control of hemorrhage and/or infection is intended to allow for further resuscitation and correction of acidosis, coagulopathy, and hypothermia, while also preventing abdominal compartment syndrome, permitting reevaluation of potentially compromised bowel, and facilitating further exploration for missed injury after an initial trauma operation. Although many patients have clear indications for DCL, DCL seems to be overused in a minority of patients who could likely be closed at their index operation.[39,40] From an abdominal wall perspective, the likelihood of primary fascial closure decreases with the length of time that the abdomen remains open after DCL.[41] In addition, use of DCL in patients who likely could have been closed has been associated with an increase in ventilator, intensive care unit, and hospital days.[42] Therefore, the authors recommend judicious use of DCL in general and prompt abdominal closure when it is used.

RECOVERY AND REHABILITATION

Postoperatively, many surgeons use abdominal binders with the expectation that these will reduce postoperative pain, allow patients to mobilize more easily, and potentially reduce risk of abdominal wall complications. Although there are some data to suggest that patients have reduced pain and/or increased comfort in the early postoperative period, as well as increased mobility, there are no data to suggest a benefit with regard to FD or incisional hernia development.[43–45]

DIAGNOSIS OF FASCIAL DEHISCENCE

Several signs and symptoms should raise concern for the possibility of FD, including delayed return of bowel function, new onset of postoperative bowel obstruction symptoms after operation, unexpected incisional pain, serous drainage from an incision, or development of new bulging at the site of an incision. When such symptoms occur, they should lead to prompt evaluation for FD. If patients develop new incisional drainage and the clinical picture is unclear, initial evaluation may occur with removal of skin staples or sutures and probing the wound with a sterile cotton applicator for a fascial defect, or cross-sectional imaging may be performed. If frank evisceration occurs, bowel should be covered with a moist gauze while arrangements are made for urgent return to the OR. Occasionally, FD may be noted on imaging obtained for another reason in an otherwise asymptomatic patient (eg, reimaging a known fluid collection). It is worthwhile to look for these on imaging so that further decisions can be made regarding their management.

MANAGEMENT

In contrast with fairly substantial data regarding optimal closure of primary abdominal incisions, data to guide management of FD when it occurs is of significantly lower quality. Again, the uncommon and often emergent nature of FD makes RCTs on FD management difficult to perform. Many recommendations from the 2018 EHS guidelines on management of FD are extrapolated from retrospective studies of FD or from evidence regarding primary fascial closure, and the quality of evidence for all key questions regarding FD management in these guidelines was considered very low.[1]

If the overlying skin closure is intact, there does not seem to be radiographic bowel obstruction or compromise, and the patient is not having symptoms related to FD, then nonoperative management may be appropriate with a low threshold to return to the OR should symptoms develop. A nonoperative approach is likely most appropriate for patients in whom FD was discovered incidentally during imaging for another reason. This approach may also be borne out of necessity for patients with hostile abdomens or those who are severely ill and might not tolerate return to the OR. There are little to no data to guide this decision.

However, for many patients with FD, return to the OR will be necessary based on presence of symptoms. An assessment of the reason that FD occurred should be made. If there is a clear and isolated technical cause for failure, such as a knot becoming unraveled, consideration could be given to repeating the same closure method. However, in most cases, it is likely that FD has occurred secondary to a combination of both technical and patient-related factors, which may include poor tissue quality at baseline, infection, and tissue necrosis. In these cases, it is important to obtain source control for any ongoing infectious process and to debride any devitalized tissue until healthy tissue is reached. At this point, the surgeon must determine whether fascial reapproximation will be possible.

The 2018 EHS guidelines recommend that, when definitive primary fascial closure is possible, continuous monofilament sutures with an SL/WL ratio of greater than or equal to 4:1 should be used to close after FD; however, this is based on very limited data and is extrapolated from some of the data on closure of abdominal wall incisions in general. In clinical practice, it is unclear how many patients who experience FD would be able to be closed without tension and have healthy tissue to facilitate such an approach. In addition, for surgeons not familiar with this technique, it is not advisable to start in this challenging clinical scenario.

Similar to the approach for initial fascial closure as described earlier, most patients who would experience an FD at our institution would undergo closure with interrupted figure-of-eight slowly absorbable monofilament sutures if fascial reapproximation under minimal tension were possible, and closure with a polyglactin mesh inlay if fascial reapproximation were not possible or possible only under a great deal of tension.

The EHS guidelines recommend mesh reinforcement in procedures where fascial closure is possible after FD based on significantly decreased pooled rates of incisional hernia after fascial closure with mesh reinforcement (12.5%) as opposed to fascial closure alone (32.9%). Of note, the rate of surgical site occurrences was higher in the mesh group (48.8%) than for fascial closure alone (23.5%).[1] No data were available regarding incidence of fascial redehiscence, nor for fistula formation. The ultimate conclusion in these guidelines is that the decision to use mesh, the type of mesh used, and the location of the mesh used should be considered by the surgeon. A more recent meta-analysis further supports the use of mesh for closure after FD, suggesting lower rates of incisional hernia and equivalent rates of SSI.[3] Again, although mesh may reduce hernia formation, it is unclear how many patients might go on to develop infected mesh after these frequently contaminated procedures, subsequently requiring further surgical intervention and likely developing hernia at a later time point.

In general, the authors advise caution regarding the use of advanced AWR techniques such as component separation techniques (CSTs) for management of FD. Many of these patients are malnourished, have other ongoing catabolic issues, have fixed and noncompliant edematous abdominal walls, and cannot tolerate a major AWR. In particular, the goal with patients with FD is to prevent fistula formation and not necessarily prevent eventual incisional hernia formation. If surgeons do not regularly use CSTs in elective settings, there is greater risk of poor outcomes when CSTs are applied acutely after a patient has already had an unexpected complication and where there is frequently contamination. Potential complications of CSTs include bleeding, skin necrosis, SSI, abdominal wall denervation, and flank hernias. In addition, attempts at a CST can make future hernia repair more challenging if native anatomic planes are violated.

An intriguing technique for abdominal closure in the context of an open abdomen or after FD when primary closure is not possible is vacuum-assisted mesh-mediated fascial traction (VAWCM). A perforated polyethylene sheet with a thin central sponge is placed into the abdomen to protect the viscera. Two halves of a polypropylene mesh are then sewn to the fascial edges on each side of the abdominal wall and then sewn together in the midline. In addition, an additional sponge is placed on top of the polypropylene mesh to act as a wound VAC (vacuum-assisted closure). Every 2 to 3 days, the patient is taken back to the OR for exchange of the vacuum system and mesh tightening. Fascial closure is then considered when 3 to 7 cm of fascial separation are achieved.[46] This technique yields a high reported rate of fascial closure (89%); however, at 1 year, up to 66% of these patients develop incisional hernias.[47]

Attempting to perform component separation or returning to the OR for serial VAC changes and mesh tightening in the context of VAWCM are clear indicators that surgeons want to be aggressive in returning patients to their predisease quality of life. However, these interventions are not benign, and the patients receiving them have already had at least 1 major postoperative setback. In our opinion, it is likely most prudent to give patients a safe and prompt abdominal closure with Vicryl mesh to get them out of trouble, accepting that this will result in a hernia, and refer them to a specialist in AWR in a few months once they have recovered from their acute illness.

SUMMARY

Secure fascial closure is a fundamental technical step of any abdominal operation. Using optimal primary closure techniques may reduce the risk of FD and subsequent incisional hernia formation. Adjuncts such as PM may further reduce the risk of these adverse outcomes in appropriately selected patients. In selected patients who already have hernias, a combined operation with definitive mesh-based hernia repair can allow avoidance of a subsequent hernia recurrence. Although FD is an uncommon complication, it happens most often in acutely ill and debilitated patients and is frequently related to intra-abdominal infection. Multiple closure strategies after FD exist with few data to guide clinicians. In general, safe abdominal closure should be prioritized with absorbable mesh interposition if needed, accepting that hernia formation is likely but avoiding additional returns to the OR and further abdominal wall complications.

CLINICS CARE POINTS

- Closure with a greater than or equal to 4:1 suture to wound length ratio using small bites with a running, slowly absorbable monofilament suture is the current recommendation for abdominal closure.

- In patients with existing ventral hernias undergoing elective abdominal surgery, consideration can be given to concomitant ventral hernia repair.

- There are substantial data that PM reduces incisional hernia rates and may reduce risk of FD, although questions remain regarding the optimal mesh, placement within the abdominal wall, and secondary complications associated with mesh placement offsetting its advantages. Deciding whether to use this depends on the clinical context and surgeon and patient preference.

- DCL can be lifesaving for selected patients who are not stable for definitive abdominal closure. Risk for incisional hernia increases with the duration of time that the abdomen remains open, so prompt closure is recommended.

- Avoiding advanced AWR techniques in the acute setting is advisable. The value of knowing when to come back another day cannot be overstated in the management of these complex patients.

DISCLOSURE

S.J. Zolin has nothing to disclose. M.J. Rosen has received salary support for his leadership position in the Abdominal Core Health Quality Collaborative, is a board member and has stock/stock options from Ariste Medical, and has research grants from Pacira Pharmaceuticals Inc. and Intuitive Inc.

REFERENCES

1. López-Cano M, García-Alamino JM, Antoniou SA, et al. EHS clinical guidelines on the management of the abdominal wall in the context of the open or burst abdomen. Hernia 2018;22(6):921–39.
2. Kenig J, Richter P, Lasek A, et al. The efficacy of risk scores for predicting abdominal wound dehiscence: a case-controlled validation study. BMC Surg 2014;14(1):1–6.
3. Denys A, Monbailliu T, Allaeys M, et al. Management of abdominal wound dehiscence: update of the literature and meta-analysis. Hernia 2020;25(2):449–62.

4. Israelsson LA, Millbourn D. Prevention of incisional hernias. How to close a midline incision. Surg Clin North Am 2013;93(5):1027–40.
5. van Ramshorst GH, Eker HH, van der Voet JA, et al. Long-term outcome study in patients with abdominal wound dehiscence: a comparative study on quality of life, body image, and incisional hernia. J Gastrointest Surg 2013;17(8):1477–84.
6. Henriksen NA, Deerenberg EB, Venclauskas L, et al. Meta-analysis on materials and techniques for laparotomy closure: the MATCH review. World J Surg 2018; 42(6):1666–78.
7. Harris HW, Hope WH, Adrales G, et al. Contemporary concepts in hernia prevention: selected proceedings from the 2017 International Symposium on Prevention of Incisional Hernias. Surgery 2018;164(2):319–26.
8. Webster C, Neumayer L, Smout R, et al. Prognostic models of abdominal wound dehiscence after laparotomy. J Surg Res 2003;109(2):130–7.
9. Van Ramshorst GH, Nieuwenhuizen J, Hop WCJ, et al. Abdominal wound dehiscence in adults: development and validation of a risk model. World J Surg 2010; 34(1):20–7.
10. Lima HVG, Rasslan R, Novo FCF, et al. Prevention of fascial dehiscence with onlay prophylactic mesh in emergency laparotomy: a randomized clinical trial. J Am Coll Surg 2020;230(1):76–87.
11. Petro CC, Rosen MJ. Fight or flight: the role of staged approaches to complex abdominal wall reconstruction. Plast Reconstr Surg 2018;142(3S):38S–44S.
12. Privitera GP, Costa AL, Brusaferro S, et al. Skin antisepsis with chlorhexidine versus iodine for the prevention of surgical site infection: a systematic review and meta-analysis. Am J Infect Control 2017;45(2):180–9.
13. Noorani A, Rabey N, Walsh SR, et al. Systematic review and meta-analysis of preoperative antisepsis with chlorhexidine versus povidone-iodine in clean-contaminated surgery. Br J Surg 2010;97(11):1614–20.
14. Muysoms FE, Antoniou SA, Bury K, et al. European Hernia Society guidelines on the closure of abdominal wall incisions. Hernia 2015;19(1):1–24.
15. Kang S II, Oh HK, Kim MH, et al. Systematic review and meta-analysis of randomized controlled trials of the clinical effectiveness of impervious plastic wound protectors in reducing surgical site infections in patients undergoing abdominal surgery. Surgery 2018;164(5):939–45.
16. Edwards JP, Ho AL, Tee MC, et al. Wound protectors reduce surgical site infection: a meta-analysis of randomized controlled trials. Ann Surg 2012;256(1):53–9.
17. van 't Riet M, Steyerberg EW, Nellensteyn J, et al. Meta-analysis of techniques for closure of midline abdominal incisions. Br J Surg 2002;89(11):1350–6.
18. Hewin DF, Osther PJ, Gottrup F. Randomized comparison of polyglycolic acid and polyglyconate sutures for abdominal fascial closure after laparotomy in patients with suspected impaired wound healing. Br J Surg 1995;82(12):1698–9.
19. Millbourn D, Cengiz Y, Israelsson LA. Effect of stitch length on wound complications after closure of midline incisions: a randomized controlled trial. Arch Surg 2009;144(11):1056–9.
20. Deerenberg EB, Harlaar JJ, Steyerberg EW, et al. Small bites versus large bites for closure of abdominal midline incisions (STITCH): A double-blind, multicentre, randomised controlled trial. Lancet 2015;386(10000):1254–60.
21. Israelsson LA. Bias in clinical trials: The importance of suture technique. Eur J Surg 1999;165(1):3–7.
22. Patel SV, Paskar DD, Nelson RL, et al. Closure methods for laparotomy incisions for preventing incisional hernias and other wound complications. Cochrane Database Syst Rev 2017;2017(11):CD005661.

23. Fischer JP, Harris HW, López-Cano M, et al. Hernia prevention: practice patterns and surgeons' attitudes about abdominal wall closure and the use of prophylactic mesh. Hernia 2019;23(2):329–34.

24. Tolstrup MB, Watt SK, Gögenur I. Reduced rate of dehiscence after implementation of a standardized fascial closure technique in patients undergoing emergency laparotomy. Ann Surg 2017;265(4):821–6.

25. Thorup T, Tolstrup MB, Gögenur I. Reduced rate of incisional hernia after standardized fascial closure in emergency laparotomy. Hernia 2019;23(2):341–6.

26. Lewis RH, Sharpe JP, Croce MA, et al. How soon is too soon?: optimal timing of split-thickness skin graft following polyglactin 910 mesh closure of the open abdomen. J Trauma Acute Care Surg 2020;89(2):377–81.

27. Renard Y, de Mestier L, Henriques J, et al. Absorbable polyglactin vs. non-cross-linked porcine biological mesh for the surgical treatment of infected incisional hernia. J Gastrointest Surg 2020;24(2):435–43.

28. Fischer PE, Fabian TC, Magnotti LJ, et al. A ten-year review of enterocutaneous fistulas after laparotomy for trauma. J Trauma - Inj Infect Crit Care 2009;67(5):924–8.

29. Jernigan TW, Fabian TC, Croce MA, et al. Staged management of giant abdominal wall defects: acute and long-term results. Ann Surg 2003;238(3):349–57.

30. Dayton MT, Buchele BA, Shirazi SS, et al. Use of an absorbable mesh to repair contaminated abdominal-wall defects. Arch Surg 1986;121(8):954–60.

31. Ivatury RR, Nallathambi M, Rao PM, et al. Open management of the septic abdomen: therapeutic and prognostic considerations based on APACHE II. Crit Care Med 1989;17(6):511–7.

32. Mayberry JC, Burgess EA, Goldman RK, et al. Enterocutaneous fistula and ventral hernia after absorbable mesh prosthesis closure for trauma: the plain truth. J Trauma 2004;57(1):157–62.

33. Bee TK, Croce MA, Magnotti LJ, et al. Temporary abdominal closure techniques: a prospective randomized trial comparing polyglactin 910 mesh and vacuum-assisted closure. J Trauma 2008;65(2):337–42.

34. Khorgami Z, Shoar S, Laghaie B, et al. Prophylactic retention sutures in midline laparotomy in high-risk patients for wound dehiscence: a randomized controlled trial. J Surg Res 2013;180(2):238–43.

35. Rink AD, Goldschmidt D, Dietrich J, et al. Negative side-effects of retention sutures for abdominal wound closure. A prospective randomised study. Eur J Surg 2000;166(12):932–7.

36. Borab ZM, Shakir S, Lanni MA, et al. Does prophylactic mesh placement in elective, midline laparotomy reduce the incidence of incisional hernia? A systematic review and meta-analysis. Surgery 2017;161(4):1149–63.

37. Jairam AP, López-Cano M, Garcia-Alamino JM, et al. Prevention of incisional hernia after midline laparotomy with prophylactic mesh reinforcement: a meta-analysis and trial sequential analysis. BJS Open 2020;4(3):357–68.

38. AlMarzooqi R, Petro C, Tish S, et al. Patient perceptions on mesh use in hernia repair: a prospective, questionnaire-based study. Surgery 2020;167(4):751–6.

39. Hatch QM, Osterhout LM, Podbielski J, et al. Impact of closure at the first take back: complication burden and potential overutilization of damage control laparotomy. J Trauma 2011;71(6):1503–11.

40. Harvin JA, Sharpe JP, Croce MA, et al. Better understanding the utilization of damage control laparotomy: a multi-institutional quality improvement project. J Trauma Acute Care Surg 2019;87(1):27–34.

41. Pommerening MJ, Dubose JJ, Zielinski MD, et al. Time to first take-back operation predicts successful primary fascial closure in patients undergoing damage control laparotomy. Surgery 2014;156(2):431–8.
42. Harvin JA, Sharpe JP, Croce MA, et al. Effect of damage control laparotomy on major abdominal complications and lengths of stay: a propensity score matching and Bayesian analysis. J Trauma Acute Care Surg 2019;87(2):282–8.
43. Bouvier A, Rat P, Drissi-Chbihi F, et al. Abdominal binders after laparotomy: review of the literature and French survey of policies. Hernia 2014;18(4):501–6.
44. Clay L, Gunnarsson U, Franklin KA, et al. Effect of an elastic girdle on lung function, intra-abdominal pressure, and pain after midline laparotomy: a randomized controlled trial. Int J Colorectal Dis 2014;29(6):715–21.
45. Arici E, Tastan S, Can MF. The effect of using an abdominal binder on postoperative gastrointestinal function, mobilization, pulmonary function, and pain in patients undergoing major abdominal surgery: a randomized controlled trial. Int J Nurs Stud 2016;62:108–17.
46. Petersson U, Acosta S, Björck M. Vacuum-assisted wound closure and mesh-mediated fascial traction - A novel technique for late closure of the open abdomen. World J Surg 2007;31(11):2133–7.
47. Bjarnason T, Montgomery A, Ekberg O, et al. One-year follow-up after open abdomen therapy with vacuum-assisted wound closure and mesh-mediated fascial traction. World J Surg 2013;37(9):2031–8.
48. Pans A, Elen P, Dewé W, et al. Long-term results of polyglactin mesh for the prevention of incisional hernias in obese patients. World J Surg 1998;22(5):479–82 [discussion: 482–3].
49. Gutiérrez de la Peña C, Medina Achirica C, Domínguez-Adame E, et al. Primary closure of laparotomies with high risk of incisional hernia using prosthetic material: analysis of usefulness. Hernia 2003;7(3):134–6.
50. Strzelczyk JM, Szymański D, Nowicki ME, et al. Randomized clinical trial of postoperative hernia prophylaxis in open bariatet alric surgery. Br J Surg 2006;93(11):1347–50.
51. El-Khadrawy OH, Moussa G, Mansour O, et al. Prophylactic prosthetic reinforcement of midline abdominal incisions in high-risk patients. Hernia 2009;13(3):267–74.
52. Bevis PM, Windhaber RA, Lear PA, et al. Randomized clinical trial of mesh versus sutured wound closure after open abdominal aortic aneurysm surgery. Br J Surg 2010;97(10):1497–502.
53. Abo-Ryia MH, El-Khadrawy OH, Abd-Allah HS. Prophylactic preperitoneal mesh placement in open bariatric surgery: a guard against incisional hernia development. Obes Surg 2013;23(10):1571–4.
54. Caro-Tarrago A, Olona Casas C, Jimenez Salido A, et al. Prevention of incisional hernia in midline laparotomy with an onlay mesh: a randomized clinical trial. World J Surg 2014;38(9):2223–30.
55. Sarr MG, Hutcher NE, Snyder S, et al. A prospective, randomized, multicenter trial of Surgisis Gold, a biologic prosthetic, as a sublay reinforcement of the fascial closure after open bariatric surgery. Surgery 2014;156(4):902–8.
56. Bali C, Papakostas J, Georgiou G, et al. A comparative study of sutured versus bovine pericardium mesh abdominal closure after open abdominal aortic aneurysm repair. Hernia 2015;19(2):267–71.
57. García-Ureña MÁ, López-Monclús J, Hernando LA, et al. Randomized controlled trial of the use of a large-pore polypropylene mesh to prevent incisional hernia in colorectal surgery. Ann Surg 2015;261(5):876–81.

Management of Postcholecystectomy Complications

Xiaoxi (Chelsea) Feng, MD, MPH[a], Edward Phillips, MD[a],
Daniel Shouhed, MD[b],*

KEYWORDS

- Cholecystectomy • Complications • Gallbladder • Cholecystitis • Surgery

KEY POINTS

- Proper surgical technique, knowledge of potential aberrant anatomy, achieving the critical view of safety, and use of cholangiography are all measures that can help prevent bile duct injury.
- Early recognition of bile duct injury and prompt referral to a tertiary hepatobiliary referral center is key.
- Techniques such as cholangiogram and ERCP should be used to avoid retained common bile duct stones.

INTRODUCTION
Epidemiology

Gallstone disease affects 12% to 15% of the population in the United States. Stones can be found in the gallbladder (cholelithiasis) or the common bile duct (choledocholithiasis). Although most patients with gallstones remain asymptomatic, it is estimated that 20% will develop symptoms or complications over a 20-year period.[1] Risk factors for gallstone disease include female sex, increased age, pregnancy, obesity, diabetes, and genetics, among others.

Imaging Studies

Ultrasound is useful as a first test for gallbladder disease, as it is noninvasive, inexpensive, readily available, and can give information about the gallbladder and the biliary tree. Computed tomography (CT) can also identify gallbladder wall edema, thickness, and adjacent fluid associated with cholecystitis but is less accurate in identifying choledocholithiasis. Nuclear scintigraphy is the most sensitive and specific imaging

[a] Department of Surgery, Cedars Sinai Medical Center, 8635 W Third Street, West Medical Office Tower, Suite 795, Los Angeles, CA 90048, USA; [b] Department of Surgery, Cedars Sinai Medical Center, 459 North Croft Avenue, Los Angeles, CA 90048, USA
* Corresponding author. Department of Surgery, 250 North Robertson Boulevard Suite 106 Beverly Hills, CA 90211
E-mail address: Daniel.shouhed@cshs.org

Surg Clin N Am 101 (2021) 889–910
https://doi.org/10.1016/j.suc.2021.06.012
0039-6109/21/© 2021 Elsevier Inc. All rights reserved.

modality for identifying cystic duct obstruction, which is often associated cholecystitis. However, it does not give anatomic information, and is a time-intensive study. Magnetic resonance cholangiopancreatography (MRCP) is more sensitive than both ultrasound and CT for choledocholithiasis and delineation of biliary anatomy.

Indications for Surgery

Indications for cholecystectomy range from benign to malignant, elective to urgent. The most common reasons include biliary colic, acute and chronic calculous cholecystitis, biliary dyskinesia, and acalculous cholecystitis. Other presentations include gangrenous cholecystitis, gallstone pancreatitis, choledocholithiasis with or without cholangitis, gallbladder fistulae (duodenum, colon), and gallbladder carcinoma. Gallbladder polyps are also an indication for cholecystectomy, with several different considerations: size over 10 mm, smaller size (6-9 mm) but with risk factors for gallbladder carcinoma, polyp(s) with biliary symptoms, and increase in size on interval imaging.

Patients presenting with choledocholithiasis should be referred for cholecystectomy, especially if the patient has experienced complications, such as biliary pancreatitis or cholangitis. If the patient presents with cholangitis in the setting of common bile duct (CBD) stones, urgent decompression of the biliary tree is indicated. If the patient presents with evidence of biliary pancreatitis, the degree of pancreatitis should be assessed. If the pancreatitis is mild, it is advised to perform cholecystectomy during the same admission, rather than deferring for an interval cholecystectomy.[2,3] Cholecystectomy during the same admission was not found to be associated with increased intraoperative or postoperative complications, but has been found to decrease hospital length of stay, as well as readmissions in patients who had mild gallstone pancreatitis.[3-5] In severe acute pancreatitis with peripancreatic collections, some authors advocate waiting 3 weeks or longer.[6] The current International Association of Pancreatology/American Pancreatic Association recommendations state that cholecystectomy after severe acute pancreatitis should be delayed until the collections either resolve or after 6 weeks.[2,7]

EARLY SURGICAL COMPLICATIONS
Adjacent Organ Injury

Injuries to nearby organs during cholecystectomy, including the duodenum, colon, and liver, have all been described. In addition to bowel and vascular injury occurring during the course of abdominal entry, an injury can occur during dissection, especially in an inflamed surgical field seen in acute superimposed on chronic cholecystitis. The incidence of injury to nearby organs ranges between 0.2% and 1.1%.[8,9]

Duodenum

The overall incidence of duodenal injuries during cholecystectomy is rare (0.07% to 0.2%).[10,11] One review cited the following causes for injury to the duodenum during cholecystectomy: 46% due to cautery, 39% due to dissection, and 14% due to retraction.[10] Duodenal injury has been noted in the first, second, and third portions. Pain after surgery may be nonspecific, and laboratory values such as liver function tests may also have nonspecific elevations. However, pain that persists or worsens after 24 hours should raise suspicion. Ultrasound imaging may be considered, as well as contrast study with gastrograffin or CT scan with oral contrast. In a patient with clinical suspicion or deteriorating status, re-exploration is indicated. Delayed presentation may be due to thermal injury and eschar sloughing.

Management of the duodenal injury depends on the timing of identification, size of the defect, as well as the location. If identified at the time of the index operation, direct suture repair with omental patch can be performed. Delays in diagnosis may result in the tissue becoming inflamed and edematous, thus precluding primary repair. If the injury is small or self-sealing, conservative management with external drainage and broad-spectrum antibiotics may be sufficient. For larger defects or longer time to diagnosis, mucosal or serosal or seromuscular patches can be performed, as well as wide drainage (duodenostomy tube) with pyloric exclusion and gastrojejunostomy, gastric resection with duodenal stump closure, or even duodenopancreatectomy resection.[10] The same review found an increase in mortality rate with delayed detection of the duodenal injury.[10]

Colon

Colonic injuries have also been described during cholecystectomy. One study reported 2 cases of colonic injury during laparoscopic cholecystectomy (LC): one injury was attributed to electrocautery and grasping forceps, and the other case due to blunt dissection around an adherent, acutely inflamed gallbladder.[12] Colonic injuries can also occur at the time of laparoscopic entry. On-table identification typically allows for primary repair, possibly with drainage.

Liver

A variety of presentations of liver injury after cholecystectomy have been described. There is a paucity of published reports and the true incidence is unknown. Intrahepatic and/or subcapsular hematomas or bilomas and even hemobilia have been reported. Most of these case reports describe patients presenting in delayed fashion with right-sided chest or right upper quadrant abdominal pain with fever.[13–15] Diagnosis is typically made with CT, and treatment may require percutaneous or surgical drainage, with or without endoscopic retrograde cholangiopancreatography (ERCP)/ transampullary stenting. Bilomas were attributed to injuries of small biliary radicals near the gallbladder or in the gallbladder bed at the index operation. Traction injuries to the liver are also possible and have led to subcapsular hematomas.[16,17]

Bleeding

Bleeding during cholecystectomy can occur from trocar sites or other forms of iatrogenic trauma to the liver or liver bed, hepatic arteries or veins, portal vein, mesentery, omentum, and other major vessels (aorta, vena cava, middle colic, iliac vessels). A pooled data analysis of cholecystectomies reported a 0.79% prevalence of bleeding, although this complication may be hard to capture as the definitions vary from study to study.[18] There does not seem to be a significant difference between risk of bleeding for open versus laparoscopic cholecystectomy,[19] although bleeding was cited as one of the more frequent reasons prompting emergent conversion to laparotomy.[20]

Bleeding during dissection can be avoided by having an appreciation for possible anatomic variations of the vascular anatomy. There can be superficial and deep branches of the cystic artery, with up to 8.9% of patients having multiple cystic arteries.[21] There can also be small anastomotic vessels between the cystic artery to intrahepatic branches of the right or left hepatic artery, occurring in approximately 12% of postmortem models.[22] Injury to the middle hepatic vein may also be encountered, with up to 10% of patients having a large middle hepatic vein adjacent to the gallbladder bed[23–25] (also see below in Vascular Complications).

Bile Duct Injury

Bile duct injury (BDI) is a very serious complication of cholecystectomy. After the initial learning curve of laparoscopy, more current studies of the rates of BDI during laparoscopic cholecystectomy estimates between 0.08% and 0.5% is generally higher than the reported rates for open cholecystectomy (0.1%–0.2%) though BDI may be under-reported when occurring in open surgery.[26–31] Most of the BDI injuries are due to errors in visual perception (97%), with errors due to faults in technical skill accounting for only 3%.[33] Twenty-five percent of injuries in this study were recognized at the index operation.[33] Factors that contribute to iatrogenic injury include excessive retraction distorting anatomy, anatomic aberrancies, presence of inflammation, improper use of cautery, or problems related to control of intraoperative hemorrhage, to name a few.[28] In addition, higher severity grades of acute cholecystitis are associated with a higher risk of BDI.[32] Management depends on when the injury is recognized, the location of the injury, and whether or not there is concurrent vascular injury.

Prevention

Proper surgical technique, knowledge of potential aberrant anatomy, achieving the critical view of safety, converting to open and use of radiographic and/or florescent cholangiography are all measures that can help avoid BDI. The critical view of safety was first described by Strasberg and colleagues as a method of consistent identification of the cystic duct and artery. However, it can be difficult to obtain in some cases with severe inflammation. It consists of fulfilling 3 criteria: (1) the hepatocystic triangle is cleared of fat and fibrous tissue, (2) the lower third of the gallbladder is separated from the liver to expose the cystic plate, and (3) two and only two structures should be seen entering the gallbladder[34] (**Fig. 1**). These two structures should be viewed anteriorly and posteriorly with an angled laparoscope or by "waving" the fundus. The critical view of safety has been largely supported by expert opinion to be the most reliable method of anatomic identification, and therefore is recommended as a strong guideline for laparoscopic cholecystectomies.[35]

If there is uncertainty about biliary anatomy, or suspicion for anatomic aberrations, cholangiography via the gallbladder itself or cystic duct should be used if possible to clarify structures.[36] Reports have shown that the use of cholangiography can reduce the risk of bile duct injuries, but there are also studies that have found no association.[35] However, if a biliary injury is suspected intraoperatively, intraoperative cholangiogram is effective for increasing the odds of early recognition, which improves outcomes in the treatment of BDI.[35] The Society of American Gastrointestinal and Endoscopic Surgeons recommends "liberal use" of cholangiography or other modalities to accurately delineate surgical anatomy.[34] There are some proponents for the use of routine

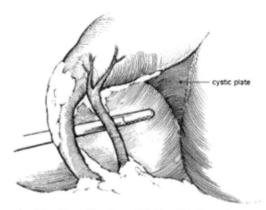

cystic plate

Fig. 1. Critical view of safety. (*From* Strasberg SM, Hertl M, Soper NJ. An analysis of the problem of biliary injury during laparoscopic cholecystectomy. J Am Coll Surg 1995;180(1):113.)

cholangiography, citing not just a lower rate of BDI but the avoidance of excisional injuries which are more serious.[35,37–39] Biliary anatomy can also be imaged using intraoperative ultrasound if the expertise is available.

Presentation

Patients typically present with abdominal pain, vomiting, ileus, fever, and/or jaundice. Subhepatic drains, when used, can allow for early detection of a leak. Laboratory values will typically show leukocytosis with liver function tests consistent with obstruction, absorption of bilirubin from the peritoneal cavity, cholestasis, and jaundice, although if the biliary system remains relatively decompressed due to an active leak or presence of a drain, liver function tests may be near normal in the early period. Left undiagnosed, intraperitoneal bile may cause peritonitis, abscess, and sepsis.

Imaging

Ultrasound is typically the first imaging modality used, as it can show a fluid collection or dilated bile ducts. A contrast-enhanced CT scan is helpful in determining the size and location of fluid collections as well as vascular anatomy. Occasionally, ultrasound and CT scan will only show free peritoneal fluid in the pelvis.[40] HIDA scan can also confirm a bile leak, evidenced by extra-biliary tracer accumulation, but does not render useful anatomic detail. MRCP is useful in that respect, giving good resolution of the biliary tree. ERCP can also be used and has the advantage of therapeutic options, such as sphincterotomy and stent placement. Similarly, percutaneous transhepatic cholangiography (PTC) can be performed, and also be followed by interventions such as drainage, balloon dilation, or stent placement. PTC has the advantage of better visualization of the proximal biliary tree than ERCP.

Classification

There are multiple classification systems for bile leaks. The Bismuth classification describes the injury according to distance from the hepatic hilum, the level of injury, the involvement of the confluence, and the right sectoral duct (**Fig. 2**). The more commonly used system is the Strasberg classification (**Fig. 3**).

The "classical" BDI that has been described by Davidoff and colleagues is where the common bile duct is mistaken for the cystic duct and divided. This is often followed by the common hepatic duct being mistaken for an "accessory duct" and also divided[41] (**Fig. 4**). It can occur as a result of excessive cephalad retraction of the fundus or insufficient lateral retraction of the infundibulum. The right hepatic artery is near, often passing either posterior or anterior to the common hepatic duct, and thus is also at risk for injury from dissection during this process (see *Vascular Injury* section).

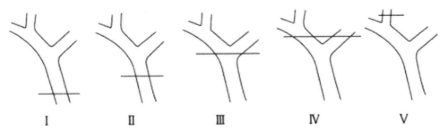

I   II   III   IV   V

Fig. 2. Bismuth classification. (*Adapted from* Jarnagin WR, Blumgart LH. Benign biliary strictures. In: Blumgart LH, editor. Surgery of the liver, biliary tract, and pancreas. 4th edition. Philadelphia: Saunders; 2007. p. 634.)

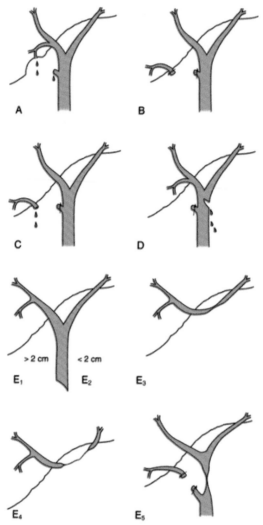

Fig. 3. Strasberg classification. (Strasberg SM, Hertl M, Soper NJ, et al. AN analysis of the problem of biliary injury during laparoscopic cholecystectomy, J Am Coll Surg. 1995;180:101.)

Management

If a BDI is suspected during cholecystectomy, a cholangiogram should be performed to clarify the biliary anatomy and identify the injury. Repair may require conversion to open technique. As the occurrence of a serious injury can be emotionally and psychologically difficult for the surgeon, requesting the help of a more experienced colleague is often recommended. If a BDI is suspected postoperatively, MRCP, ERCP, or PTC can all be helpful in delineating biliary anatomy and injury. The percutaneous technique can be superior to ERCP at visualizing the proximal portion of the system, which may be helpful in assessing higher-level BDIs. Referral to a center experienced in the repair of complicated biliary injuries should be considered.

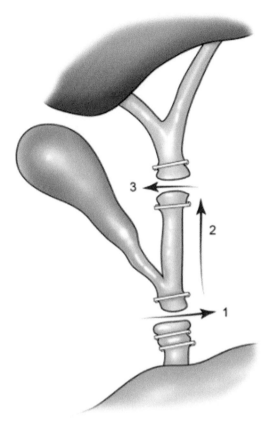

Fig. 4. Classical bile duct injury. The "classical" bile duct injury—Excessive cephalad retraction of the GB leads to dissection of the CBD low down. (1) Subsequent mobilization of the bile duct occurs. (2) Removal of the GB specimen requires further division of the bile duct. (3) In around 25% of cases, division of the RHA as well. GB, gallbladder; CBD, common bile duct; RHA, right hepatic artery.

For minor injuries (defined as involving the cystic duct or small peripheral or duct of Luschka), endoscopic stenting and intra-abdominal drainage are often sufficient for definitive treatment.[28] Major injuries that involve loss of bile duct tissue or long complex strictures will usually require surgery.[42]

The goal of any repair is to maintain biliary-enteric continuity. Small partial transections may be amenable to primary repair and placement of a T-tube or stent across the area of injury. Complete transection can also be treated with primary end-to-end repair over a T-tube if there is minimal loss of tissue, and the ends can be brought together without tension. Consideration should be given to ischemia due to transection of the biliary blood supply, which will lead to nonhealing or stricturing of the bile duct long-term. Thermal/electrocautery injuries will require debridement to normal tissues and rarely can be repaired end to end. If there is loss of tissue that precludes a tension-free anastomosis or if there is a concern for ischemia, then a loop of jejunum should be brought up in a roux-en-Y configuration for an end-to-side anastomosis. Oftentimes this is done over a temporary silastic stent for biliary decompression. Another option for low injuries is to Kocherize the duodenum and perform a choledocho-duodenostomy. Any type of biliary reconstruction should be accompanied by external drainage.

If the BDI is diagnosed in delayed fashion, surgical intervention typically should be delayed if the bile can be diverted or drained. A combination of CT-guided drainage and percutaneous transhepatic drainage, or ERCP with stenting should be undertaken to control intra-abdominal fluid collections, as well as provide biliary decompression. This will allow for temporization and adequate treatment of infection and peritonitis, both of which are risk factors for poor outcome of future reconstruction. In addition, it provides time for final demarcation of any vascular injury, which helps to ensure that the definitive repair is performed at the correct level. Finally, a delayed approach allows for nutritional and clinical optimization of the patient. One study found that intermediate repair of BDI in their cohort (which they defined as between 72 hours and 6 weeks) was significantly correlated with the development of biliary stricture, which occurred in 14% of their study group.[43]

In the event of a nonreparable injury due to anatomy, lack of expertise or equipment, the proximal biliary system should be intubated and brought out for external drainage. The surgical field should be widely and adequately drained. For management of complex BDI or any BDI that the surgeon is not equipped to address, transfer to a high-volume hepatobiliary center should be initiated. Delayed referral to a tertiary center has been demonstrated in some studies to have a negative effect on outcomes.[44,45] The treatment of BDIs is often multidisciplinary and should involve expertise from other specialties, such as gastroenterology and radiology. Suboptimal repair may lead to further tissue loss or progressively higher level of biliary stricture that prohibits reconstruction options. There is also risk of development of biliary cirrhosis or portal hypertension with unsuccessful repair and subsequent stricture. Chapman and colleagues reported on their case series, which included both primary, revisional, and multiply-revisional postcholecystectomy BDI cases, and noted that there was evidence of portal hypertension in 17.7%.[46] Johnson and colleagues reported that delayed referral, average 12 months, was associated with significant hepatic injury in 31.3% of their BDI cohort.[47] Lastly, liver transplant may be necessary if reconstruction fails or has already resulted in liver failure.

Retained Gallstones

Careful management of common bile duct stones during cholecystectomy is key in avoiding morbidity associated with retained stones, and the first step lies in recognition. The American Society for Gastrointestinal Endoscopy published guidelines for stratification of the risk of choledocholithiasis based on biochemical tests and abdominal ultrasound findings; high-risk features include choledocolithiasis on ultrasound, bilirubin > 4 mg/dL, bilirubin level 1.8 to 4.0 mg/dL plus a dilated CBD, or evidence of cholangitis. These criteria are imperfect and these guidelines are estimated to have a 74% specificity and 64% positive predictive value for choledocholithiasis.[48] Preoperative MRCP or endoscopic ultrasound (EUS) may be a consideration for identification of suspected common bile duct stones. Nonetheless, small stones (<5 mm) may be missed.[49,50] IOC is estimated to have a slightly higher sensitivity for common bile duct stones than ERCP.[51]

If common bile duct stones are identified or clinically suspected preoperatively, several approaches are feasible: LC with preoperative, intraoperative, or postoperative ERCP; and LC or open cholecystectomy with laparoscopic or open common bile duct exploration (LCBDE). A meta-analysis comparing all 4 techniques found that LC with intraoperative ERCP is the safest and most successful method of retrieval when performed by an expert team.[52] However, this technique involves the coordination of two separate operators and may not be as widely available. LCBDE had the highest probability of avoiding acute pancreatitis but was associated with a higher risk of biliary leak.[52] Transcystic laparoscopic common bile duct exploration is another approach for common bile duct stones that has proven efficacy in the treatment of choledocholithiasis and symptom resolution.[53,54]

IOC can be performed to ensure clearance of the biliary tree. The incidental discovery rate for CBD stones during IOC is estimated to be 3.4% to 4.6%.[55–57] One study followed these common bile duct stones over time to describe their natural history: 26% had a normal cholangiogram at 48 hours (raising the possibility of false-positive initial cholangiogram), 26% were found to have a negative 12-week cholangiogram (stones spontaneously passed), and 47.8% had persistent choledocholithiasis at 6 weeks after LC, which were retrieved by ERCP/ sphincterotomy.[57] While the latter group only comprised 2.2% of that total study population, failure to identify and clear the biliary tree may cause postoperative symptoms. Another study reported an incidence of 2.3% of symptomatic retained CBD stones after LC, and identified that small stone size and multiple gallstones were both risk factors for retained CBD stones.[58]

Early presentation of retained common bile duct stones is possible, and a patient representing postcholecystectomy with abdominal pain, elevated liver function tests, pancreatitis, and/or cholangitis should raise suspicion for retained common bile duct stone. On ultrasound imaging, size of the CBD may be mild to moderately dilated at 10 to 15 mm, although 10% of patients had normal-sized CBD (6 mm or less).[59] MRCP is most often used. ERCP can be used in these patients for endoscopic sphincterotomy and/or stent placement. In particular, a stent may be needed if the patient presents with cholangitis and continued drainage of the biliary tree is indicated. There are risks to performing ERCP in the acute post-LC period, in addition to the usual risks of ERCP. However, one study reported that of their cohort, 75% underwent ERCP within 1 week after LC and did not suffer immediate complications.[60]

Vascular Complications

Beyond the immediate bleeding complications that can be incurred on abdominal entry, vascular injuries can manifest in several different forms after cholecystectomy. There can be a vascular injury without concomitant biliary injury, or what is known as a vasculobiliary injury, where there is injury to a bile duct as well as a hepatic artery and/or portal vein. Either case may or may not be associated with hepatic ischemia. The most commonly injured vessel is the right hepatic artery (or aberrant right hepatic artery), followed by the portal vein.[61]

Right hepatic artery

There are anatomic variations to the origin and course of the right hepatic artery (RHA), which can complicate dissection in Calot's triangle and predispose to iatrogenic injury. Dandekar and colleagues found an aberrant replaced right hepatic artery in 18.3% of their cadaver study population, and an aberrant accessory right hepatic artery in 3.4%.[62] It tends to cross posterior to the common hepatic duct (71.6%), although can cross anteriorly as well (8.3%).[62] One anatomic variant is known as the caterpillar or Moynihan's hump, which describes a tortuosity in the right hepatic artery that can cause it to occupy a large part of Calot's triangle, lying very close to the gallbladder neck and cystic duct. There is also usually a very short cystic artery in this variant, which is estimated to be found in 1.3% to 13.3% of patients.[62–65] The right hepatic artery can be mistaken for the cystic artery in these situations and be inadvertently injured or ligated, thus highlighting the importance of adherence to tenets of the critical view of safety.

Strasberg and Helton postulate that isolated right hepatic artery injury without associated biliary injury may not always clinically manifest, especially if the right hepatic artery is occluded.[61] They reason that when there is an associated biliary injury, reports of occlusion are more common than pseudoaneurysms, whereas with reports of arterial injury without biliary injury, pseudoaneurysms predominate. Supporting this idea is a cadaveric study of 71 patients who had undergone cholecystectomies, where 7% had an injury to the right hepatic artery but with no evidence of liver or bile duct abnormalities.[66]

In addition to occlusion, injury to the right hepatic artery can manifest as a pseudoaneurysm. This is most often accompanied by a biliary leak, but can also happen in isolation.[67–69] They are thought to form due to unrecognized mechanical or thermal trauma to the vessel during the initial operation, or due to a local inflammatory milieu (eg, bile leak or infected fluid collection) causing erosion of the arterial wall. Time from cholecystectomy to clinical manifestation of the pseudoaneurysm can range anywhere from 6 days to 5 years, with a mean time of 36 days.[68,70] Presentation is usually due to rupture, causing intra-abdominal bleeding, intraluminal bleeding, or hemobilia (hemorrhage into the biliary tract). If stable with resuscitation, CT scan with IV contrast can be considered, and if a pseudoaneurysm is identified, transarterial embolization is usually effective in occlusion of the sac (94.5% success rate).[68,71] Endovascular stent placement is another possibility, although rarely used. Failure of angiography or hemodynamic instability should prompt surgical intervention and ligation of the artery or excision of the pseudoaneurysm.

Cystic artery

Cystic artery pseudoaneurysms after cholecystectomy can occur by the same pathophysiology as described earlier.[72–74] This is the second most common vessel susceptible to pseudoaneurysm formation after the right hepatic artery.[68,75] Other vessels such as the common hepatic and gastroduodenal artery have also been described but are even less common.

Portal vein

Direct injury to the portal vein is a rare occurrence as it is a posterior structure; Strasberg and Helton reviewed 16 such cases, and the majority were associated with concurrent injury to a major hepatic artery.[61] Almost all of these patients suffered some sequelae of hepatic ischemia, ranging from hepatic abscess, to hepatic necrosis requiring right hepatectomy, and in some cases, liver transplant. Mortality is estimated to increase by 56% when a portal vein injury occurs with a BDI.[76]

Portal vein thrombosis is estimated to occur in about 1.4% or less of patients. Patients typically present anywhere from 6 days to 2 months after cholecystectomy with nausea, bloating, and diffuse abdominal pain.[77–79] Diagnosis can be made with ultrasound, or more commonly, CT imaging with IV contrast. There may be associated infarction of the liver.[77]

Formation of portal vein thrombosis is likely multifactorial. Patients may have procoagulation risk factors, such as oral contraceptive use or a known hypercoagulable disorder.[77,78,80,81] Pneumoperitoneum from the laparoscopy also changes portal venous blood flow. Lastly, there can be direct injury to the vessel, but this is less likely given its posterior position. For treatment, anticoagulation should be started, and other interventions such as percutaneous transhepatic portal vein thrombectomy have been reported with success.[77]

Combined vasculobiliary injury

Oftentimes, a BDI occurs together with a vascular injury, with the bile leak and the concurrent compromised blood supply compounding morbidity. These vasculobiliary injuries are estimated to occur during 12% to 61% of bile duct injuries.[61] There is conflicting data on whether or not vascular injury affects long-term outcomes of biliary injuries, such as future stricture rates.[82–85] Strasberg and Helton hypothesize that these differences may be due to the difference in outcomes of early versus late repair in the presence of a vessel injury.[61]

The rate of associated liver infarction with a vasculobiliary injury is about 10%.[61] Liver parenchymal morbidities include abscess, necrosis, and atrophy. There are some case reports of extreme injuries requiring right hepatectomy, or even liver transplant.[86–88] In the event of a high BDI that is at risk for concurrent vascular injury, or a recognized complex vasculobiliary injury, referral to a tertiary hepatobiliary center is recommended. Angiography or cross-sectional imaging with arterial and portal venous phases can be used to delineate the location and extent of the vascular injury.

LATE COMPLICATIONS
Retained Gallstones—Late

Retained common bile duct stones can also have a delayed presentation, ranging between 6 days and 18 years, with a median time of 152 days after index cholecystectomy.[59,89] Similar to earlier presentation of retained CBD stones, patients can present with abdominal pain, fevers, jaundice, and deranged liver function tests. In fact, some patients experience what is described as recurrent biliary colic, highlighting that retained common bile duct stones (or retained gallbladder stones) should be on the differential for recurrent postcholecystectomy symptoms.[90]

Ultrasound, MRCP, or CT can all be used in the diagnosis of retained stones. ERCP is usually effective for clearance of the duct, and may be urgently indicated if the patient presents with cholangitis. If initial ERCP is unsuccessful or incomplete at ductal clearance, a stent can be placed and ERCP reattempted at a later time, as was reported to be performed in 2 case series.[59,89] In fact, in a study of the second attempt of ERCP performed for retained CBD stones, the authors found that 37% of patients had spontaneous stone passage, and another 49% underwent successful stone extraction, all avoided further surgical intervention.[91] Another alternative to ERCP is laparoscopic or open common bile duct exploration, where the cystic duct stump can be identified and used for transcystic exploration, or a choledochotomy can be created. One series of laparoscopic CBDE for retained CBD stones reported that cystic duct stump identification was possible in 84% of cases.[92] Finally, a nonsurgical technique that has been reported is shockwave lithotripsy, but this depends on institutional expertise.[90]

Outside of two years after cholecystectomy, the possibility of primary bile duct stones should be considered, especially if pigment stones are found. Primary biliary stones are usually light brown and soft, and are hypothesized to be related to biliary stasis, rather than originating from the gallbladder.[93] A drainage procedure is usually indicated if primary stones are suspected.

Spilled Gallstones

Spillage of stones can occur with gallbladder perforation, during intraoperative dissection or specimen extraction.[94] With an incidence of 5.7% to 33%,[95–98] retained spilled gallstones have the potential to cause a variety of complications if lost within the surgical field. The incidence of a lost gallstone leading to complication can range from 7% to 8.5%.[96,99]

Most manifest in the first several months after cholecystectomy, although delayed presentation up to several years have been reported. Intra-abdominal abscess is the most common complication, cited to account for approximately 60% in one review.[96] The second-most common complication was wound sinus or fistula, accounting for approximately 30%.[96] Fistulas have been reported to the skin, umbilicus, colon, and bladder.[99–101] Other reports include empyema, bowel obstruction, and erosion through the flank.[96] Systemic complications such as septicemia and recurrent bacteremia are also possible.[102,103] A search of the literature will reveal a plethora of interesting case reports of long-term consequences of spilled gallstones, including mimicking a retroperitoneal sarcoma,[104] resembling pleural metastases and subsequently expectorated,[105] discovery in a direct inguinal hernia sac,[106] and causing a transdiaphragmatic abscess.[107]

All authors of these case reports and reviews emphasize the importance of prevention of spillage of gallstones, and in the event of spillage, thorough retrieval and irrigation. Placing a Raytec sponge in the subhepatic space can help limit spilled stones to the subhepatic space, also making retrieval easier. Loss of gallstones and retention in the abdominal cavity should certainly be documented in the operative report, for future reference.[108] Some advocate for a short course of antibiotics.[97] As this is a rare complication, conversion to open is not generally not recommended for retrieval of stones.

Postcholecystectomy Syndrome

Postcholecystectomy syndrome (PCS) describes the persistence or development of new gastrointestinal symptoms after cholecystectomy, and has been estimated to occur in anywhere from 4% to 18% of patients.[109,110] Symptoms can include abdominal pain, indigestion, fatty food intolerance, heartburn, vomiting, and diarrhea. Pain is estimated to persist in 19%-26% of patients postcholecystectomy, whereas nonpain symptoms can persist in up to 43%-57%.[111–113] In one study, diarrhea was the most common nonpain symptom that was new or not found to be significantly decreased after surgery.[111,113] Another study found that pre-existing belching, flatulence, and heartburn were all symptoms that had suboptimal improvement after LC.[114]

There are multiple, varied causes of PCS that have been described, which can generally be divided into biliary and extra-biliary. Biliary etiologies include retained stones, primary bile duct stones, biliary stenosis, and sphincter of Oddi dysfunction. One hypothesis for patients having similar symptoms postsurgery despite the removal of the gallbladder is dilation of the biliary tree and increased common bile duct pressure.[115] Patients could have extra-biliary disease such as gastroesophageal reflux disease, hiatal hernia, pancreatitis, intestinal disorders, and intercostal neuritis, to name a few.[116] Patients presenting with such complaints should undergo a renewed workup, possibly including upper endoscopy, liver function tests, imaging such as ultrasound or MRCP, HIDA, ERCP, etc.

Hernias

Hernias can occur at any port site or incision, and for laparoscopic procedures, rates vary from 0.2% to 1.7%.[117–121] In laparoscopic procedures, the periumbilical (midline) location was the most common site (76%) and most (86.3%) were from ports that were 10 mm in size or larger.[122] However, incarceration can occur through 5 mm and 8 mm trocar sites as well, if placed through the midline.[123–127] Risk factors include older age (>70 years), body mass index over 30 kg/m^2, duration of surgery, diabetes mellitus, incision enlargement, and wound infection.[119]

About one-third of trocar site hernias present soon after the operation, while the rest occurred more than 30 days after surgery.[128] 76% of early-onset cases presented with bowel obstruction, and thus a high degree of suspicion for incarceration for early-onset trocar site hernias and a low threshold to surgical intervention is encouraged.[128] Authors have observed that Richter's hernias tend to present more so with early-onset cases.[129,130] Patients can present with vomiting and abdominal pain and require prompt surgical intervention to avoid ischemia and perforation. The median interval for late-onset cases was 5.5 months. These tend to present with a bulge instead of obstructive symptoms.[128] Various preventative measures have been proposed, such as routine closure of trocar sites over 10 mm, but currently, there are no definitive recommendations.[128,131]

Rates of hernia after open cholecystectomies are estimated to be around 3.3% to 6%.[132–134] Another technique of cholecystectomy, the single-incision laparoscopic cholecystectomy, was introduced in the 1990s and is suggested to have better incisional cosmesis. Some studies and reviews have not found a difference in the rate of incisional hernias between single-incision LC versus conventional LC.[135,136] Other studies have indeed found a statistically significant difference, with a higher rate in the single-incision LC (5.8% to 13.3%) versus conventional LC (0.9% to 4.7%).[137–139]

Stricture

Strictures are one of the most common long-term outcomes of BDI, and occur after biliary reconstruction as well. Postsurgical strictures are often the result of direct thermal injury, ischemia, or clipping. They can also occur due to chronic or recurrent choledocholithiasis causing local inflammation. Strictures typically present with signs of cholestasis and biliary obstruction, including jaundice, pruritus, cholangitis, or intrahepatic abscess formation. Time to manifestation can vary anywhere between 3 days and 190 months after the BDI, with one study reporting a median of 35 months.[140] Thus, some recommend a 2- to 3-year minimum follow-up after BDI repair, up to 7 to 10 years, to truly assess the risk of stricture formation.[46]

The typical surgical approach for postcholecystectomy benign biliary stricture is roux-en-Y hepaticojejunostomy depending on biliary anatomy. Other nonsurgical techniques such as percutaneous transhepatic stenting, catheter balloon dilation, or endoscopic stenting can also be used as either primary therapies or adjuncts to surgery. Risk factors that predict poor outcomes of the bilioenteric anastomosis include previous failed repairs, repair in the presence of a fistula (perhaps due to inflammation or lack of a dilated ductal system), presence of peritonitis, and presence of cirrhosis and portal hypertension.[140]

In BDI patients with concurrent vascular injury, roux-en-Y bilio-enteric anastomosis may not offer optimal long-term results. This may be due to compromised blood supply to the repaired ducts. If such cases include parenchymal pathology, such as liver atrophy/fibrosis or abscess, then hepatic resection with biliary reconstruction or transplant may be a better option.[83,141,142]

SUMMARY

Cholecystectomy is one of the most common general surgery procedures performed worldwide but can be fraught with potential pitfalls. The Society for American Gastrointestinal Endoscopic Surgeons Safe Cholecystectomy Task Force identified multiple important factors for safety in laparoscopic cholecystectomy[31]:

- Establishing the critical view of safety
- Understanding the anatomy
- Obtaining adequate exposure
- Calling a senior colleague for help
- Recognizing when to convert or abandon

Complications after cholecystectomy include bile duct injuries or leaks, bleeding, combined vasculobiliary injuries, retained gallstones, spilled gallstones, abscesses, strictures, hernias, and PCS. Although the rates of these complications are generally very low, awareness and high clinical suspicion when a patient presents a week, a month, or years after cholecystectomy can help with diagnosis and appropriate treatment.

CLINICS CARE POINTS

- Safe laparoscopic abdominal entry techniques are critical in avoiding hollow viscus and vascular injuries.

- Bile duct injury is a dreaded complication; vigilance for distorted anatomy, knowledge of anatomic variations, judicious use of thermal energy and clipping, application of the critical view of safety, use of intraoperative cholangiography, and prudent conversion to open can all help to decrease the risk.

- Bile duct injuries diagnosed in delayed fashion usually benefit from delayed repair, after adequate treatment of intra-abdominal infection, clinical and nutritional optimization of the patient, and demarcation of any concurrent vascular injury causing ischemia.

- Prompt referral to a high volume hepatobiliary referral center in the event of a bile duct injury that is outside the scope of the surgeon is critical in optimizing patient outcome.

- There is no consensus on whether intraoperative cholangiogram should be used routinely versus selectively; any clinical suspicion of choledocholithiasis should prompt an intraoperative cholangiogram to avoid retained common bile duct stones. ERCP can also be used preoperatively, intraoperatively, or postoperatively to address choledocholithiasis.

- The most commonly injured vessel in a cholecystectomy is the right hepatic artery.

- Bile duct injury can occur in conjunction with a vascular injury; these combined vasculobiliary injuries typically require complex, multimodal treatment algorithms.

- Postcholecystectomy syndrome can occur because of both biliary causes, thought to be due to distention of the biliary tree, or extra-biliary causes.

DISCLOSURE

The authors have nothing to disclose.

REFERENCES

1. Shabanzadeh DM, Sørensen LT, Jørgensen T. A Prediction Rule for Risk Stratification of Incidentally Discovered Gallstones: Results From a Large Cohort Study. Gastroenterology 2016;150(1):156–67.e1.
2. Working Group IAP/APA Acute Pancreatitis Guidelines. IAP/APA evidence-based guidelines for the management of acute pancreatitis. Pancreatol Off J Int Assoc Pancreatol IAP Al 2013;13(4 Suppl 2):e1–15.
3. da Costa DW, Bouwense SA, Schepers NJ, et al. Same-admission versus interval cholecystectomy for mild gallstone pancreatitis (PONCHO): a multicentre randomised controlled trial. Lancet Lond Engl 2015;386(10000):1261–8.
4. Moody N, Adiamah A, Yanni F, et al. Meta-analysis of randomized clinical trials of early versus delayed cholecystectomy for mild gallstone pancreatitis. Br J Surg 2019;106(11):1442–51.
5. Gurusamy KS, Nagendran M, Davidson BR. Early versus delayed laparoscopic cholecystectomy for acute gallstone pancreatitis. Cochrane Database Syst Rev 2013;9:CD010326.

6. Uhl W, Müller CA, Krähenbühl L, et al. Acute gallstone pancreatitis: timing of laparoscopic cholecystectomy in mild and severe disease. Surg Endosc 1999;13(11):1070–6.

7. Nealon WH, Bawduniak J, Walser EM. Appropriate timing of cholecystectomy in patients who present with moderate to severe gallstone-associated acute pancreatitis with peripancreatic fluid collections. Ann Surg 2004;239(6):741–9, discussion 749-751.

8. Schrenk P, Woisetschläger R, Rieger R, et al. Mechanism, management, and prevention of laparoscopic bowel injuries. Gastrointest Endosc 1996;43(6): 572–4.

9. Fletcher E, Seabold E, Herzing K, et al. Laparoscopic cholecystectomy in the Acute Care Surgery model: risk factors for complications. Trauma Surg Acute Care Open 2019;4(1):e000312.

10. Machado NO. Duodenal injury post laparoscopic cholecystectomy: Incidence, mechanism, management and outcome. World J Gastrointest Surg 2016;8(4): 335–44.

11. Croce E, Golia M, Russo R, et al. Duodenal perforations after laparoscopic cholecystectomy. Surg Endosc 1999;13(5):523–5.

12. El-Banna M, Abdel-Atty M, El-Meteini M, et al. Management of laparoscopic-related bowel injuries. Surg Endosc 2000;14(9):779–82.

13. Cervantes J, Rojas GA, Ponte R. Intrahepatic subcapsular biloma. A rare complication of laparoscopic cholecystectomy. Surg Endosc 1994;8(3):208–10.

14. Leppard WM, Chavin KD, McGillicuddy JW. A what? Subcapsular biloma after laparoscopic cholecystectomy. Am Surg 2011;77(7):E131–2.

15. Stathopoulos V, Georganas M, Stratakis K, et al. Hepatic Subcapsular Biloma: A Rare Complication of Laparoscopic Cholecystectomy. Case Rep Surg 2014. https://doi.org/10.1155/2014/186819.

16. de Castro SMM, Reekers JA, Dwars BJ. Delayed intrahepatic subcapsular hematoma after laparoscopic cholecystectomy. Clin Imaging 2012;36(5):629–31.

17. Alexander HC. Two unusual hemorrhagic complications during laparoscopic cholecystectomy. Surg Laparosc Endosc 1993;3(4):346–8.

18. Pucher PH, Brunt LM, Davies N, et al. Outcome trends and safety measures after 30 years of laparoscopic cholecystectomy: a systematic review and pooled data analysis. Surg Endosc 2018;32(5):2175–83.

19. Suuronen S, Kivivuori A, Tuimala J, et al. Bleeding complications in cholecystectomy: a register study of over 22,000 cholecystectomies in Finland. BMC Surg 2015;15:97.

20. Lengyel BI, Azagury D, Varban O, et al. Laparoscopic cholecystectomy after a quarter century: why do we still convert? Surg Endosc 2012;26(2):508–13.

21. Andall RG, Matusz P, du Plessis M, et al. The clinical anatomy of cystic artery variations: a review of over 9800 cases. Surg Radiol Anat SRA 2016;38(5): 529–39.

22. Bergamaschi R, Ignjatovic D. Anatomic rationale for arterial bleeding from the liver bed during and/or after laparoscopic cholecystectomy: a postmortem study. Surg Laparosc Endosc Percutan Tech 1999;9(4):267–70.

23. Levi Sandri GB, Eugeni E, Bufo A, et al. Unexpected bleeding during laparoscopic cholecystectomy: a hepatic vein injury. Surg Radiol Anat 2017;39(9): 1061–2.

24. Ball CG, MacLean AR, Kirkpatrick AW, et al. Hepatic vein injury during laparoscopic cholecystectomy: the unappreciated proximity of the middle hepatic

vein to the gallbladder bed. J Gastrointest Surg Off J Soc Surg Aliment Tract 2006;10(8):1151–5.

25. Bharatam KK. An unspoken threat hiding behind the gall bladder in laparoscopic cholecystectomy - The middle hepatic vein. Clin Med Rev Case Rep 5:229.

26. Mangieri CW, Hendren BP, Strode MA, et al. Bile duct injuries (BDI) in the advanced laparoscopic cholecystectomy era. Surg Endosc 2019;33(3):724–30.

27. Halbert C, Pagkratis S, Yang J, et al. Beyond the learning curve: incidence of bile duct injuries following laparoscopic cholecystectomy normalize to open in the modern era. Surg Endosc 2016;30(6):2239–43.

28. Nuzzo G, Giuliante F, Giovannini I, et al. Bile duct injury during laparoscopic cholecystectomy: results of an Italian national survey on 56 591 cholecystectomies. Arch Surg Chic Ill 1960 2005;140(10):986–92.

29. Rystedt J, Lindell G, Montgomery A. Bile Duct Injuries Associated With 55,134 Cholecystectomies: Treatment and Outcome from a National Perspective. World J Surg 2016;40(1):73–80.

30. Roslyn JJ, Binns GS, Hughes EF, et al. Open cholecystectomy. A contemporary analysis of 42,474 patients. Ann Surg 1993;218(2):129–37.

31. Pucher PH, Brunt LM, Fanelli RD, et al. SAGES expert Delphi consensus: critical factors for safe surgical practice in laparoscopic cholecystectomy. Surg Endosc 2015;29(11):3074–85.

32. Törnqvist B, Waage A, Zheng Z, et al. Severity of Acute Cholecystitis and Risk of Iatrogenic Bile Duct Injury During Cholecystectomy, a Population-Based Case-Control Study. World J Surg 2016;40(5):1060–7.

33. Way LW, Stewart L, Gantert W, et al. Causes and prevention of laparoscopic bile duct injuries: analysis of 252 cases from a human factors and cognitive psychology perspective. Ann Surg 2003;237(4):460–9.

34. The SAGES Safe Cholecystectomy Program - Strategies for Minimizing Bile Duct Injuries. SAGES. Available at: https://www.sages.org/safe-cholecystectomy-program/. Accessed January 8, 2021.

35. Brunt LM, Deziel DJ, Telem DA, et al. Safe Cholecystectomy Multi-society Practice Guideline and State of the Art Consensus Conference on Prevention of Bile Duct Injury During Cholecystectomy. Ann Surg 2020;272(1):3–23.

36. Carroll BJ, Friedman RL, Liberman MA, et al. Routine cholangiography reduces sequelae of common bile duct injuries. Surg Endosc 1996;10(12):1194–7.

37. Fletcher R, Deal R, Kubasiak J, et al. Predictors of Increased Length of Hospital Stay Following Laparoscopic Sleeve Gastrectomy from the National Surgical Quality Improvement Program. J Gastrointest Surg Off J Soc Surg Aliment Tract 2018;22(2):274–8.

38. Buddingh KT, Weersma RK, Savenije RAJ, et al. Lower rate of major bile duct injury and increased intraoperative management of common bile duct stones after implementation of routine intraoperative cholangiography. J Am Coll Surg 2011;213(2):267–74.

39. Nickkholgh A, Soltaniyekta S, Kalbasi H. Routine versus selective intraoperative cholangiography during laparoscopic cholecystectomy: a survey of 2,130 patients undergoing laparoscopic cholecystectomy. Surg Endosc 2006;20(6):868–74.

40. Walker AT, Shapiro AW, Brooks DC, et al. Bile duct disruption and biloma after laparoscopic cholecystectomy: imaging evaluation. AJR Am J Roentgenol 1992;158(4):785–9.

41. Davidoff AM, Pappas TN, Murray EA, et al. Mechanisms of major biliary injury during laparoscopic cholecystectomy. Ann Surg 1992;215(3):196–202.

42. Vitale GC, Tran TC, Davis BR, et al. Endoscopic management of postcholecystectomy bile duct strictures. J Am Coll Surg 2008;206(5):918–23, discussion 924-925.

43. Sahajpal AK, Chow SC, Dixon E, et al. Bile duct injuries associated with laparoscopic cholecystectomy: timing of repair and long-term outcomes. Arch Surg Chic Ill 1960 2010;145(8):757–63.

44. Martinez-Lopez S, Upasani V, Pandanaboyana S, et al. Delayed referral to specialist centre increases morbidity in patients with bile duct injury (BDI) after laparoscopic cholecystectomy (LC). Int J Surg Lond Engl 2017;44:82–6.

45. Fischer CP, Fahy BN, Aloia TA, et al. Timing of referral impacts surgical outcomes in patients undergoing repair of bile duct injuries. HPB 2009;11(1):32–7.

46. Chapman WC, Halevy A, Blumgart LH, et al. Postcholecystectomy bile duct strictures. Management and outcome in 130 patients. Arch Surg Chic Ill 1960 1995;130(6):597–602, discussion 602-604.

47. Johnson SR, Koehler A, Pennington LK, et al. Long-term results of surgical repair of bile duct injuries following laparoscopic cholecystectomy. Surgery 2000;128(4):668–77.

48. He H, Tan C, Wu J, et al. Accuracy of ASGE high-risk criteria in evaluation of patients with suspected common bile duct stones. Gastrointest Endosc 2017; 86(3):525–32.

49. Kondo S, Isayama H, Akahane M, et al. Detection of common bile duct stones: comparison between endoscopic ultrasonography, magnetic resonance cholangiography, and helical-computed-tomographic cholangiography. Eur J Radiol 2005;54(2):271–5.

50. Venneman NG, Buskens E, Besselink MGH, et al. Small gallstones are associated with increased risk of acute pancreatitis: potential benefits of prophylactic cholecystectomy? Am J Gastroenterol 2005;100(11):2540–50.

51. Gurusamy KS, Giljaca V, Takwoingi Y, et al. Endoscopic retrograde cholangiopancreatography versus intraoperative cholangiography for diagnosis of common bile duct stones. Cochrane Database Syst Rev 2015;(2):CD010339.

52. Ricci C, Pagano N, Taffurelli G, et al. Comparison of Efficacy and Safety of 4 Combinations of Laparoscopic and Intraoperative Techniques for Management of Gallstone Disease With Biliary Duct Calculi: A Systematic Review and Network Meta-analysis. JAMA Surg 2018;153(7):e181167.

53. Giurgiu DI, Margulies DR, Carroll BJ, et al. Laparoscopic common bile duct exploration: long-term outcome. Arch Surg Chic Ill 1960 1999;134(8):839–43, discussion 843-844.

54. Phillips EH, Toouli J, Pitt HA, et al. Treatment of common bile duct stones discovered during cholecystectomy. J Gastrointest Surg Off J Soc Surg Aliment Tract 2008;12(4):624–8.

55. MacFadyen BV. Intraoperative cholangiography: past, present, and future. Surg Endosc 2006;20(Suppl 2):S436–40.

56. Kakos GS, Tompkins RK, Turnipseed W, et al. Operative cholangiography during routine cholecystectomy: a review of 3,012 cases. Arch Surg Chic Ill 1960 1972;104(4):484–8.

57. Collins C, Maguire D, Ireland A, et al. A prospective study of common bile duct calculi in patients undergoing laparoscopic cholecystectomy: natural history of choledocholithiasis revisited. Ann Surg 2004;239(1):28–33.

58. Andrews S. Gallstone size related to incidence of post cholecystectomy retained common bile duct stones. Int J Surg Lond Engl 2013;11(4):319–21.
59. Cox MR, Budge JPO, Eslick GD. Timing and nature of presentation of unsuspected retained common bile duct stones after laparoscopic cholecystectomy: a retrospective study. Surg Endosc 2015;29(7):2033–8.
60. Danilewitz MD. Early postoperative endoscopic sphincterotomy for retained common bile duct stones. Gastrointest Endosc 1989;35(4):298–9.
61. Strasberg SM, Helton WS. An analytical review of vasculobiliary injury in laparoscopic and open cholecystectomy. HPB 2011;13(1):1–14.
62. Dandekar U, Dandekar K, Chavan S. Right Hepatic Artery: A Cadaver Investigation and Its Clinical Significance. Anat Res Int 2015;2015.
63. Marano L, Bartoli A, Polom K, et al. The unwanted third wheel in the Calot's triangle: Incidence and surgical significance of caterpillar hump of right hepatic artery with a systematic review of the literature. J Minimal Access Surg 2019; 15(3):185–91.
64. Jansirani D, Mugunthan N, Shivadeep S. Caterpillar hump of right hepatic artery: incidence and surgical significance. National Journal of Clinical Anatomy 2012;1:121–4.
65. Kavitha Kamath B. An anatomical study of Moynihan's hump of right hepatic artery and its surgical importance. J Anat Soc India 2016;65:S65–7.
66. Halasz NA. Cholecystectomy and hepatic artery injuries. Arch Surg Chic Ill 1960 1991;126(2):137–8.
67. Rencuzogullari A, Okoh AK, Akcam TA, et al. Hemobilia as a result of right hepatic artery pseudoaneurysm rupture: An unusual complication of laparoscopic cholecystectomy. Int J Surg Case Rep 2014;5(3):142–4.
68. Machado NO, Al-Zadjali A, Kakaria AK, et al. Hepatic or Cystic Artery Pseudoaneurysms Following a Laparoscopic Cholecystectomy: Literature review of aetiopathogenesis, presentation, diagnosis and management. Sultan Qaboos Univ Med J 2017;17(2):e135–46.
69. Masannat YA, Al-Naser S, Al-Tal Y, et al. A rare complication of a common operation: hepatic artery pseudo aneurysm following cholecystectomy report of a case. Ir J Med Sci 2008;177(4):397–8.
70. Senthilkumar MP, Battula N, Perera M, et al. Management of a pseudo-aneurysm in the hepatic artery after a laparoscopic cholecystectomy. Ann R Coll Surg Engl 2016;98(7):456–60.
71. Rivitz SM, Waltman AC, Kelsey PB. Embolization of an hepatic artery pseudoaneurysm following laparoscopic cholecystectomy. Cardiovasc Intervent Radiol 1996;19(1):43–6.
72. Saldinger PF, Wang JY, Boyd C, et al. Cystic artery stump pseudoaneurysm following laparoscopic cholecystectomy. Surgery 2002;131(5):585–6.
73. De Molla Neto OL, Ribeiro MaF, Saad WA. Pseudoaneurysm of cystic artery after laparoscopic cholecystectomy. HPB 2006;8(4):318–9.
74. Petrou A, Brennan N, Soonawalla Z, et al. Hemobilia due to cystic artery stump pseudoaneurysm following laparoscopic cholecystectomy: case presentation and literature review. Int Surg 2012;97(2):140–4.
75. Madanur MA, Battula N, Sethi H, et al. Pseudoaneurysm following laparoscopic cholecystectomy. Hepatobiliary Pancreat Dis Int HBPD INT 2007;6(3):294–8.
76. Keleman AM, Imagawa DK, Findeiss L, et al. Associated vascular injury in patients with bile duct injury during cholecystectomy. Am Surg 2011;77(10): 1330–3.

77. Preventza OA, Habib FA, Young SC, et al. Portal vein thrombosis: an unusual complication of laparoscopic cholecystectomy. JSLS 2005;9(1):87–90.
78. Ikoma N, Anderson CL, Ohanian M, et al. Portal vein thrombosis after laparoscopic cholecystectomy. JSLS 2014;18(1):125–7.
79. Rusznak M, Kuttner R, Greim C-A. [Extrahepatic portal vein thrombosis following laparoscopic cholecystectomy]. Chir Z Alle Geb Oper Medizen 2003;74(3): 244–7.
80. Gul W, Abbass K, Qazi AM, et al. Thrombosis of portal venous system after laparoscopic cholecystectomy in a patient with prothrombin gene mutation. JSLS 2012;16(1):166–8.
81. James AW, Rabl C, Westphalen AC, et al. Portomesenteric venous thrombosis after laparoscopic surgery: a systematic literature review. Arch Surg Chic Ill 1960 2009;144(6):520–6.
82. Schmidt SC, Settmacher U, Langrehr JM, et al. Management and outcome of patients with combined bile duct and hepatic arterial injuries after laparoscopic cholecystectomy. Surgery 2004;135(6):613–8.
83. Alves A, Farges O, Nicolet J, et al. Incidence and consequence of an hepatic artery injury in patients with postcholecystectomy bile duct strictures. Ann Surg 2003;238(1):93–6.
84. Tzovaras G, Dervenis C. Vascular injuries in laparoscopic cholecystectomy: an underestimated problem. Dig Surg 2006;23(5–6):370–4.
85. Pulitanò C, Parks RW, Ireland H, et al. Impact of concomitant arterial injury on the outcome of laparoscopic bile duct injury. Am J Surg 2011;201(2):238–44.
86. Felekouras E, Megas T, Michail OP, et al. Emergency liver resection for combined biliary and vascular injury following laparoscopic cholecystectomy: case report and review of the literature. South Med J 2007;100(3):317–20.
87. Truant S, Boleslawski E, Lebuffe G, et al. Hepatic resection for postcholecystectomy bile duct injuries: a literature review. HPB 2010;12(5):334–41.
88. Leale I, Moraglia E, Bottino G, et al. Role of Liver Transplantation in Bilio-Vascular Liver Injury After Cholecystectomy. Transpl Proc 2016;48(2):370–6.
89. Lee D-H, Ahn YJ, Lee HW, et al. Prevalence and characteristics of clinically significant retained common bile duct stones after laparoscopic cholecystectomy for symptomatic cholelithiasis. Ann Surg Treat Res 2016;91(5):239–46.
90. Walsh RM, Ponsky JL, Dumot J. Retained gallbladder/cystic duct remnant calculi as a cause of postcholecystectomy pain. Surg Endosc 2002;16(6): 981–4.
91. Attaallah W, Cingi A, Karpuz S, et al. Do not rush for surgery; stent placement may be an effective step for definitive treatment of initially unextractable common bile duct stones with ERCP. Surg Endosc 2016;30(4):1473–9.
92. Chiappetta Porras LT, Nápoli ED, Canullán CM, et al. Laparoscopic bile duct re-exploration for retained duct stones. J Gastrointest Surg Off J Soc Surg Aliment Tract 2008;12(9):1518–20.
93. Tazuma S. Epidemiology, pathogenesis, and classification of biliary stones (common bile duct and intrahepatic). Best Pract Res Clin Gastroenterol 2006; 20(6):1075–83.
94. Hui TT, Giurgiu DI, Margulies DR, et al. Iatrogenic gallbladder perforation during laparoscopic cholecystectomy: etiology and sequelae. Am Surg 1999;65(10): 944–8.
95. Schäfer M, Suter C, Klaiber C, et al. Spilled gallstones after laparoscopic cholecystectomy. A relevant problem? A retrospective analysis of 10,174 laparoscopic cholecystectomies. Surg Endosc 1998;12(4):305–9.

96. Woodfield JC, Rodgers M, Windsor JA. Peritoneal gallstones following laparo-scopic cholecystectomy: incidence, complications, and management. Surg Endosc 2004;18(8):1200–7.

97. Manukyan MN, Demirkalem P, Gulluoglu BM, et al. Retained abdominal gall-stones during laparoscopic cholecystectomy. Am J Surg 2005;189(4):450–2.

98. Fitzgibbons RJ, Annibali R, Litke BS. Gallbladder and gallstone removal, open versus closed laparoscopy, and pneumoperitoneum. Am J Surg 1993;165(4): 497–504.

99. Zehetner J, Shamiyeh A, Wayand W. Lost gallstones in laparoscopic cholecys-tectomy: all possible complications. Am J Surg 2007;193(1):73–8.

100. Stevens JL, Laliotis A, Gould SWT. Hepatocolonic fistula: a rare consequence of retained gallstones after laparoscopic cholecystectomy. Ann R Coll Surg Engl 2013;95(8):e139–41.

101. Gaster RS, Berger AJ, Ahmadi-Kashani M, et al. Chronic cutaneous chest wall fistula and gallstone empyema due to retained gallstones. BMJ Case Rep 2014; 2014.

102. Van Mierlo PJWB, De Boer SY, Van Dissel JT, et al. Recurrent staphylococcal bacteraemia and subhepatic abscess associated with gallstones spilled during laparoscopic cholecystectomy two years earlier. Neth J Med 2002;60(4): 177–80.

103. Botterill ID, Davides D, Vezakis A, et al. Recurrent septic episodes following gall-stone spillage at laparoscopic cholecystectomy. Surg Endosc 2001;15(8):897.

104. Kim B-S, Joo S-H, Kim H-C. Spilled gallstones mimicking a retroperitoneal sar-coma following laparoscopic cholecystectomy. World J Gastroenterol 2016; 22(17):4421–6.

105. Heron P, Manzelli A. Back to the gallstone: a mischievous cause of morbidity. BMJ Case Rep 2016;2016.

106. Bolat H, Teke Z. Spilled gallstones found incidentally in a direct inguinal hernia sac: Report of a case. Int J Surg Case Rep 2020;66:218–20.

107. Preciado A, Matthews BD, Scarborough TK, et al. Transdiaphragmatic abscess: late thoracic complication of laparoscopic cholecystectomy. J Laparoendosc Adv Surg Tech A 1999;9(6):517–21.

108. Gerlinzani S, Tos M, Gornati R, et al. Is the loss of gallstones during laparo-scopic cholecystectomy an underestimated complication? Surg Endosc 2000; 14(4):373–4.

109. Isherwood J, Oakland K, Khanna A. A systematic review of the aetiology and management of post cholecystectomy syndrome. Surg J R Coll Surg Edinb Irel 2019;17(1):33–42.

110. Anand AC, Sharma R, Kapur BM, et al. Analysis of symptomatic patients after cholecystectomy: is the term post-cholecystectomy syndrome an anachronism? Trop Gastroenterol Off J Dig Dis Found 1995;16(2):126–31.

111. Lublin M, Crawford DL, Hiatt JR, et al. Symptoms before and after laparoscopic cholecystectomy for gallstones. Am Surg 2004;70(10):863–6.

112. Fenster LF, Lonborg R, Thirlby RC, et al. What symptoms does cholecystectomy cure? Insights from an outcomes measurement project and review of the litera-ture. Am J Surg 1995;169(5):533–8.

113. Lamberts MP, Lugtenberg M, Rovers MM, et al. Persistent and de novo symp-toms after cholecystectomy: a systematic review of cholecystectomy effective-ness. Surg Endosc 2013;27(3):709–18.

114. Niranjan B, Chumber S, Kriplani AK. Symptomatic outcome after laparoscopic cholecystectomy. Trop Gastroenterol Off J Dig Dis Found 2000;21(3):144–8.

115. Tanaka M, Ikeda S, Nakayama F. Change in bile duct pressure responses after cholecystectomy: loss of gallbladder as a pressure reservoir. Gastroenterology 1984;87(5):1154–9.
116. Girometti R, Brondani G, Cereser L, et al. Post-cholecystectomy syndrome: spectrum of biliary findings at magnetic resonance cholangiopancreatography. Br J Radiol 2010;83(988):351–61.
117. Gorsi U, Gupta P, Kalra N, et al. Multidetector computed tomography evaluation of post cholecystectomy complications: A tertiary care center experience. Trop Gastroenterol Off J Dig Dis Found 2015;36(4):236–43.
118. Owens M, Barry M, Janjua AZ, et al. A systematic review of laparoscopic port site hernias in gastrointestinal surgery. Surg J R Coll Surg Edinb Irel 2011; 9(4):218–24.
119. Nofal MN, Yousef AJ, Hamdan FF, et al. Characteristics of Trocar Site Hernia after Laparoscopic Cholecystectomy. Sci Rep 2020;10(1):2868.
120. Bunting DM. Port-site hernia following laparoscopic cholecystectomy. JSLS 2010;14(4):490–7.
121. Chatzimavroudis G, Papaziogas B, Galanis I, et al. Trocar site hernia following laparoscopic cholecystectomy: a 10-year single center experience. Hernia J Hernias Abdom Wall Surg 2017;21(6):925–32.
122. Montz FJ, Holschneider CH, Munro MG. Incisional hernia following laparoscopy: a survey of the American Association of Gynecologic Laparoscopists. Obstet Gynecol 1994;84(5):881–4.
123. Khurshid N, Chung M, Horrigan T, et al. 5-millimeter trocar-site bowel herniation following laparoscopic surgery. JSLS 2012;16(2):306–10.
124. Wicks A, Voyvodic F, Scroop R. Incisional hernia and small bowel obstruction following laparoscopic surgery: computed tomography diagnosis. Australas Radiol 2000;44(3):331–2.
125. Reardon PR, Preciado A, Scarborough T, et al. Hernia at 5-mm laparoscopic port site presenting as early postoperative small bowel obstruction. J Laparoendosc Adv Surg Tech A 1999;9(6):523–5.
126. Dulskas A, Lunevičius R, Stanaitis J. A case report of incisional hernia through a 5 mm lateral port site following laparoscopic cholecystectomy. J Minimal Access Surg 2011;7(3):187–9.
127. Cho WT, Yoo T, Kim SM. Is the 8-mm robotic port safe? A case of trocar site hernia after robotic cholecystectomy using the da Vinci Xi system. Wideochirurgia Inne Tech Maloinwazyjne Videosurgery Miniinvasive Tech 2019;14(1):137–40.
128. Tonouchi H, Ohmori Y, Kobayashi M, et al. Trocar site hernia. Arch Surg Chic Ill 1960 2004;139(11):1248–56.
129. Boughey JC, Nottingham JM, Walls AC. Richter's hernia in the laparoscopic era: four case reports and review of the literature. Surg Laparosc Endosc Percutan Tech 2003;13(1):55–8.
130. Chorti A, AbuFarha S, Michalopoulos A, et al. Richter's hernia in a 5-mm trocar site. SAGE Open Med Case Rep 2019;7. 2050313X18823413.
131. Singal R, Zaman M, Mittal A, et al. No Need of Fascia Closure to Reduce Trocar Site Hernia Rate in Laparoscopic Surgery: A Prospective Study of 200 Non-Obese Patients. Gastroenterol Res 2016;9(4–5):70–3.
132. Sanz-López R, Martínez-Ramos C, Núñez-Peña JR, et al. Incisional hernias after laparoscopic vs open cholecystectomy. Surg Endosc 1999;13(9):922–4.
133. Howie A, Sandblom G, Enochsson L, et al. Incisional hernias following gallstone surgery. A population-based study. HPB 2020;22(12):1775–81.

134. Glavic Z, Begic L, Simlesa D, et al. Treatment of acute cholecystitis. A comparison of open vs laparoscopic cholecystectomy. Surg Endosc 2001;15(4): 398–401.

135. Garg P, Thakur JD, Garg M, et al. Single-incision laparoscopic cholecystectomy vs. conventional laparoscopic cholecystectomy: a meta-analysis of randomized controlled trials. J Gastrointest Surg Off J Soc Surg Aliment Tract 2012;16(8): 1618–28.

136. Trastulli S, Cirocchi R, Desiderio J, et al. Systematic review and meta-analysis of randomized clinical trials comparing single-incision versus conventional laparoscopic cholecystectomy. Br J Surg 2013;100(2):191–208.

137. Sun N, Zhang J, Zhang C, et al. Single-site robotic cholecystectomy versus multi-port laparoscopic cholecystectomy: A systematic review and meta-analysis. Am J Surg 2018;216(6):1205–11.

138. Balachandran B, Hufford TA, Mustafa T, et al. A Comparative Study of Outcomes Between Single-Site Robotic and Multi-port Laparoscopic Cholecystectomy: An Experience from a Tertiary Care Center. World J Surg 2017;41(5):1246–53.

139. Hoyuela C, Juvany M, Guillaumes S, et al. Long-term incisional hernia rate after single-incision laparoscopic cholecystectomy is significantly higher than that after standard three-port laparoscopy: a cohort study. Hernia J Hernias Abdom Wall Surg 2019;23(6):1205–13.

140. Pottakkat B, Vijayahari R, Prakash A, et al. Factors predicting failure following high bilio-enteric anastomosis for post-cholecystectomy benign biliary strictures. J Gastrointest Surg Off J Soc Surg Aliment Tract 2010;14(9):1389–94.

141. Perini MV, Herman P, Montagnini AL, et al. Liver resection for the treatment of post-cholecystectomy biliary stricture with vascular injury. World J Gastroenterol 2015;21(7):2102–7.

142. Laurent A, Sauvanet A, Farges O, et al. Major hepatectomy for the treatment of complex bile duct injury. Ann Surg 2008;248(1):77–83.

Management of Complications Following Lung Resection

Paul A. Toste, MD[a,b,*], Sha'shonda L. Revels, MD[a]

KEYWORDS

- Postoperative complications • Lung resection • Thoracic surgery

KEY POINTS

- Complications after lung resection typically involve the cardiac and/or respiratory systems.
- Adequate preoperative evaluation is key to anticipating and minimizing complications of lung resection.
- Prompt recognition and treatment of complications after lung resection is essential to optimize outcomes.

Lung cancer is the leading cause of cancer-related deaths in the United States, and anatomic lung resection is the mainstay of treatment of early stage lung cancer.[1] Apart from lunger cancer, other indications for lung resection include diagnosis of nodules, resection of selected metastatic tumors, tissue diagnosis in interstitial disease, removal of blebs and bullae, and medically refractory infectious processes. Lung resections can be approached with a variety of surgical techniques, including open thoracotomy, thoracoscopy, and robotics. Despite many advances in thoracic surgery, lung resections continue to be associated with a variety of potential postoperative complications. Most complications after lung surgery involve either the cardiac or respiratory systems (**Table 1**). As a result, much of the preoperative planning and postoperative care focus on assessing and optimizing cardiopulmonary function.[2,3]

PREOPERATIVE EVALUATION

A major key to minimizing postoperative complications is a thorough assessment and optimization of patient risk factors preoperatively. Many lung resection patients are

[a] Division of Thoracic Surgery, David Geffen School of Medicine at UCLA, Box 957313, Room 64-128 CHS, 10833 Le Conte Avenue, Los Angeles, CA 90095-7313, USA; [b] Division of Thoracic Surgery, Ronald Reagan UCLA Medical Center, Box 957313, Room 64-128 CHS, 10833 Le Conte Avenue, Los Angeles, CA 90095-7313, USA
* Corresponding author.
E-mail address: ptoste@mednet.ucla.edu

Surg Clin N Am 101 (2021) 911–923
https://doi.org/10.1016/j.suc.2021.06.013
0039-6109/21/Published by Elsevier Inc.

Table 1
Summary of complications after lung resection

Complication	Definition	Prevention and Management
Atelectasis	Parenchymal opacification with shift of structures toward abnormality on chest radiograph	Ambulation, incentive spirometry, chest physiotherapy, hyperinflation therapy, pain control.
Pneumonia	Lung infiltrate with associated infectious signs/symptoms (fever, leukocytosis, positive culture)	As per atelectasis, mucolytic therapy, bronchoscopy, antibiotics.
Respiratory failure	$Pao_2<60$ or O2 saturation<90% on room air	Treatment of underlying cause, supplemental oxygen, noninvasive ventilation, intubation.
Pleural effusion	Collection of fluid in the pleural space	Diuresis, drainage.
Postoperative hemorrhage	Bleeding requiring transfusion and causing hemodynamic changes	Resuscitation and transfusion, correction of coagulopathy, reoperation.
Chylothorax	Pleural fluid triglyceride >110	NPO, very low fat diet, octreotide, TPN.
Pneumothorax	Air in the pleural space	Drainage.
Prolonged air leak	Air leak that persists beyond postoperative day 7	Prolonged drainage, blood patch, endobronchial valve, pleurodesis, reoperation.
Bronchopleural fistula	Communication between a central airway and the pleural space	Avoid devascularization of airway stump, cover stump with muscle flap. Drainage, repair, open window thoracostomy.
Empyema	Infection of the pleural space	Drainage, antibiotics, decortication, open window thoracostomy.
Bronchospasm	Reversible airway constriction that results in obstructive physiology	Resume/replace home asthma/COPD medications. Bronchodilators, anticholinergics, steroids.
Cardiac tamponade	Pericardial effusion that causes elevation and equalization of intracardiac pressures	Volume resuscitation, pericardiocentesis, pericardial window.
Cardiac herniation	Displacement of heart through a pericardial defect	Patch closure of large pericardiotomies, reoperation and reduction.
Lobar torsion	Twisting of a lobe around its bronchovascular axis	Assure normal reexpansion of remaining lobes after resection. Reoperation and reduction, resection if needed.

(continued on next page)

Table 1 (continued)		
Complication	**Definition**	**Prevention and Management**
Atrial fibrillation	Irregularly irregular heart rate resulting from rapid, inefficient atrial contractions	Rate or rhythm control (β-blockers, calcium channel blockers, digoxin, amiodarone), correct volume and electrolyte disturbances, cardioversion if unstable, consider anticoagulation if persists.
Heart failure	Inadequate systemic perfusion secondary to cardiac insufficiency	Diuresis, inotropic support.
Myocardial infarction	Myocardial ischemia resulting from impaired coronary blood flow	Continue preoperative β-blockers, statins, and aspirin. Prompt recognition of symptoms, cardiology consultation, antiplatelet therapy/anticoagulation, cardiac catheterization.
Venous thromboembolism	Blood clots in the deep venous system with or with embolization to the pulmonary arterial system	Prophylactic anticoagulation. Therapeutic anticoagulation, thrombectomy in select severe cases.

Abbreviations: COPD, chronic obstructive pulmonary disease; TPN, total parenteral nutrition.

current or former smokers.[4] All patients should be counseled to stop smoking preoperatively. The history of smoking also puts lung resection patients at high risk for chronic obstructive pulmonary disease and cardiovascular disease. Pulmonary function tests (PFTs) are essential to assess patient's preoperative and postoperative predicted lung function. Forced expiratory volume in 1 second (FEV1) and diffusing capacity for carbon monoxide (DLCO) are the most commonly followed PFT parameters. Guidelines vary on exact cutoffs, but postoperative predicted FEV1 and DLCO greater than 40% of predicted based on age and size typically indicate that a patient can tolerate the proposed resection. If either value is lower than 40%, risk is higher, and further testing such as stair climbing, cardiopulmonary exercise testing, and perfusion scanning may be indicated.[2,3,5] Functional status and exercise tolerance in addition to medical risk factors should be assessed. Significant underlying cardiovascular disease and/or symptoms such as exertional dyspnea, angina, or limited exercise tolerance should prompt further cardiac evaluation with echocardiogram and stress testing.[6,7]

PULMONARY COMPLICATIONS

Not surprisingly, pulmonary complications make up the most significant category of problems following lung resection. By its very nature, operating in the thorax to remove pulmonary parenchyma induces a variety of physiologic changes such as atelectasis, effusion, air leak, and pneumothorax that can become complications in and of themselves as well as contribute to the development of other complications. Optimal care of the postoperative lung resection patient requires active prevention measures to reduce the risk of the pulmonary complications as well as prompt recognition and treatment of complications when they do occur.

Atelectasis and Pneumonia

Atelectasis, defined as lung opacification with shift of the mediastinum, diaphragm, or hilum toward the affected area, is present to some degree in all postoperative lung resection patients.[8] Management of this known consequence of lung surgery is important to prevent further complications. Early and frequent ambulation is probably the single most important intervention to treat atelectasis and prevent respiratory complications.[9,10] By ambulating, the patient reduces dependent atelectasis that is present in the recumbent position. The patient also naturally breathes more deeply during ambulation. Additional recruitment maneuvers to minimize atelectasis such as incentive spirometry, flutter valves, and hyperinflation therapy can be useful adjuncts. Pulmonary clearance therapies such as percussive therapy, mucolytic nebulizers, and frequent coughing are also useful, particularly in patients with underlying difficulty managing secretions such as patients with chronic obstructive pulmonary disease (COPD) and smokers. Adequate pain control following thoracic surgery is also necessary for the management of atelectasis. Minimally invasive surgery has the potential to reduce postoperative pain and positively affect recovery.[11–13]

Pneumonia is typically characterized by fever, productive cough, lung infiltrate, and leukocytosis.[8] Atelectasis is a major contributing factor to the development of pneumonia owing to the poor clearance that occurs in atelectatic areas. Patients with COPD are more prone to respiratory infections at baseline and after surgery.[14] Aspiration can also lead to pneumonitis and pneumonia, and precautions must be taken postoperatively to avoid this complication. Pneumonia following lung resection generally falls into the category of hospital acquired pneumonia, given that it typically occurs over 48 hours after hospital admission. Antibiotics and airway clearance are the mainstays of pneumonia treatment. Empirical antibiotic choices are made based on

Not Ventilator-associated	Ventilator-associated
Initial agents (choose one)	**Initial agents (choose one)**
• Piperacillin-tazobactam	• Piperacillin-tazobactam
• Fluoroquinolone	• Anti-pseudomonal cephalosporin
• Carbapenem	• Carbapenem
Additional as indicated:	**Additional as indicated:**
MRSA Risk Factors[a]	**MRSA Risk Factors[a]**
• Vancomycin or linezolid	• Vancomycin or linezolid
Resistant Pseudomonas Risk[b]	**Resistant Pseudomonas Risk[b]**
• Second anti-pseudomonal agent	• Second anti-pseudomonal agent
Broad coverage in septic shock	**Broad coverage in septic shock**

Fig. 1. Antibiotic selection for postoperative pneumonia. [a]Major risk factors for MRSA include IV antibiotics in the past 90 days, high rate of MRSA isolates in the treating unit, and screening positivity for MRSA. [b]Major risk factors for resistant pseudomonas include IV antibiotics within the past 90 days, structural lung disease, and high rate of resistant organisms in the treating unit. IV, intravenous; MRSA, methicillin-resistant *Staphylococcus aureus*.

disease severity and risk of resistant organisms.[15] A simplified algorithm for treating hospital-acquired and ventilator-associated pneumonias based on the 2016 Infectious Diseases Society of America/American Thoracic Society guidelines is presented in **Fig. 1**. Obtaining sputum samples for microbiology allows more tailored antibiotic choices. Flexible bronchoscopy is an option for obtaining high-quality samples. Bronchoscopy is also therapeutic for airway clearance, can be performed in the awake patient, and should be used liberally in patients whose secretions are difficult to manage with less invasive interventions.

Respiratory Failure

Acute respiratory failure following lung resection is typically hypoxemic in nature and defined by room air Pao_2 less than 60 or room air O2 saturation less than 90%, which is quite common.[8] Respiratory failure can manifest along a wide spectrum of severity. Mild disease is characterized by an adequate response to simple supplemental oxygen. Moderate disease is characterized by an inadequate response to supplemental oxygen requiring noninvasive or invasive ventilatory support. Severe disease is characterized by frank acute respiratory distress syndrome (ARDS).[16]

Mild respiratory failure is managed with supplemental oxygen and maneuvers aimed at improving respiratory mechanics, ventilation, and oxygenation. Many of these treatments are described earlier, including ambulation, recruitment methods, secretion mobilization, and treatment of underlying infections. Addressing any other factors that may be contributing to poor respiratory function such as volume overload, pleural effusion, and pneumothorax are also important considerations. For most patients, such an approach will be successful.

When respiratory failure does progress in severity, prompt management is essential. Noninvasive ventilation is typically only useful as a short-term bridge to definitive therapy. For example, a patient with pulmonary edema may benefit from short-duration noninvasive ventilation while diuresis is initiated. For those patients without a quickly reversible problem, intubation is needed to obtain a secure airway and provide adequate ventilation and oxygenation, and this allows the treatment team to stabilize the patient while further diagnostics and treatments are pursued. In patients with severe respiratory failure and ARDS, a ventilator strategy that uses lung protective measures including low tidal volumes, higher positive end expiratory pressure, and permissive hypercapnia can be beneficial.[17,18] Careful fluid management with avoidance of volume overload in the postoperative setting is important to reduce the risk of ARDS, and treatment of pulmonary edema when it does develop is necessary.[19] This concept is particularly important in patients who have undergone pneumonectomy. Patients who are being mechanically ventilated should be assessed frequently for their progress toward extubation with spontaneous breathing trials.

Pleural Effusion

Pleural effusion is a blanket term for fluid that accumulates in the pleural space. Accumulation of simple serous fluid is common after lung resection; this is typically managed expectantly and resolves spontaneously. Small effusions can usually be managed with observation with or without the addition of diuretics. When effusions are moderate to large in size, they can begin to cause symptoms such as dyspnea and increasing supplemental oxygen requirements. In these cases, drainage is warranted. Depending on the size and location of the effusion, drainage can be performed at the bedside or using interventional radiology techniques. Small bore drainage catheters are typically sufficient to treat simple effusions.

Less commonly, effusions may be related to other processes such as bleeding or leakage of lymphatic fluid (chylothorax). Postoperative bleeding is managed with close monitoring, reversal of coagulopathy, and resuscitation with fluid and blood products as needed. Patients whose bleeding requires more than 1 to 2 units of red blood cells or results in hemodynamic instability typically require reoperation. Bloody chest tube output greater than 200 mL/h for several hours is another sign that reoperation is likely needed.[20] Although reoperation is never desired, quickly taking a bleeding patient back to the operating room is the safest and most effective method to address significant bleeding.

Chylothorax is a rare complication of pulmonary resection.[21] It is diagnosed by milky appearing chest tube output and confirmed by a pleural triglyceride fluid level greater than 110. Triglyceride levels between 50 and 110 are equivocal. In such cases, pleural chylomicron detection can be used to confirm if chylothorax is present. Chylothorax can result from injury to the thoracic duct or smaller lymphatic channels. Management begins with making the patient nil per os. Patients whose output decreases with this maneuver can be transitioned to very low-fat diets or total parenteral nutrition until the leak heals. The addition of octreotide is sometimes helpful. In patients with persistently high output (greater than 500-1000ml daily) pleurodesis, thoracic duct ligation, and/or thoracic duct embolization is indicated. Patients with more modest output are more likely to respond to simple pleurodesis without reoperation.[21–23]

Prolonged Air Leak and Pneumothorax

Air leaks after pulmonary resection are exceedingly common and typically resolve with simple chest tube drainage. Prolonged air leak is generally defined as air leakage that persists beyond the seventh postoperative day.[24] Most of such air leaks are best described as alveolar-pleural fistulas, which contrasts to the more serious complication of bronchopleural fistula. Air leaks can contribute to pneumothorax after lung resection. It is important to make a distinction between a pneumothorax that results from air leakage and a postoperative space that results from incomplete filling of the hemithorax following parenchymal resection. A postoperative space without air leakage does not require any specific treatment and typically decreases in size or resolves with time as the patient's hemidiaphragm and mediastinum move toward the space. Air leakage can also contribute to subcutaneous emphysema when the air tracks through the subcutaneous tissues of the chest and, at times, to other parts of the body. This process is benign but can be quite distressing to the patient. In patients with an air leak and concurrent air space, the suction setting on the chest tube can be increased to assess whether increased suction resolves or reduces the space. If it does, the increased suction may help aid in healing of the air leak by promoting pleural apposition. An optimal strategy for managing chest tube suction has never been definitively established. A reasonable approach is to use the minimum amount of suction needed to maximize lung expansion and manage any subcutaneous emphysema. In addition, in patients with persistent large pneumothorax or subcutaneous emphysema, assessment of whether the pleural space is adequately drained should be made. Targeted placement of an additional tube can be useful in cases where existing tubes are not sufficient. Computed tomography (CT) scanning can be helpful to identify loculated regions that would benefit from drainage. Most prolonged air leaks can be managed conservatively. Patients can be sent home with tubes connected to one-way valve systems. Endobronchial valves, autologous blood patch, and bedside pleurodesis are occasionally useful for persistent leaks.[25–27] Rarely, reoperation is required and typically consists of removing the area that is leaking and/or performing pleurodesis.[24,25]

Bronchopleural Fistula and Empyema

Bronchopleural fistula (BPF) occurs when there is a connection between the bronchial tree and the pleural space. Postoperative BPF is a dreaded and serious complication that is most commonly encountered following pneumonectomy.[28] BPF may be suspected when a patient has a refractory large air leak. After pneumonectomy, a drop in the postoperative air fluid level on chest radiograph may be the first sign. The diagnosis of BPF is confirmed by bronchoscopy. In patients who underwent lobar or sublobar resection, small BPFs can be minimally symptomatic and managed conservatively. However, BPFs can cause pneumothorax as well as retrograde aspiration of pleural contents into the lungs. If a BPF is suspected after pneumonectomy, the patient should be positioned with the remaining lung up to protect it from aspiration. Tube drainage of the postpneumonectomy space and antibacterial treatment is then instituted, and bronchoscopy is performed to confirm the diagnosis. Larger BPFs typically require repair if diagnosed early or open drainage if diagnosed late.[29]

Empyema is infection of the pleural space. Prolonged air leakage can lead to pleural soiling and predispose to empyema formation.[30] Initial empyema management consists of drainage via tube thoracostomy and antibiotics. Patients with postoperative empyema should also be evaluated for evidence of BPF both with cross-sectional imaging (CT scan) and bronchoscopy when they are stable. In patients who develop empyema after lobectomy or lesser resection, simple drainage and antibiotics may be sufficient. In the setting of a persistent space after drainage, open window thoracostomy (Eloesser flap or Clagett window) may be needed. Open drainage is typically required in postpneumonectomy empyema, although repair and antibiotic irrigation of the pleural space has been successful in BPF diagnosed in the early postoperative setting.[31,32]

Bronchospasm and Chronic Obstructive Pulmonary Disease Exacerbation

Given the frequent history of smoking in patients with lung cancer, chronic obstructive pulmonary disease COPD is a common comorbidity in lung resection patients.[33] Patients without underlying COPD may also be more prone to bronchospasm in the postoperative setting. In patients with underlying COPD, it is important to continue the use of inhaled bronchodilators or substitute for equivalent nebulized formulations. It is also essential to closely monitor all postoperative patients for changes in respiratory rate, accessory muscle usage, and development of wheezing that may signal worsening bronchospasm. These patients need to be treated promptly with bronchodilators such as albuterol. Anticholinergic medications such as ipratropium are also useful.

Vocal Cord Paralysis

Although much more common after esophageal surgery, vocal cord paralysis can occur after lung resection. Potential causes include direct injury from intubation and recurrent laryngeal nerve injury, typically on the left side. The left recurrent laryngeal nerve passes under the aortic arch and along the left tracheoesophageal groove. Operations that involve dissection in the aortopulmonary window or the left paratracheal space can result in injury to the left recurrent laryngeal nerve. The right recurrent laryngeal nerve passes under the right subclavian artery and takes a more lateral course to the larynx. Although less common than left-sided injuries, the right recurrent laryngeal nerve is at risk during operations involving the right thoracic inlet and high right paratracheal space. Patients with vocal cord paralysis present with a hoarse voice and weak cough. In the postoperative thoracic surgical patient, such symptoms should be evaluated endoscopically. If vocal cord paralysis is found, early medialization by a head and neck surgeon is preferred to allow the patient to produce an adequate cough and reduce the risk of pneumonia.[34] The patient should also be assessed for aspiration. A diet that includes thickened liquids may be necessary to prevent aspiration.

Cardiac Tamponade and Cardiac Herniation

Cardiac tamponade is a rare occurrence after lung resection. It presents with recurrent hypotension along with elevation and equalization of central venous pressure and pulmonary artery diastolic pressure. It can be readily diagnosed by echocardiogram. Patients should be kept volume replete. Typically, percutaneous drainage is technically feasible and successful. In cases that cannot be adequately managed with percutaneous drainage or that recur, pericardial window should be considered. Cardiac herniation can occur when a large portion of the pericardium is resected. This typically presents with acute hypotension. Treatment is prompt surgical exploration to correct the herniation. Patch repair of large pericardiotomies reduces the risk of this complication.

Lobar Torsion

Lobar torsion occurs when a remaining lobe twists along its bronchovascular axis. This complication is very rare but is most common in the right middle lobe after right upper lobectomy.[35] The patient may present with dyspnea, cough, tachycardia, fever, and new consolidation on chest radiograph. CT scan demonstrates twisting of the bronchovascular structures with complete obstruction. Flexible bronchoscopy demonstrates a "fish mouth" appearance of the proximal lobar bronchus that cannot be passed. Bronchoscopy is likely to be the most expeditious diagnostic modality when there is high suspicion for torsion. Treatment is emergent surgical exploration and detorsion. If the lobe is viable, it can be fixed to prevent recurrent torsion. If there is any concern for infarction/gangrene, lobectomy is the treatment. Assuring that the lung reexpands in a normal anatomic configuration at the conclusion of the original operation is key to preventing this complication.

CARDIOVASCULAR AND THROMBOTIC COMPLICATIONS
Atrial Fibrillation

Atrial fibrillation is a common complication of lung resection. More than 15% of patients undergoing major thoracic surgery develop atrial fibrillation.[36,37] Given this frequency, many surgeons routinely give prophylactic medications to reduce the risk of atrial fibrillation. Beta blockers are used most commonly and should certainly be continued perioperatively for any patients taking them before surgery. Calcium channel blockers and amiodarone are also alternative prophylactic agents.[38] When atrial fibrillation does occur postoperatively, the patient should be evaluated for precipitating factors. Factors that predispose to atrial fibrillation include hypovolemia, hypervolemia, electrolyte abnormalities, and high catecholamine states related to pain or infection. In addition to treating precipitating factors, patients with new atrial fibrillation need to be rate or rhythm controlled (**Fig. 2**). Control of the heart rate to a level less than 110 beats/min is typically the initial goal, and this can be achieved by nodal blocking agents such as intravenous β-blockers or calcium channel antagonists. Digoxin is an alternative rate control agent and may be useful in patients with underlying ventricular dysfunction. Amiodarone is a frequently used antiarrhythmic that can also achieve rate control and, at times, rhythm control. In hemodynamically unstable patients, cardioversion is the treatment of choice. In patients who continue to have atrial fibrillation

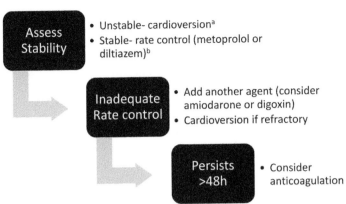

Fig. 2. Treatment algorithm for postoperative atrial fibrillation. [a]Signs of unstable atrial fibrillation include hypotension, chest pain, and ST-segment changes. [b]β-Blockers or calcium channel blockers are typical first-line agents. Digoxin and amiodarone can be considered based on patient-specific factors. The decision to anticoagulate is based on surgical bleeding risk as well as CHADS2-VASC score.

for more than 48 hours, an assessment of stroke risk (CHADS2-VASC score) should be made and anticoagulation considered.[39] Consultation with a cardiologist is useful in complicated or treatment refractory patients. Most atrial fibrillation following thoracic surgery resolves within 6 weeks.[38]

Myocardial Infarction and Heart Failure

Patients undergoing lung resection tend be older and have a smoking history. These factors result in a relatively high incidence of coronary artery disease in patient's undergoing lung resection. As mentioned previously, patients must undergo a thorough preoperative cardiac evaluation. Aspirin typically does not need to be held for thoracic operations. Patients taking β-blockers and statins should also continue those medications postoperatively. Lung resection patients should have continuous cardiac monitoring postoperatively, and changes to the tracing should prompt further evaluation with 12 lead electrocardiogram and, potentially, cardiac biomarker measurement. Chest pain is a difficult symptom to assess after chest surgery, but new onset pain that is not of the same character as the incisional pain should be evaluated. Early involvement of the cardiology service is highly beneficial in any patients suspected of having myocardial ischemia. If ischemia is diagnosed, it is treated by standard-of-care measures with high vigilance of bleeding complications.[40] Patients with preexisting cardiac dysfunction require careful postoperative management. Fluid shifts, arrhythmias, hypoxia, and ischemia can all contribute to worsening heart failure. Avoidance of excessive fluid administration during and after the operation is essential, and many of these patients will require diuresis in the postoperative period.

Deep Venous Thrombosis and Pulmonary Embolism

Lung resection patients have many potential risk factors for thromboembolism: major surgery, advanced age, cancer, and immobility. Pharmacologic prophylaxis with subcutaneous heparin (unfractionated or low-molecular-weight) is the mainstay of prevention. Intermittent leg compression devices are also beneficial.[41] Patients with unilateral leg swelling and/or pain, should be evaluated for deep venous thrombosis (DVT). Anticoagulation is the treatment of choice of DVT. Inferior vena cava filter can be considered in select patients who cannot be anticoagulated. For patients with acute onset dyspnea, tachypnea, tachycardia, and hypoxia, pulmonary embolism (PE) must be on the differential diagnosis particularly if another common postoperative cause is not present, such as atelectasis, mucous plugging, pneumonia, pulmonary edema, pleural effusion, or pneumothorax. Contrast-enhanced CT angiography is the diagnostic modality of choice. Anticoagulation is the cornerstone of treatment of PE in hemodynamically stable patients and should be initiated as soon as possible. Patients with large PE resulting in hemodynamic instability should be considered for interventional options such as catheter-directed therapies. Postoperative patients are typically not good candidates for systemic thrombolysis.[42]

PAIN

Postoperative pain is not necessarily a complication per se, but it is a consequence of thoracic surgery that can lead to other complications. Pain control is essential to postoperative recovery, as it allows the patient to ambulate, breathe deeply, and cough. Acute postoperative pain should be approached from a multimodality perspective. Useful medications include narcotics, anti-inflammatories, and acetaminophen. Agents targeting neuropathic pain and muscle relaxants can be useful adjuncts. Regional anesthesia techniques such as epidural catheters or paraspinal blockade can also be very beneficial, particularly for open incisions.[43]

CLINICS CARE POINTS

- Preoperative evaluation of pulmonary and cardiac function is essential prior to lung resection.
- Measures to prevent pulmonary complications after lung resection including early ambulation, incentive spirometry, chest physiotherapy, nebulizer and airway clearance therapies can help reduce morbidity.
- Atrial fibrillation is a common an expected complication after lung resection. A systematic approach starting with beta blockers or calcium channel blockers and escalating to other medications as needed is typically effective.
- Occasionally, complications will occur that require prompt intervention such as bronchoscopy or even re-operation. Moving forward with needed invasive treatment is key to successfully managing complications after lung resection.

ACKNOWLEDGMENTS

None.

CONFLICTS OF INTEREST

The authors have no conflicts of interest to declare.

REFERENCES

1. Cancer Facts & Figures 2020. American Cancer Society. Available at: https://www.cancer.org/content/dam/cancer-org/research/cancer-facts-and-statistics/annual-cancer-facts-and-figures/2020/cancer-facts-and-figures-2020.pdf.
2. Brunelli A, Charloux A, Bolliger CT, et al. ERS/ESTS clinical guidelines on fitness for radical therapy in lung cancer patients (surgery and chemo-radiotherapy). Eur Respir J 2009;34(1):17–41.

3. Brunelli A, Kim AW, Berger KI, et al. Physiologic evaluation of the patient with lung cancer being considered for resectional surgery: Diagnosis and management of lung cancer, 3rd ed: American College of Chest Physicians evidence-based clinical practice guidelines. Chest 2013;143(5 Suppl):e166S–90S.
4. Warren GW, Alberg AJ, Kraft AS, et al. The 2014 Surgeon General's report: "The health consequences of smoking–50 years of progress": a paradigm shift in cancer care. Cancer 2014;120(13):1914–6.
5. Brunelli A, Al Refai M, Monteverde M, et al. Predictors of early morbidity after major lung resection in patients with and without airflow limitation. Ann Thorac Surg 2002;74(4):999–1003.
6. Brunelli A, Varela G, Salati M, et al. Recalibration of the revised cardiac risk index in lung resection candidates. Ann Thorac Surg 2010;90(1):199–203.
7. Lee TH, Marcantonio ER, Mangione CM, et al. Derivation and prospective validation of a simple index for prediction of cardiac risk of major noncardiac surgery. Circulation 1999;100(10):1043–9.
8. Jammer I, Wickboldt N, Sander M, et al. Standards for definitions and use of outcome measures for clinical effectiveness research in perioperative medicine: European Perioperative Clinical Outcome (EPCO) definitions: a statement from the ESA-ESICM joint taskforce on perioperative outcome measures. Eur J Anaesthesiol 2015;32(2):88–105.
9. Kaneda H, Saito Y, Okamoto M, et al. Early postoperative mobilization with walking at 4 hours after lobectomy in lung cancer patients. Gen Thorac Cardiovasc Surg 2007;55(12):493–8.
10. Khandhar SJ, Schatz CL, Collins DT, et al. Thoracic enhanced recovery with ambulation after surgery: a 6-year experience. Eur J Cardiothorac Surg 2018; 53(6):1192–8.
11. Scott WJ, Allen MS, Darling G, et al. Video-assisted thoracic surgery versus open lobectomy for lung cancer: a secondary analysis of data from the American College of Surgeons Oncology Group Z0030 randomized clinical trial. J Thorac Cardiovasc Surg 2010;139(4):976–81, discussion 981-3.
12. Whitson BA, Groth SS, Duval SJ, et al. Surgery for early-stage non-small cell lung cancer: a systematic review of the video-assisted thoracoscopic surgery versus thoracotomy approaches to lobectomy. Ann Thorac Surg 2008;86(6):2008–16, discussion 2016-8.
13. Zhang R, Ferguson MK. Video-Assisted versus Open Lobectomy in Patients with Compromised Lung Function: A Literature Review and Meta-Analysis. PLoS One 2015;10(7):e0124512.
14. Schussler O, Alifano M, Dermine H, et al. Postoperative pneumonia after major lung resection. Am J Respir Crit Care Med 2006;173(10):1161–9.
15. Kalil AC, Metersky ML, Klompas M, et al. Management of Adults With Hospital-acquired and Ventilator-associated Pneumonia: 2016 Clinical Practice Guidelines by the Infectious Diseases Society of America and the American Thoracic Society. Clin Infect Dis 2016;63(5):e61–111.
16. Ranieri VM, Rubenfeld GD, Thompson BT, et al. Acute respiratory distress syndrome: the Berlin Definition. J Am Med Assoc 2012;307(23):2526–33.
17. Brower RG, Lanken PN, MacIntyre N, et al. Higher versus lower positive end-expiratory pressures in patients with the acute respiratory distress syndrome. N Engl J Med 2004;351(4):327–36.
18. Brower RG, Matthay MA, Morris A, et al. Ventilation with lower tidal volumes as compared with traditional tidal volumes for acute lung injury and the acute respiratory distress syndrome. N Engl J Med 2000;342(18):1301–8.

19. Chau EH, Slinger P. Perioperative fluid management for pulmonary resection surgery and esophagectomy. Semin Cardiothorac Vasc Anesth 2014;18(1):36–44.

20. Dai W, Yang XJ, Zhuang X, et al. Reoperation for hemostasis within 24 hours can get a better short-term outcome when indicated after lung cancer surgery. J Thorac Dis 2017;9(10):3677–83.

21. Bryant AS, Minnich DJ, Wei B, et al. The incidence and management of postoperative chylothorax after pulmonary resection and thoracic mediastinal lymph node dissection. Ann Thorac Surg 2014;98(1):232–5, discussion 235-7.

22. Cho HJ, Kim DK, Lee GD, et al. Chylothorax complicating pulmonary resection for lung cancer: effective management and pleurodesis. Ann Thorac Surg 2014; 97(2):408–13.

23. Petrella F, Casiraghi M, Radice D, et al. Treatment of Chylothorax after Lung Resection: Indications, Timing, and Outcomes. Thorac Cardiovasc Surg 2020; 68(6):520–4.

24. Singhal S, Ferraris VA, Bridges CR, et al. Management of alveolar air leaks after pulmonary resection. Ann Thorac Surg 2010;89(4):1327–35.

25. Cerfolio RJ, Tummala RP, Holman WL, et al. A prospective algorithm for the management of air leaks after pulmonary resection. Ann Thorac Surg 1998;66(5): 1726–31.

26. Gkegkes ID, Mourtarakos S, Gakidis I. Endobronchial valves in treatment of persistent air leaks: a systematic review of clinical evidence. Med Sci Monit 2015;21:432–8.

27. Lang-Lazdunski L, Coonar AS. A prospective study of autologous 'blood patch' pleurodesis for persistent air leak after pulmonary resection. Eur J Cardiothorac Surg 2004;26(5):897–900.

28. Hu XF, Duan L, Jiang GN, et al. A clinical risk model for the evaluation of bronchopleural fistula in non-small cell lung cancer after pneumonectomy. Ann Thorac Surg 2013;96(2):419–24.

29. Berry MF, Harpole DH. Bronchopleural fistula after pneumonectomy. In: Sugarbaker DJ, Bueno R, Burt BM, et al, editors. Sugarbaker's Adult Chest Surgery, 3e. New York: McGraw-Hill Education; 2020. p. 790–7.

30. Attaar A, Luketich JD, Schuchert MJ, et al. Prolonged Air Leak After Pulmonary Resection Increases Risk of Noncardiac Complications, Readmission, and Delayed Hospital Discharge: A Propensity Score-adjusted Analysis. Ann Surg 2021;273(1):163–72.

31. Mazzella A, Pardolesi A, Maisonneuve P, et al. Bronchopleural Fistula After Pneumonectomy: Risk Factors and Management, Focusing on Open-Window Thoracostomy. Semin Thorac Cardiovasc Surg 2018;30(1):104–13. https://doi.org/10.1053/j.semtcvs.2017.10.003.

32. Zanotti G, Mitchell JD. Bronchopleural Fistula and Empyema After Anatomic Lung Resection. Thorac Surg Clin 2015;25(4):421–7. https://doi.org/10.1016/j.thorsurg.2015.07.006.

33. Durham AL, Adcock IM. The relationship between COPD and lung cancer. Lung Cancer 2015;90(2):121–7. https://doi.org/10.1016/j.lungcan.2015.08.017.

34. Bhattacharyya N, Batirel H, Swanson SJ. Improved outcomes with early vocal fold medialization for vocal fold paralysis after thoracic surgery. Auris Nasus Larynx 2003;30(1):71–5.

35. Cable DG, Deschamps C, Allen MS, et al. Lobar torsion after pulmonary resection: presentation and outcome. J Thorac Cardiovasc Surg 2001;122(6):1091–3.

36. Roselli EE, Murthy SC, Rice TW, et al. Atrial fibrillation complicating lung cancer resection. J Thorac Cardiovasc Surg 2005;130(2):438–44.

37. Vaporciyan AA, Correa AM, Rice DC, et al. Risk factors associated with atrial fibrillation after noncardiac thoracic surgery: analysis of 2588 patients. J Thorac Cardiovasc Surg 2004;127(3):779–86.

38. Frendl G, Sodickson AC, Chung MK, et al. 2014 AATS guidelines for the prevention and management of perioperative atrial fibrillation and flutter for thoracic surgical procedures. J Thorac Cardiovasc Surg 2014;148(3):e153–93.

39. Lip GY, Nieuwlaat R, Pisters R, et al. Refining clinical risk stratification for predicting stroke and thromboembolism in atrial fibrillation using a novel risk factor-based approach: the euro heart survey on atrial fibrillation. Chest 2010;137(2): 263–72.

40. Landesberg G, Beattie WS, Mosseri M, et al. Perioperative myocardial infarction. Circulation 2009;119(22):2936–44.

41. Gould MK, Garcia DA, Wren SM, et al. Prevention of VTE in nonorthopedic surgical patients: Antithrombotic Therapy and Prevention of Thrombosis, 9th ed: American College of Chest Physicians Evidence-Based Clinical Practice Guidelines. Chest 2012;141(2 Suppl):e227S–77S.

42. Kearon C, Akl EA, Ornelas J, et al. Antithrombotic Therapy for VTE Disease: CHEST Guideline and Expert Panel Report. Chest 2016;149(2):315–52.

43. Marshall K, McLaughlin K. Pain Management in Thoracic Surgery. Thorac Surg Clin 2020;30(3):339–46.

Venous Thromboembolism and Pulmonary Embolism
Strategies for Prevention and Management

Rachel R. Blitzer, MD[a], Samuel Eisenstein, MD[b],*

KEYWORDS

- Perioperative anticoagulation • Deep venous thrombosis • Pulmonary embolism
- VTE prophylaxis • Management of VTE

KEY POINTS

- VTE is a common perioperative complication
- Perioperative VTE prophylaxis depends on the nature of the procedure and patient risk stratification
- Diagnosis of postoperative DVT or PE requires prompt intervention, most commonly immediate anticoagulation extending 3 months postoperatively

INTRODUCTION

Care of the surgical patient is complex; the surgeon must not only execute the required procedure but also must be aware of the perioperative risks and address them to maximize patient outcomes. One of the most common complications for postsurgical patients is venous thromboembolism (VTE), which includes deep venous thrombosis (DVT) and pulmonary embolism (PE). VTE is the most common preventable cause of death in postsurgical patients.[1–4] VTE occurs in up to 20% of postoperative patients not receiving appropriate prophylaxis; of these an estimated 7% experience a PE, which can be fatal in a small percentage of cases.[5–7] To best prevent and manage these devastating comorbidities, surgeons must be able to risk-stratify the patient preoperatively, institute appropriate prophylactic measures, promptly diagnose signs of postoperative VTE, and understand the best course of treatment.[8]

Background

VTE is a condition in which thrombi form inappropriately within the venous system. Portions of a thrombus may detach from the endothelium and travel within the venous

[a] Department of Surgery, UC San Diego Health System, 200 W. Arbor Drive, San Diego, CA 92103, USA; [b] Department of Surgery, UC San Diego Health System, 3855 Health Sciences Drive #0987, La Jolla, CA 92037, USA
* Corresponding author.
E-mail address: seisenstein@ucsd.edu
Twitter: @DrE_UCSD (S.E.)

Surg Clin N Am 101 (2021) 925–938
https://doi.org/10.1016/j.suc.2021.06.015
0039-6109/21/© 2021 Elsevier Inc. All rights reserved.

system, at which point the detached thrombus becomes an embolus. The embolus then has the potential to occlude vasculature in distant portions of the venous system.[9]

It is estimated that 10% to 40% of hospitalized US patients experience VTE, whereas the general population is diagnosed with VTE at a rate of 0.1% to 0.2%.[10–12] Although there is likely some detection bias implicated in this discrepancy, up to 60% of hospitalized surgical patients have moderate to high risk of VTE.[13] Importantly, presence of this comorbidity significantly increases 30-day mortality rates. In addition, the annual cost of VTE within the United States is tens of billions of dollars per year.[14] Recognition of the scale of the problem has led to the widespread adoption of perioperative prophylaxis as a best practice. As such, multiple critical care and surgical societies recommend implementation of a standardized protocol to reduce VTE risk in hospitalized postsurgical patients.[15]

Pathophysiology of VTE can be explained by Virchow triad, which conceptualizes venous thrombosis as resulting from one or more of the following factors: endothelial injury, hypercoagulability, and venous stasis. In retrospective studies, more than 90% of patients with VTE have demonstrated at least one of these factors.[16,17]

Risk factors

There are multitudes of patient factors that can affect one or more aspects of Virchow triad, thus increasing VTE risk and complicating the practitioner's assessment of a patient's individual risk. These factors are typically divided between intrinsic factors, such as genetic anomalies, and extrinsic (or acquired) factors (**Box 1**). A careful patient history must be taken to assess intrinsic factors, because these conditions have not always been previously identified. Although some of the extrinsic factors are phenotypically apparent, a diligent history again plays an important role in patient risk factor

---

Box 1
Patient factors influencing VTE risk

Intrinsic factors
- Factor V Leiden
- Protein C or S deficiency
- Antithrombin deficiency
- Sickle cell trait
- Antiphospholipid antibody syndrome
- Prothrombin mutations
- Family history of thrombophilia

Extrinsic factors
- Increased age
- Elevated BMI
- Immobility
- Smoking
- Heart failure
- Malignancy
- Inflammatory bowel disease
- Trauma
- Hospitalization
- Surgery
- Central venous catheter
- Oral contraception, pregnancy
- Prior personal history of DVT
   BMI, body mass index.

assessment.[18,19] The most important of these are smoking, malignancy, inflammatory bowel disease, congestive heart failure, and history of prior VTE.[8] The last of these poses a 20% risk of recurrent perioperative VTE in the surgical patient with a greater likelihood of subsequent 30-day mortality.[18] Risk factors can be stratified into low-, moderate-, and high-risk categories, which helps inform perioperative chemoprophylaxis decision making[20,21] (**Box 2**).

Patient evaluation and overview: risk assessment

A thorough evaluation of patient risk must be undertaken before implementation of VTE prophylaxis; both VTE and bleeding risk must be taken into account as part of a preoperative VTE risk assessment.[22–25] All surgical patients are at risk, because the resultant physiologic changes and inflammatory response can affect each aspect of Virchow triad. Multiple perioperative predictive models have been proposed to estimate risk. These models can be divided into qualitative and quantitative risk assessment models (RAM).[15]

Qualitative RAMs use risk factors to categorize patients into broad risk categories, which are then used to inform perioperative prophylactic regimens. These "bucket" modules assign high-, moderate-, and low-risk categories to patient factors to place patients in one of these risk categories, which is associated with recommended prophylaxis measures[20,21] (**Fig. 1**).

Quantitative RAMs assign values to each different risk factor to create a precise scoring system predicting each patient's risk of perioperative VTE and bases treatment recommendations on a patient's score.

The Caprini model is externally validated; it is the most used quantitative model in the surgical setting, assigning weighted values to each thrombotic risk contributor.[19,26,27]

Box 2
Common VTE risk factors by risk severity

High risk
- Long bone fracture or pelvic procedure
- Trauma
- Ischemic stroke
- Spinal cord surgery
- Neurosurgery
- Malignancy
- Postoperative intubation

Moderate risk
- Thrombophilia
- Congestive heart failure
- Oral contraceptives
- Immobility greater than 3 days
- Pregnancy
- Prior major surgery less than 7 days
- Infection requiring intravenous abx

Low risk
- Laparoscopic surgery
- Surgery less than 30 minutes
- Obesity
- Smoking
- Immobility less than 3 days
- Varicose veins

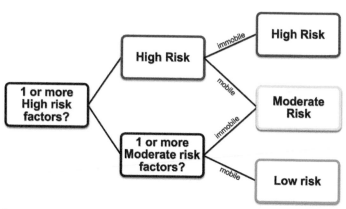

Fig. 1. Perioperative VTE risk stratification.

The Rogers, Intermountain, and International Medical Prevention Registry on Venous Thromboembolism (IMPROVE) models are all empirically derived and have not been externally validated.[23,28–31]

Both quantitative and qualitative RAMs must be weighed against the patient's risk of perioperative bleeding, and this is assessed by the surgeon based on intraoperative blood loss and hemostasis along with predisposing factors such as recent gastrointestinal or intracranial bleeding or hematologic abnormalities (bleeding diathesis disorders, thrombocytopenia, etc.).

Perioperative venous thromboembolism prevention measures

All patients should undergo nonpharmacologic prophylaxis measures such as early and frequent ambulation as well as mechanical prophylaxis when appropriate. These interventions have been shown to reduce the risk of postoperative DVT by 50% in hospitalized patients through reduction of venous stasis.[32,33] Inpatient pharmacologic DVT prevention includes subcutaneous injections of unfractionated heparin (UFH) or low-molecular-weight heparin (LMWH), although aspirin and indirect factor Xa inhibitors are occasionally used, typically in preparation for discharge. Historically, patients with malignancy are prescribed LMWH, although there is no firm consensus on the benefits of this therapy versus UFH in surgical patients with cancer at this time.[34] UFH is favored in patients with chronic kidney disease due to its rapid reversibility and lack of bioaccumulation, although LMWH has been shown to have a slightly decreased risk of postoperative bleeding.[35] In addition, LMWH is administered every 12 hours, whereas UFH is injected every 8 hours, which can be a factor in patient adherence. Timing of pharmacologic VTE prophylaxis requires weighing VTE versus postoperative bleeding risk; American College of Chest Physicians (ACCP) 10th edition guidelines suggest a decision tree in combination with a "bucket" system for risk assessment (**Figs. 2** and **3**).

Prophylaxis for patients undergoing surgery for malignancy is a well-studied cohort; use of UFH or LMWH has been intensely debated. Updated American Society of Clinical Oncology guidelines noted no difference in VTE, mortality, or bleeding, although LMWH was recommended over UFH for ambulatory settings.[35] In addition, the recommendation for at least 4 weeks of postoperative prophylaxis using LMWH, including after discharge from the hospital was confirmed without a concomitant increased risk of bleeding.[36–38] The nature and site of surgery affects the thrombosis/bleeding

1 point Risk Factors	2 point risk factors	3 point risk factors	5 point Risk Factors
Age 41–60 y	Age 61–74 y	Age >75 y	Stroke <1 mo
Swollen legs	Arthroscopic surgery	History of DVT/PE	Major lower extremity arthroplasty
Varicose veins	Malignancy	Positive Factor V Leiden	Hip, pelvis, or leg fracture <1 mo
Obesity	Laparoscopic surgery	Elevated serum Homocysteine	Acute spinal cord injury <1 mo
Minor surgery	Bed rest >72 h	Heparin-induced thrombocytopenia	
Sepsis	Immobilizing plaster cast	Elevated anti-cardiolipin antibodies	
Serious lung disease	Central Venous Access	Thrombophilia	
Hormone therapy	Major surgery <45 min	Family history of thrombosis	
Pregnancy		Positive Prothrombin 20210A	
History of unexplained prenatal complications		Positive Lupus Anticoagulant	
Acute Myocardial Infarction			
Congestive Heart Failure			
Bed rest (current)			
Inflammatory Bowel Disease			
Recent Major Surgery			
Congestive Obstructive Pulmonary Disease			

Total Risk Factor Score	Risk Level	Incidence of DVT	Prophylaxis Regimen
0–1	Low	2%	early ambulation
2	Moderate	10%–20%	SCDS OR UFH 5000 U SQ TID
3–4	Higher Risk	20%–40%	SCDS +/- UFH 5000 U SQ TID or weight-based LMWH dosing
5 or more	Highest Risk	40%–80%	SCDS AND UFH 5000 U SQ TID or weight-based LMWH dosing

Fig. 2. Caprini VTE risk factor assessment tool.

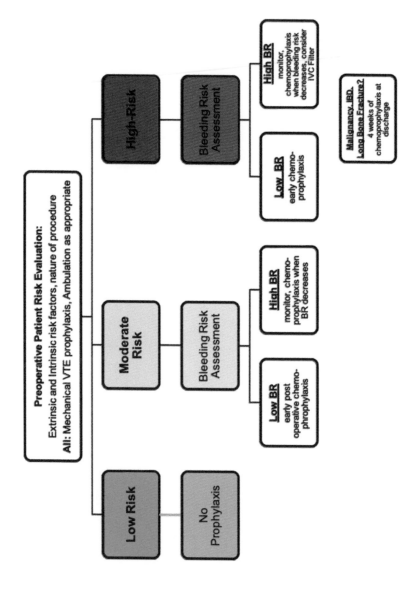

Fig. 3. Perioperative VTE prophylaxis decision tree (BR, bleeding risk assessment).

risk; for example, thromboprophylaxis is not recommended for breast surgery, where the risk of bleeding outweighs the risk of VTE.

Diagnosis of postoperative venous thromboembolism

Suspicion for VTE in the postoperative period should be high. Presenting symptoms of chest pain, dyspnea, leg swelling, skin changes, and leg pain all suggest VTE; however, the differential diagnosis is broad and must be confirmed with imaging. Postoperative DVT is commonly asymptomatic, and PE symptoms may be the first indication of underlying DVT. These symptoms include chest pain, dyspnea, tachypnea, tachycardia, desaturation, cardiac rhythm abnormalities, and sudden cardiopulmonary collapse. The modified Wells score for DVT can be used to predict pretest probability[39] (**Table 1**).

The true gold standard for the diagnosis of DVT is contrast venography, but it is more often diagnosed on duplex ultrasonographic studies with a sensitivity and specificity of greater than 90%.[40,41] Ultrasound resolution can be limited by obesity, tissue swelling, or patient intolerance of probe compression. Pelvic venous thrombosis is not diagnosed by lower extremity ultrasonography and should be suspected in cases in which PE occurs and ultrasonography does not show DVT in the lower extremities. Adjunct imaging studies include venous phase contrast computed tomography (CT) or MRI, depending on patient comorbidities.

Clinical risk predictors for PE include the Wells and Geneva scores[39,42] (**Tables 2 and 3**). CT angiography of the chest is the gold standard for diagnosis of postoperative PE. If the patient cannot tolerate intravenous contrast, ventilation-perfusion scintigraphic perfusion scanning or MRI pulmonary angiography can be obtained; both tests are highly sensitive but have lower specificity than CT angiography, which has a sensitivity of 83% and specificity of 96%.[43-45]

Critically ill or unstable patients with high suspicion for PE may undergo empirical treatment. In addition, these patients can be diagnosed with transthoracic or transesophageal echocardiography, which is unlikely to show embolic material but will reveal right-sided heart strain that is characteristic of a massive or submassive PE. Conventional angiography may also be used and has the benefit of both diagnostic and treatment potentials for DVT and PE and can be used in selected clinical scenarios.

Table 1
The Modified Wells Score for Deep Vein Thrombosis

Clinical Feature	Points
Active cancer (<6 mo)	1
Paralysis	1
>3 d immobilization or major surgery <3 mo	1
Tenderness in deep venous system	1
Entire leg swollen	1
Calf swelling 3 cm larger than the asymptomatic side	1
Pitting edema in affected leg	1
History of DVT	1
Alternative diagnosis as least as likely as DVT	−2

Score	Points
DVT likely	2 or more
DVT unlikely	1 or less

Table 2
Modified Wells Score for Pulmonary Embolism

Clinical Feature	Points
Clinical signs and symptoms of DVT	3
Alternative diagnosis less likely than PE	3
Heart rate >100 beats per minute	1.5
>3 d immobilization or major surgery <3 mo	1.2
Hemoptysis	1
Malignancy	1
History of VTE	1.5

Score	Points
PE likely	>4 points
PE unlikely	4 or less

Treatment options: venous thromboembolism

Treatment of DVT aims to prevent further clot formation and embolization. Fresh thrombus is fragile, but over time, cross-linking of fibrin stabilizes the thrombus. Early recognition and treatment prevent PE while minimizing recurrence and morbidity in the long term. Risk of recurrent DVT decreases with the duration of anticoagulation. According to ACCP guidelines, patients with postoperative DVT or PE are recommended to have at least 3 months of anticoagulant therapy, considered long term[1] (**Fig. 4**). Others continue therapy for an extended period with no defined stop date (**Fig. 5**). Options for treatment of established DVT/PE anticoagulation include adjusted dose UFH; LMWH; newer anticoagulants, including rivaroxaban, apixaban, dabigatran, and edoxaban; and vitamin K antagonists, such as warfarin.[4,6,46,47] The most common inpatient medications are heparin and LMWH. For prophylaxis, the same agents are available, plus aspirin. Historically, if the patient requires only limited treatment,

Table 3
The Revised Geneva Score

Risk Factors	Points
Age >65 y	1
Malignancy	1
>3 d immobilization or major surgery <1 mo	1
Signs and Symptoms	
Unilateral lower limb pain	1
Hemoptysis	1
Heart rate 75–94 beats per minute	1
Heart rate 95 or greater beats per minute	1
Pain on palpation and unilateral edema	−2

Probability	Total Points
Low	0–3
Intermediate	4–10
High	11 or greater

Phases of anticoagulation

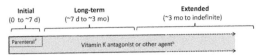

Fig. 4. Phases of anticoagulation treatment for VTE. [a]Heparin, LMWH, fondaparinux. [b]Includes LMWH, dabigatran, rivaroxaban.

LMWH has been used opposed to warfarin, primarily because of the reversibility.[48,49] Of note, dabigatran and edoxaban require initial parenteral prophylaxis, whereas rivaroxaban and apixaban do not. Adjunct catheter-directed thrombolysis and/or inferior vena cava filter placement is not recommended except in cases in which thrombotic risk is high and there are absolute contraindications to anticoagulation.[1,50,51] In patients without preexisting comorbidities, postsurgical prophylaxis can be brief. High-risk patients may have been on anticoagulation chronically before surgery.

Nonpharmacologic or surgical/interventional treatment options

Treatment is primarily pharmacologic for isolated DVT; previous recommendations had indicated compression stockings to prevent recurrent DVT or postphlebitic syndrome; however, this has not been borne out in subsequent studies. Stockings may be used for symptom management.[52–54]

Pulmonary embolism treatment

Treatment of postoperative PE depends on the clinical status of the patient. For hemodynamically stable patients, therapeutic anticoagulation is initiated with either LMWH or UFH with subsequent transition to a long-term anticoagulation for a minimum of 3 months; this algorithm is similar to that for DVTs outlined in **Fig. 5**.[55,56] For patients with hypotension and low to moderate bleeding risk, systemic thrombolytic therapy is recommended. Per ACCP guidelines, catheter-based thrombectomy is recommended in cases in which bleeding risk is high, there is prior failed thrombolysis, or the patient is likely to deteriorate before onset of systemic thrombolytic effect. There are no randomized studies of this intervention, and observational studies have few sample sizes; there is little evidence to support this intervention.

Treatment resistance/complications

The most common complication of VTE treatment is bleeding, usually from surgical incisions; this may be managed with careful monitoring, pressure, and cessation of anticoagulation, although some patients can require return to the operating room to achieve hemostasis. If anticoagulation is supratherapeutic, chances of spontaneous hemorrhage are increased and can occur in the intracranial and retroperitoneal spaces. The intensity of anticoagulation can readily be measured only with heparin or warfarin; measures for other agents, like Xa activity, may not be available. For heparin anticoagulation (both UFH and LMWH), up to 5% of patients experience heparin-induced thrombocytopenia, which is caused by an autoantibody directed against platelet factor 4 complexed with heparin.[57,58] In this case, the heparin product must be stopped and an alternate anticoagulant must be started.

Post–venous thromboembolism morbidity

DVT and PE are not always life-threatening, whereas multiple studies have shown that postoperative patients with VTE have a lower quality of life than their peers who do not

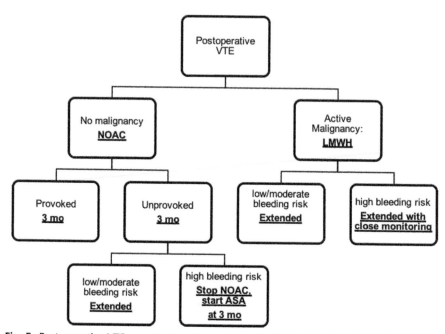

Fig. 5. Postoperative VTE treatment. ASA, Aspirin; NOAC, Novel oral anticoagulant.

experience this complication[59] In addition, patients with VTE have been shown to have double the Length of stay (LOS) of their similar counterparts.[14] Late recognition and treatment leads to incomplete resolution of clot with resultant symptoms. Postthrombotic syndrome occurs in up to 40% of patients with DVT and can cause pain, skin changes, and ulceration in the distal extremities.[60] Other patients experience venous insufficiency in the form of varicose veins, which can also cause pain. Survivors of a PE can have chronic pulmonary hypertension or right-sided heart failure.[53,61]

Long-term recommendations

Patients experiencing postoperative VTE require closer postoperative management than their peers, particularly if prescribed extended anticoagulant therapy. These patients should be followed by both a primary care physician and/or an anticoagulation clinic to ensure proper titration of medications and periodic evaluation of continued anticoagulant therapy.

Summary/discussion/future directions

Perioperative VTE is a common, costly, and morbid complication in the surgical population. Patients with malignancy, inflammatory bowel disease, and long bone fractures are particularly likely to experience VTE and may require longer duration of prophylaxis. Perioperative prophylaxis is essential in the surgical patient and typically consists of subcutaneous heparin therapy along with mechanical prophylaxis where appropriate. Should postoperative VTE occur, long-term therapy is prescribed depending on the level of bleeding risk as well as the diagnosed cause of the thrombus. Patients experiencing postoperative VTE must be monitored closely and may experience long-term complications even after resolution of thrombus.

CLINICS CARE POINTS

- Perioperative VTE is a common and costly complication in the surgical population.
- Perioperative prophylaxis is essential in the surgical patient and typically consists of subcutaneous heparin therapy along with mechanical prophylaxis
- Patients with malignancy, inflammatory bowel disease, and long bone fractures have an increased risk of postoperative VTE
- Should postoperative VTE occur, long-term therapy is prescribed depending on the level of bleeding risk

DISCLOSURE

S. Eisenstein is a consultant for Ethicon Surgical robotics, Takeda, and Prescient Surgical.

REFERENCES

1. Kearon C, Akl EA, Ornelas J, et al. Antithrombotic therapy for VTE disease: CHEST guideline and expert panel report. Chest 2016;149(2):315–52.
2. Granziera S, Cohen AT. VTE primary prevention, including hospitalised medical and orthopaedic surgical patients. Thromb Haemost 2015;113(6):1216–23.
3. O'Donnell M, Weitz JI. Thromboprophylaxis in surgical patients. Can J Surg 2003; 46(2):129–35.
4. Eikelboom JW, Kearon C, Guyatt G, et al. Perioperative aspirin for prevention of venous thromboembolism. Surv Anesthesiol 2017;61(2):1121–9.
5. Geerts WH, Heit JA, Clagett GP, et al. Prevention of venous thromboembolism. Chest 2001;119:132S–75S.
6. Mismetti P, Quenet S, Levine M, et al. Enoxaparin in the treatment of deep vein thrombosis with or without pulmonary embolism: an individual patient data meta-analysis. Chest 2005;128(4):2203–10.
7. Tooher R, Middleton P, Pham C, et al. A systematic review of strategies to improve prophylaxis for venous thromboembolism in hospitals. Ann Surg 2005;241(3):397–415.
8. Kearon C, Kahn SR, Agnelli G, et al. Antithrombotic therapy for venous thrombo-embolic disease: American College of Chest Physicians evidence-based clinical practice guidelines (8th edition). Chest 2008;133(6 SUPPL. 6):454S–545S.
9. Vazquez-Garza E, Jerjes-Sanchez C, Navarrete A, et al. Venous thromboembolism: thrombosis, inflammation, and immunothrombosis for clinicians. J Thromb Thrombolysis 2017;44(3):377–85.
10. Heit JA, Cohen AT, Anderson FA. Estimated annual number of incident and recurrent, non-fatal and fatal venous thromboembolism (VTE) events in the US. Blood 2005;106(11):910.
11. Heit JA, Silverstein MD, Mohr DN, et al. Risk factors for deep vein thrombosis and pulmonary embolism: a population-based case-control study. Arch Intern Med 2002;160(6):809–15.
12. Anderson FA, Wheeler HB, Goldberg RJ, et al. A population-based perspective of the hospital incidence and case-fatality rates of deep vein thrombosis and pulmonary embolism: the worcester DVT study. Arch Intern Med 1991;151(5):933–8.
13. Bergmann J-F, Cohen AT, Victor, et al. Blood coagulation, fibrinolysis and cellular haemostasis venous thromboembolism risk and prophylaxis in hospitalised

medically ill patients the ENDORSE global survey 2010. Thromb Haemost 2010;103:736–48.

14. Fernandez MM, Hogue S, Preblick R, et al. Review of the cost of venous thromboembolism. Clin Outcomes Res 2015;7:451–62.

15. Chapter 4. Choose the model to assess VTE and bleeding risk | Agency for Healthcare Research and Quality. Available at: https://www.ahrq.gov/patient-safety/resources/vtguide/guide4.html. Accessed April 11, 2021.

16. Wolberg AS, Aleman MM, Leiderman K, et al. Procoagulant activity in hemostasis and thrombosis: Virchow's triad revisited. Anesth Analg 2012;114(2):275–85.

17. Brotman DJ, Deitcher SR, Lip GYH, et al. Virchow's triad revisited. South Med J 2004;97(2):213–5. Available at: https://go.gale.com/ps/i.do?p=AONE&sw=w&issn=00384348&v=2.1&it=r&id=GALE%7CA114134751&sid=googleScholar&linkaccess=fulltext. Accessed April 13, 2021.

18. Spencer FA, Emery C, Lessard D, et al. The Worcester Venous Thromboembolism study: a population-based study of the clinical epidemiology of venous thromboembolism. J Gen Intern Med 2006;21(7):722–7.

19. Bahl V, Hu HM, Henke PK, et al. A validation study of a retrospective venous thromboembolism risk scoring method. Ann Surg 2010;251(2):344–50.

20. Jenkins IH, White RH, Amin AN, et al. Reducing the incidence of hospital-associated venous thromboembolism within a network of academic hospitals: findings from five University of California medical centers. J Hosp Med 2016;11:S22–8.

21. Streiff M, Carolan H, Hobson D, et al. Lessons from the Johns Hopkins multidisciplinary venous thromboembolism (VTE) prevention collaborative. bmj.com. 2012. Available at: https://www.bmj.com/content/344/bmj.e3935.full. Accessed April 13, 2021.

22. Park MY, Fletcher JP, Hoffmann C, et al. Prevention of venous thromboembolism through the implementation of a risk assessment tool: a comparative study in medical and surgical patients. Int Angiol 2018;37(5).

23. Nazarenko GI, Kleymenova EB, Payushik SA, et al. Decision support systems in clinical practice: the case of venous thromboembolism prevention. Int J Risk Saf Med 2016;27(s1):S104–5.

24. Erem HH, Aytac E. The use of surgical care improvement projects in prevention of venous thromboembolism. Adv Exp Med Biol 2017;906:15–22.

25. Muntz JE, Michota FA. Prevention and management of venous thromboembolism in the surgical patient: options by surgery type and individual patient risk factors. Am J Surg 2010;199(1 Suppl):S11–20.

26. Segon YS, Summey RD, Slawski B, et al. Surgical venous thromboembolism prophylaxis: clinical practice update. Hosp Pract (1995) 2020;48(5):248–57.

27. Caprini J, Arcelus J, Hasty J, et al. Clinical assessment of venous thromboembolic risk in surgical patients. europepmc.org. 1991. Available at: https://europepmc.org/article/med/1754886. Accessed April 13, 2021.

28. Spyropoulos A Jr, Chest GF. Predictive and associative models to identify hospitalized medical patients at risk for VTE. Elsevier; 2011. Available at: https://www.sciencedirect.com/science/article/pii/S0012369211604777?casa_token=TnOGutndam0AAAAA:McoFpfViNq1F7f8-UArgxLLfibvO4Nh_fFxcOsVpBfPnobEUzc586nRnSjo8Hpl1fOeUjiU4U3gL. Accessed April 13, 2021.

29. Rogers Jr S, Kilaru R, Hosokawa P, et al. Multivariable predictors of postoperative venous thromboembolic events after general and vascular surgery: results from the patient safety in surgery study. Elsevier; 2007. Available at: https://www.sciencedirect.com/science/article/pii/S1072751507003274?casa_token=vvkvN4

HXSVMAAAAA:FxBGeMZHHeEGqRnKPpbJ3XNFArSpexyby2S1OmZekrbOFYo
9QgwiBPRgU53heRgKdVj_810YPlN4. Accessed April 13, 2021.

30. Woller S, Stevens S, Jones J, et al. Derivation and validation of a simple model to identify venous thromboembolism risk in medical patients. Elsevier; 2011. Available at: https://www.sciencedirect.com/science/article/pii/S0002934311004797? casa_token=4Aiaj97gZDQAAAAA:MhrbjwtULz8wwLor2B0jYm9fmo6nUQ irWAwJ1o8y2SkjxDSuMlnZY9P4zc9QDqSrAnCUwFLzTAm-. Accessed April 13, 2021.

31. Obi A, Pannucci C, Nackashi A, et al. Validation of the Caprini venous thromboembolism risk assessment model in critically ill surgical patients. jamanetwork.com. 2015. Available at: https://jamanetwork.com/journals/jamasurgery/article-abstract/2426414. Accessed April 13, 2021.

32. Vanek VW. Meta-analysis of effectiveness of intermittent pneumatic compression devices with a comparison of thigh-high to knee-high sleeves. Am Surg 1998; 64(11):1050–8.

33. Urbankova J, Quiroz R, Kucher N, et al. Intermittent pneumatic compression and deep vein thrombosis prevention: a meta-analysis in postoperative patients. Thromb Haemost 2005;94(6):1181–5.

34. Akl EA, Kahale LA, Sperati F, et al. Low molecular weight heparin versus unfractionated heparin for perioperative thromboprophylaxis in patients with cancer. Cochrane Database Syst Rev 2014;6:CD009447

35. Key NS, Khorana AA, Kuderer NM, et al. Venous thromboembolism prophylaxis and treatment in patients with cancer: ASCO clinical practice guideline update. J Clin Oncol 2020;38(5):496–520.

36. Vedovati M, Becattini C, Rondelli F, et al. A randomized study on 1-week versus 4-week prophylaxis for venous thromboembolism after laparoscopic surgery for colorectal cancer. journals.lww.com. 2014. Available at: https://journals.lww.com/annalsofsurgery/Fulltext/2014/04000/A_Randomized_Study_on_1_Week_Versus_4_Week.9.aspx. Accessed April 14, 2021.

37. Pai A, Hurtuk M, Park J, et al. A randomized study on 1-week versus 4-week prophylaxis for venous thromboembolism after laparoscopic surgery for colorectal cancer. journals.lww.com. 2016. Available at: https://journals.lww.com/annalsofsurgery/fulltext/2016/04000/a_randomized_study_on_1_week_versus_4_week.31.aspx. Accessed April 14, 2021.

38. Felder S, Rasmussen MS, King R, et al. Prolonged thromboprophylaxis with low molecular weight heparin for abdominal or pelvic surgery. Cochrane Database Syst Rev 2019. https://doi.org/10.1002/14651858.cd004318.pub5.

39. Wells P, Anderson DR, Bormanis J, et al. Value of assessment of pretest probability of deep-vein thrombosis in clinical management. Lancet 1997;350(9094): 1795–8.

40. Le Gal G, Righini M. Controversies in the diagnosis of venous thromboembolism. J Thromb Haemost 2015;13(S1):S259–65.

41. Zitek T, Baydoun J, Yepez S, et al. Mistakes and pitfalls associated with Two-Point compression ultrasound for deep vein thrombosis. West J Emerg Med 2016; 17(2):201–8.

42. goire Le Gal G, Righini M, Roy P-M, et al. Prediction of pulmonary embolism in the emergency department: the revised Geneva score 2006. Available at: www.annals.org. Accessed April 12, 2021.

43. Moore AJE, Wachsmann J, Chamarthy MR, et al. Imaging of acute pulmonary embolism: an update. Cardiovasc Diagn Ther 2018;8(3):225–43.

44. Stein PD, Woodard PK, Weg JG, et al. Diagnostic pathways in acute pulmonary embolism: recommendations of the PIOPED II Investigators. Am J Med 2006; 119(12):1048–55.
45. Grosse C, Grosse A. CT findings in diseases associated with pulmonary hypertension: a current review. Radiographics 2010;30(7):1753–74.
46. Mavrakanas T, Bounameaux H. The potential role of new oral anticoagulants in the prevention and treatment of thromboembolism. Pharmacol Ther 2011; 130(1):46–58.
47. Leizorovicz A. Comparison of the efficacy and safety of low molecular weight heparins and unfractionated heparin in the initial treatment of deep venous thrombosis. an updated meta-analysis. Drugs 1996;52(SUPPL. 7):30–7.
48. Barnes GD, Li Y, Gu X, et al. Periprocedural bridging anticoagulation in patients with venous thromboembolism: a registry-based cohort study. J Thromb Haemost 2020;18(8):2025–30.
49. van Veen JJ, Maclean RM, Hampton KK, et al. Protamine reversal of low molecular weight heparin. Blood Coagul Fibrinolysis 2011;22(7):565–70.
50. Muriel A, Jiménez D, Aujesky D, et al. Survival effects of inferior vena cava filter in patients with acute symptomatic venous thromboembolism and a significant bleeding risk. J Am Coll Cardiol 2014;63(16):1675–83.
51. Martinez C, Cohen AT, Bamber L, et al. Epidemiology of first and recurrent venous thromboembolism: a population-based cohort study in patients without active cancer. Thromb Haemost 2014;112(2):255–63.
52. Kahn SR, Kearon C, Julian JA, et al. Predictors of the post-thrombotic syndrome during long-term treatment of proximal deep vein thrombosis. J Thromb Haemost 2005;3(4):718–23.
53. Stain M, Schonauer V, Minar E, et al. The post-thrombotic syndrome: risk factors and impact on the course of thrombotic disease. J Thromb Haemost 2005;3(12):2671–6.
54. Anderson FA, Brecht JG, Cohen AT, et al. Venous thromboembolism (VTE) in Europe. The number of VTE events and associated morbidity and mortality Ve nous thromboembolism (VTE) in Europe The number of VTE events and associated morbidity and mortality Meyer-Michel Samama 12 ,MichaelSpannagl 13 forthe VTEImpact Assessment Group in Europe (Blood Coagulation, Fibrinolysis and CellularHaemostasis. ThrombHaemost 2007;98:756–64.
55. Bauersachs R. Oral rivaroxaban for symptomatic venous thromboembolism. N Engl J Med 2010;363(26):2499–510.
56. Bailey AL. Oral rivaroxaban for the treatment of symptomatic pulmonary embolism. Cardiol Rev 2012;28(3):1287–97.
57. Alasfar FS, Badgett D, Comerota AJ. Deep venous thrombosis. In: Vascular surgery: cases, Questions and commentaries. Switzerland (Cham): Springer; 2018. https://doi.org/10.1007/978-3-319-65936-7_48.
58. Matar CF, Kahale LA, Hakoum MB, et al. Anticoagulation for perioperative thromboprophylaxis in people with cancer. Cochrane Database Syst Rev 2018; 2018(7):CD009447.
59. Lamping DL. Measuring health-related quality of life in venous disease: Practical and scientific considerations. Angiology 1997;48:51–7.
60. Hansson PO, Sörbo J, Eriksson H. Recurrent venous thromboembolism after deep vein thrombosis: incidence and risk factors. Arch Intern Med 2002. https://doi.org/10.1001/archinte.160.6.769.
61. Kahn SR, Solymoss S, Lamping DL, et al. Long-term outcomes after deep vein thrombosis: postphlebitic syndrome and quality of life. J Gen Intern Med 2000; 15(6):425–9.

UNITED STATES POSTAL SERVICE ®

Statement of Ownership, Management, and Circulation
(All Periodicals Publications Except Requester Publications)

1. Publication Title	2. Publication Number	3. Filing Date
SURGICAL CLINICS OF NORTH AMERICA	529 – 800	9/18/2021

4. Issue Frequency	5. Number of Issues Published Annually	6. Annual Subscription Price
FEB, APR, JUN, AUG, OCT, DEC	6	$443.00

7. Complete Mailing Address of Known Office of Publication (Not printer) (Street, city, county, state, and ZIP+4®)

ELSEVIER INC.
230 Park Avenue, Suite 800
New York, NY 10169

Contact Person
Malathi Samayan

Telephone (Include area code)
91-44-4299-4507

8. Complete Mailing Address of Headquarters or General Business Office of Publisher (Not printer)

ELSEVIER INC.
230 Park Avenue, Suite 800
New York, NY 10169

9. Full Names and Complete Mailing Addresses of Publisher, Editor, and Managing Editor (Do not leave blank)

Publisher (Name and complete mailing address)

DOLORES MELONI, ELSEVIER INC.
1600 JOHN F KENNEDY BLVD. SUITE 1800
PHILADELPHIA, PA 19103-2899

Editor (Name and complete mailing address)

JOHN VASSALLO, ELSEVIER INC.
1600 JOHN F KENNEDY BLVD. SUITE 1800
PHILADELPHIA, PA 19103-2899

Managing Editor (Name and complete mailing address)

PATRICK MANLEY, ELSEVIER INC.
1600 JOHN F KENNEDY BLVD. SUITE 1800
PHILADELPHIA, PA 19103-2899

10. Owner (Do not leave blank. If the publication is owned by a corporation, give the name and address of the corporation immediately followed by the names and addresses of all stockholders owning or holding 1 percent or more of the total amount of stock. If not owned by a corporation, give the names and addresses of the individual owners. If owned by a partnership or other unincorporated firm, give its name and address as well as those of each individual owner. If the publication is published by a nonprofit organization, give its name and address.)

Full Name	Complete Mailing Address
WHOLLY OWNED SUBSIDIARY OF REED/ELSEVIER, US HOLDINGS	1600 JOHN F KENNEDY BLVD. SUITE 1800 PHILADELPHIA, PA, 19103-2899

11. Known Bondholders, Mortgagees, and Other Security Holders Owning or Holding 1 Percent or More of Total Amount of Bonds, Mortgages, or Other Securities. If none, check box. → ☐ None

Full Name	Complete Mailing Address
N/A	

12. Tax Status (For completion by nonprofit organizations authorized to mail at nonprofit rates) (Check one)
The purpose, function, and nonprofit status of this organization and the exempt status for federal income tax purposes:
☒ Has Not Changed During Preceding 12 Months
☐ Has Changed During Preceding 12 Months (Publisher must submit explanation of change with this statement)

PS Form **3526**, July 2014 [Page 1 of 4 (see instructions page 4)] PSN 7530-01-000-9931 PRIVACY NOTICE: See our privacy policy on www.usps.com.

---

13. Publication Title	14. Issue Date for Circulation Data Below
SURGICAL CLINICS OF NORTH AMERICA	JUNE 2021

15. Extent and Nature of Circulation			Average No. Copies Each Issue During Preceding 12 Months	No. Copies of Single Issue Published Nearest to Filing Date
a. Total Number of Copies (Net press run)			399	332
b. Paid Circulation (By Mail and Outside the Mail)	(1)	Mailed Outside-County Paid Subscriptions Stated on PS Form 3541 (Include paid distribution above nominal rate, advertiser's proof copies, and exchange copies)	186	156
	(2)	Mailed In-County Paid Subscriptions Stated on PS Form 3541 (Include paid distribution above nominal rate, advertiser's proof copies, and exchange copies)	0	0
	(3)	Paid Distribution Outside the Mails Including Sales Through Dealers and Carriers, Street Vendors, Counter Sales, and Other Paid Distribution Outside USPS®	169	136
	(4)	Paid Distribution by Other Classes of Mail Through the USPS (e.g., First-Class Mail®)	0	0
c. Total Paid Distribution (Sum of 15b (1), (2), (3), and (4))		▶	355	292
d. Free or Nominal Rate Distribution (By Mail and Outside the Mail)	(1)	Free or Nominal Rate Outside-County Copies included on PS Form 3541	24	19
	(2)	Free or Nominal Rate In-County Copies Included on PS Form 3541	0	0
	(3)	Free or Nominal Rate Copies Mailed at Other Classes Through the USPS (e.g., First-Class Mail)	0	0
	(4)	Free or Nominal Rate Distribution Outside the Mail (Carriers or other means)	24	19
e. Total Free or Nominal Rate Distribution (Sum of 15d (1), (2), (3) and (4))		▶	24	19
f. Total Distribution (Sum of 15c and 15e)		▶	379	311
g. Copies not Distributed (See Instructions to Publishers #4 (page #3))		▶	20	21
h. Total (Sum of 15f and g)		▶	399	332
i. Percent Paid (15c divided by 15f times 100)			93.66%	93.89%

* If you are claiming electronic copies, go to line 16 on page 3. If you are not claiming electronic copies, skip to line 17 on page 3.

PS Form **3526**, July 2014 (Page 2 of 4)

16. Electronic Copy Circulation		Average No. Copies Each Issue During Preceding 12 Months	No. Copies of Single Issue Published Nearest to Filing Date
a. Paid Electronic Copies	▶		
b. Total Paid Print Copies (Line 15c) + Paid Electronic Copies (Line 16a)	▶		
c. Total Print Distribution (Line 15f) + Paid Electronic Copies (Line 16a)	▶		
d. Percent Paid (Both Print & Electronic Copies) (16b divided by 16c × 100)	▶		

☒ I certify that 50% of all my distributed copies (electronic and print) are paid above a nominal price.

17. Publication of Statement of Ownership
☒ If the publication is a general publication, publication of this statement is required. Will be printed in the OCTOBER 2021 issue of this publication. ☐ Publication not required.

18. Signature and Title of Editor, Publisher, Business Manager, or Owner

Malathi Samayan - Distribution Controller

Malathi Samayan

Date 9/18/2021

I certify that all information furnished on this form is true and complete. I understand that anyone who furnishes false or misleading information on this form or who omits material or information requested on the form may be subject to criminal sanctions (including fines and imprisonment) and/or civil sanctions (including civil penalties).

PS Form **3526**, July 2014 (Page 3 of 4) PRIVACY NOTICE: See our privacy policy on www.usps.com.

Moving?

Make sure your subscription moves with you!

To notify us of your new address, find your **Clinics Account Number** (located on your mailing label above your name), and contact customer service at:

Email: journalscustomerservice-usa@elsevier.com

800-654-2452 (subscribers in the U.S. & Canada)
314-447-8871 (subscribers outside of the U.S. & Canada)

Fax number: 314-447-8029

Elsevier Health Sciences Division
Subscription Customer Service
3251 Riverport Lane
Maryland Heights, MO 63043

*To ensure uninterrupted delivery of your subscription, please notify us at least 4 weeks in advance of move.

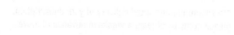

CPI Antony Rowe
Eastbourne, UK
October 29, 2021